Chiropractic and Manual Therapies

Editor: Pete Edner

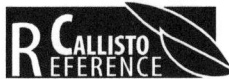

R CALLISTO REFERENCE

www.callistoreference.com

Callisto Reference,
118-35 Queens Blvd., Suite 400,
Forest Hills, NY 11375, USA

Visit us on the World Wide Web at:
www.callistoreference.com

ISBN: 978-1-63239-884-0 (Hardback)

The publisher's policy is to use permanent paper from mills that operate a sustainable forestry policy. Furthermore, the publisher ensures that the text paper and cover boards used have met acceptable environmental accreditation standards.

Printed in the United States of America.

Cataloging-in-Publication Data

Chiropractic and manual therapies / edited by Pete Edner.
    p. cm.
Includes bibliographical references and index.
ISBN 978-1-63239-884-0
1. Chiropractic. 2. Pain--Chiropractic treatment. 3. Therapeutics. 4. Chiropractic clinics.
I. Edner, Pete.
RZ241 .C45 2017
615.534--dc23

Table of Contents

Preface

This book aims to highlight the current researches and provides a platform to further the scope of innovations in this area. This book is a product of the combined efforts of many researchers and scientists from different parts of the world. The objective of this book is to provide the readers with the latest information in the field.

Chiropractic and manual therapies are medical treatment that diagnoses mechanical diseases related to the musculoskeletal system. Manual therapies of medicine have managed to treat problems that general medicine has found difficult to treat. This book attempts to understand the multiple branches that fall under the discipline of manual therapies and chiropractic. It includes some of the vital pieces of work being conducted across the globe, on various topics related to this field. This book will serve as a reference to a board spectrum of readers. It is appropriate for students seeking detailed information in the area as well as for experts.

I would like to express my sincere thanks to the authors for their dedicated efforts in the completion of this book. I acknowledge the efforts of the publisher for providing constant support. Lastly, I would like to thank my family for their support in all academic endeavors.

Editor

Exploring the construct validity of the Patient Perception Measure – Osteopathy (PPM-O) using classical test theory and Rasch analysis

Jane Mulcahy[1†] and Brett Vaughan[1,2,3*†]

Abstract

Background: Evaluation of patients' experience of their osteopathic treatment has recently been investigated leading to the development of the Patient Perception Measure – Osteopathy (PPM-O). The aim of the study was to investigate the construct validity of the PPM-O.

Methods: Patients presenting to osteopathy student-led teaching clinics at two Australian universities were asked to complete two questionnaires after their treatment: a demographic questionnaire and the PPM-O. Confirmatory factor analysis (CFA) and Rasch analysis were used to investigate the construct validity of the PPM-O.

Results: Data from the present study did not fit the *a-priori* 6-domain structure in the CFA. Modifications to the 6-domain model were then made based on the CFA results, and this analysis identified two factors: 1) Education & Information (9 items); and 2) Cognition & Fatigue (6 items). These two factors were Rasch analysed individually. Two items were removed from the Cognition & Fatigue factor during the analysis. The two factors independently were unidimensional.

Conclusions: The study produced a 2-factor, 13-item questionnaire that assesses the patients' perception of their osteopathic treatment using the items from a previous questionnaire. The results of the current study provide evidence for the construct validity of the PPM-O and the small number of items makes it feasible to implement into both clinical and research settings. Further research is now required to establish the measures' validity in a variety of patient populations.

Background

A common concern of clinicians and clinical educators working directly with patients is the significant variance in individual treatment efficacy of patients. The proposed causes for this variability in patients' experiences of their health encounters are complex and multidimensional. Demographic factors such as: gender, age, social gradient [1], education, ethnicity and geographic location have all been identified as factors that affect general health and disease status [2], as well as access to, and utilisation of, treatments and health services [2]. While nuances of the clinician and the clinical environment contribute to aspects of treatment outcome such as patient satisfaction [3], the patients' beliefs about their health and wellbeing, their illness or disease and expectations of treatment would also appear to have a significant effect [4,5].

Patient experience and expectations

Research investigating patients' experiences during, and as a result of, their treatment has tended to focus on the: patient-therapist interaction [6,7], clinical environment [8], satisfaction with treatment [9], and, efficacy of treatment outcomes [7,10]. The patients' physical experience of their treatment (i.e. sensations that the patient experiences during or after their treatment) are seldom described in manual therapy research. This aspect of the patients' experiences of a treatment requires further exploration to develop a more global picture of the patient experience during and after their consultation.

* Correspondence: brett.vaughan@vu.edu.au
†Equal contributors
[1]Centre for Chronic Disease Prevention & Management, College of Health & Biomedicine, Victoria University, Melbourne, Australia
[2]Institute of Sport, Exercise & Active Living, Victoria University, Melbourne, Australia
Full list of author information is available at the end of the article

Recently Cross et al. [4] used a qualitative approach to investigate patients' expectations of osteopathic treatment in private United Kingdom practices and concluded these expectations are primarily related to the patient-therapist interaction. Further, patients identified professional expertise and customer service as expectations of osteopathic treatment. Drawing on this work, Leach et al. [11] used a quantitative approach to identify patient expectations of their osteopathic care. The top three aspects of care highlighted by patients in this study were the ability to ask questions of the practitioner, active listening and respect. Again, the focus was very much on the patient-therapist interaction. Although, these two studies provide valuable insights into what patients expect from an osteopathic treatment, patients' cognitive, emotional and sensory responses to osteopathic treatment have not previously been established or included in commonly utilised patient reported outcomes measures (PROMs). Previous work by Mulcahy & Vaughan [12] investigated the patient-reported sensory experiences of Osteopathy in the Cranial Field (OCF) treatment. However these sensory experiences have not been validated in patients receiving general osteopathic treatment.

The Patient Perception Measure – Osteopathy (PPM-O) was developed to enhance clinicians and clinical educators understanding of what patients perceive during osteopathic treatment. Items for inclusion in the PPM-O were based on those used in a previous study to explore patient perception of OCF [12,13].

Confirmatory factor analysis

The CFA was used to determine if the data fitted the 6 domains identified by Mulcahy et al. [13]. CFA produces a variety of fit statistics indicating how well the data collected fits the proposed *a-priori* factor structure [14]. A range of fit statistics should be generated because each statistic has different measurement properties [15,16]. The chi-square statistic is used to report the fit of the data to the model and *p*-values less then 0.05 indicate a fit [17]. Whilst there is no agreement as to which type of fit statistics should be presented, in the current study the authors present a range of statistics to provide the reader with a more comprehensive representation of the data fit. Fit statistics in the present study were in line with those suggested by DiStefano & Hess [15] and included: the goodness of fit index (GFI), comparative fit index (CFI), normed fit index (NFI), Tucker-Lewis index (TLI), root mean square residual (RMR) and the root mean square error of approximation (RMSEA). The use of these fit statistics is also supported by other authors [17,18] and ensures that a range of global fit and relative fit indices are presented [15].

Rasch analysis

Rasch analysis is part of the modern test theory (MTT) statistical technique group and is widely used in the development and analysis of questionnaires and measures. The approach was developed by Dutch mathematician George Rasch [19] and fit of the data to the Rasch model is the desired outcome of the analysis [20]. Rasch analysis is sample-independent compared to the sample-dependent analyses in classical test theory. In Rasch analysis the data is fitted to a mathematical model to determine if all respondents are responding to each item in a manner dictated by the Rasch model. A range of statistics related to the interaction between the questionnaire items and the person responses (item-trait interaction) is generated. The item-trait statistics demonstrate the overall fit of the items and persons to the Rasch model [21]. This statistic analyses how each item on the PPM-O relates to all other items, and how each person is responding to each item on the PPM-O. These statistics indicate how the responses fit those expected by the Rasch model. A Bonferonni-adjusted non-statistically significant chi-square indicates an overall fit of all persons and items to the Rasch model [21]. Rasch model item and person fit is indicated by a fit residual standard deviation (SD) of ± 1.5. Fit residual SDs outside of this range suggests that issues exist with the model fit of the items and/or persons. A Person Separation Index (PSI) is also generated to indicate the internal consistency of the questionnaire being analysed and is interpreted in the same way as Cronbach's alpha [22].

Fit of the individual items to the Rasch model is analysed to ascertain whether misfitting items are impacting upon the overall model fit. Poor individual item fit is indicated by a fit residual of ± 2.5 and/or a statistically significant chi-square probability [23]. In the case of the PPM-O it may be that the probability of a patient selecting a particular response on the Likert-type scale is not equal for all possible responses on the scale – this is referred to as a disordered threshold. The threshold is the point at which there is a 50% chance of a person selecting response 1 or response 2 on a scale [21,23]. Where the threshold is disordered, respondents are selecting scale responses in a manner that is not consistent with the trait under investigation. A disordered threshold may also result from persons answering the item having trouble differentiating between the scale responses (i.e. likely, very likely, highly likely). It is possible to rescore the item to resolve the threshold disorder [21,24]. The category probability curves are used to ensure that each response on the scale is being used in an ordered manner. Each response option for the item should have the highest probability of being selected at some point along the person location.

Differential item functioning (DIF) is the investigation of how an item functions with respect to a person factor such as age or gender. In the present study, age, gender, satisfaction with life [12] and meaningful daily activity [12,25] were investigated to see if they had an impact on the way a person answers an item or items on the PPM-O. Each person factor is investigated separately to ascertain the impact of it on the fit of the data to the Rasch model. Where an item demonstrates DIF (through a statistically significant Bonferroni adjusted chi-square probability), it can be removed or recalibrated (e.g. those under 20 years of age can be split from those above 20 years of age).

Misfit of individual persons to the Rasch model is indicated by a fit residual of ± 2.5 [23]. A person is said to misfit when their response to each of the item on a questionnaire, in this case on items on the PPM-O, does not follow the prediction of the Rasch model for how that person should have responded to the item. Misfitting persons can impact on the Rasch model [21] and they will often be removed from further analysis.

The dimensionality of the measure is important because this demonstrates whether it is measuring a single underlying construct [26]. Local dependency is where the response to one item dictates the response to another item [23,26] and this can inflate the PSI [27]. Where local dependency is identified (the PSI decreases) one of the correlating items will need to be deleted. Next, the dimensionality is assessed using a Principal Components Analysis (PCA). The PCA is used to generate the 'Rasch factor' (factor 1) and display the positively and negatively loaded items. These items are then analysed using a paired t-test to examine whether the positive and negative loaded items are statistically significantly different [21]. Where no statistically significant difference exists, the questionnaire is thought to be unidimensional [21].

Study aim
The aim of the present study is to explore the construct validity of the Patient Perception Measure - Osteopathy (PPM-O) using both confirmatory factor analysis and Rasch analysis.

Methods
This study was approved by the Victoria University (VU, Melbourne, Australia) and Southern Cross University (SCU, Lismore, Australia) Human Research Ethics Committees.

Participants
Patients attending the student-led osteopathy teaching clinics at VU and SCU were invited to participate in the study. At the conclusion of their treatment, patients were invited to complete the PPM-O questionnaire by the reception staff. An Information to Participants sheet was provided to each potential participant and consent to participate was implied by completing the questionnaire. Completed PPM-O and demographic questionnaires were placed in a secure box in the reception area and collected by one of the authors weekly. Only the authors had access to the collected data.

Measure
The Patient Perception Measure – Osteopathy (PPM-O) is based on the items from a previously developed 22-item questionnaire divided into 6 domains based on an *a-priori* theoretical structure [13]. The domains identified were Education & Information, Cognition & Fatigue, Effectiveness of Osteopathic Treatment, Perceived Emotional Responses to Osteopathic Treatment, Perceived Physical Responses to Osteopathic Treatment, and Application of Osteopathic Principles.

Participants were also asked to complete a single-page demographic questionnaire. Items on the demographic questionnaire included age, gender, employment status, current medication usage and whether the participant suffers, or suffered from, one of the seven major illnesses identified by the Australian Institute of Health and Welfare [2]. Participants were also asked about 2 global items; satisfaction with life (SWL) and meaningfulness of daily activity (MDA) [25]. These global items were rated on a Likert-type scale from 0 to 6, anchored at each end. The anchors for SWL were 'not at all satisfied' (0) and 'extremely satisfied' (6), and the MDA anchors were 'not at all meaningful' (0) and 'extremely meaningful' (6). Higher scores on these global items indicated greater satisfaction with life and meaningfulness of daily activity respectively. Elements of the demographic data were used to examine the differential item function in the Rasch analysis.

Data analysis
Data were entered into SPSS Version 21 (IBM Corp, USA) for analysis. The analysis of the PPM-O took place in two stages: 1) confirmatory factor analysis (CFA); and 2) Rasch analysis. The CFA was conducted with AMOS Version 21 (IBM Corp, USA) using the Maximum Likelihood Method approach. The recommended fit statistic cut-off values for each analysis used in the present study are presented in Table 1. As the data were not normally distributed, a bootstrapping procedure was applied for each of the two models (22 item PPM-O & 13-item PPM-O), and 1000 iterations of the data were generated. Data were exported from SPSS to RUMM2030 [28] to perform the Rasch analysis using the Partial Credit Model [21] as the 'distance' between the response categories for each item were thought not to be equal. This was confirmed with a statistically significant Likelihood

Table 1 CFA fit statistics for the two versions of the PPM-O

Statistic	Recommended value	22-item PPM-O	13-item PPM-O
χ2	NA	357.23	130.46
χ2 p-value	<0.05	>0.0001	>0.0001
df	NA	194	64
χ2/df	< or = 2	1.84	2.04
Goodness of fit index (GFI)	> or = 0.9	0.828	0.879
Comparative fit index (CFI)	> or = 0.9	0.841	0.855
Normed fit index (NFI)	> or = 0.9	0.717	0.757
Tucker-Lewis index (TLI)	> or = 0.9	0.811	0.824
Root mean square residual (RMR)	As close to 0 as possible	0.048	0.054
Root mean square error of approximation (RMSEA)	< or = 0.08	0.075 (CI 0.062-0.087)	0.083 (CI 0.062-0.103)

Ratio Test (p < 0.05). Graphical and numerical threshold maps, and graphical category probability curves were produced in addition to the statistical analysis. In the present study, the decision to remove items demonstrating DIF was made *a priori* to make the PPM-O easy to administer and interpret.

Results

One hundred and eighty four questionnaires were received however 32 (18%) contained incomplete data and were subsequently removed from the CFA - 152 questionnaires were analysed in the CFA. Data from all 184 questionnaires were entered into RUMM for the Rasch analysis however one questionnaire did not contain enough data to be able to analysed and was removed. One hundred and eighty three responses (n = 183) were analysed in the Rasch analysis.

The mean age of the respondents was 35.8 years (+/- 15.1 years) and 60.5% (n = 92) were female. Employment status was shared between employed (n = 63, 41.4%) and students who were employed (n = 55, 36.2%). Participants were generally satisfied with their life (4.03 +/- 0.73) and found their daily activity moderately meaningful (3.96 +/- 0.78). No participant indicated they were not satisfied with their life or that their daily activity was not meaningful (corresponding to a score of 0). Data were collected related to the seven major Australian illnesses [2], and prevalence of these disorders were: cardiovascular disease (n = 9, 5.9%); cancer (n = 3, 2.0%); mental health disorder (n = 19, 12.5%); diabetes (n = 4, 2.6%); chronic respiratory complaint (n = 13, 8.6%); and the combined arthritis and musculoskeletal complaints (n = 65, 42.8%).

Descriptive statistics for the participant responses to the PPM-O are presented in Table 2.

Confirmatory factor analysis 1

Data were initially fitted to the *a-priori* 6 domain structure proposed by Mulcahy et al. [13]. The path diagram

for this model is presented in Figure 1 and the fit statistics are presented in Table 1. The data did not fit the model as indicated by the statistically significant chi-square probability (p < 0.001) however the GFI was approaching the recommended value.

Rasch analysis 1

The data for the 22 item PPM-O did not fit the Rasch model (χ2 = 171.95, df = 44, p < 0.0001). The PSI was 0.783 indicating borderline internal consistency. The standard deviation fit residuals for both items (1.22) and persons (0.82) were not greater than 1.5. A poor fit residual (>2.5) was identified for item 18 and statistically significant χ2 values for items 2 and 15, indicating a poor fit of these items to the Rasch model. Disordered thresholds were demonstrated for all items except 5–7, 11 and 15. The completed questionnaire from one person did not contain enough data and was removed, therefore 183 responses were analysed. DIF was identified for SWL and MDA at item 20 (I feel alone after osteopathic treatment). Those participants with low SWL and MDA scores were more likely to endorse this item highly (agree or strongly agree). Assessment of dimensionality indicated that the 22-item questionnaire was not unidimensional.

PPM-O Modification

Confirmatory factor analysis

Given the lack of model fit in the first CFA and the multidimensional nature of the 22-item PPM-O, confirmed through the initial Rasch analysis, the CFA model was modified to establish a multifactorial structure. Item covariances were analysed in order to modify the 22-item PPM-O. An item was removed if the covariance with another item was greater than 10 or did not fit onto a factor. Figure 2 demonstrates the correlation between each of the 6 domains. Strong relationships were identified between the Education, Effectiveness, Physical and Osteopathic Principles factors. The items in these

Table 2 Descriptive statistics for the 22-item Patient Perception Measure – Osteopathy (PPM-O)

Item	Response options	Min	Max	Mean	Std. Dev.
1. The way that my osteopath explains my osteopathic treatment is	Poor, fair, good, very good, excellent	3	5	4.52	0.57
2. The way my osteopath answers all of my questions is	Poor, fair, good, very good, excellent	3	5	4.59	0.54
3. My osteopath treats me with respect	Never, rarely, sometimes, mostly, always	3	5	4.97	0.21
4. The instructions my osteopath gives me regarding my home exercise program are	Poor, fair, good, very good, excellent	1	5	4.30	0.71
5. Osteopathic treatment has helped my condition	Never, rarely, sometimes, mostly, always	3	5	4.40	0.60
6. The way my management plan was explained to me was	Poor, fair, good, very good, excellent	2	5	4.26	0.71
7. The osteopathic treatment I have received has improved my quality of life	Never, rarely, sometimes, mostly, always	2	5	4.34	0.65
8. As a result of osteopathic treatment, my general health is	Poor, fair, good, very good, excellent	2	5	3.89	0.72
9. During my treatment, the questions my osteopath asked were	Poor, fair, good, very good, excellent	3	5	4.34	0.63
10. After my osteopathic treatment I felt like my whole body was treated rather than just one area	Never, rarely, sometimes, mostly, always	2	5	4.25	0.79
11. Osteopaths at this clinic talk about the body's ability to heal itself	Never, rarely, sometimes, mostly, always	1	5	3.80	0.94
12. Osteopathic treatment makes me feel vague	Never, rarely, sometimes, mostly, always	1	12	2.15	1.24
13. I cannot focus on tasks after my osteopathic treatment	Never, rarely, sometimes, mostly, always	1	5	1.86	0.92
14. I feel calmer after my osteopathic treatment	Never, rarely, sometimes, mostly, always	1	5	4.28	0.72
15. Osteopathic treatment makes no difference to my frame of mind	Never, rarely, sometimes, mostly, always	1	5	2.14	1.11
16. How helpful is osteopathic treatment in managing your condition	Poor, fair, good, very good, excellent	2	5	4.22	0.69
17. I feel sad after osteopathic treatment	Never, rarely, sometimes, mostly, always	1	5	1.22	0.58
18. I feel tired after osteopathic treatment	Never, rarely, sometimes, mostly, always	1	5	2.48	1.04
19. I am anxious after osteopathic treatment	Never, rarely, sometimes, mostly, always	1	3	1.16	0.38
20. I feel alone after osteopathic treatment	Never, rarely, sometimes, mostly, always	1	4	1.11	0.37
21. I feel less pain after osteopathic treatment	Never, rarely, sometimes, mostly, always	1	5	4.05	0.81
22. I find it hard to concentrate after my osteopathic treatment	Never, rarely, sometimes, mostly, always	1	4	1.82	0.88

Note: negatively phrased items are in italics and require rescoring prior to analysis.
Legend – response option scoring.
Poor (1), fair (2), good (3), very good (4), excellent (5).
Never (1), rarely (2), sometimes (3), mostly (4), always (5).
NB these scores are reversed for negatively phrased items.

domains were combined into a single factor called Education & Effectiveness. The items remaining in the Cognition and Emotion factors were combined to form the Cognition & Fatigue factor. This process produced a 2-factor, 15 item version of the PPM-O (Figure 2).

Rasch analysis
The revised 2-factor, 15-item PPM-O was Rasch analysed. As two factors had been identified, they were independently analysed in order for each factor to fit the Rasch model.

Rasch analysis of the education & effectiveness factor
The Education & Effectiveness factor demonstrated fit to the Rasch model ($\chi2 = 35.47$, df = 18, p = 0.008). The PSI was 0.763. The fit residual SD for items was 0.77 and 0.95 for persons. None of the items demonstrated statistically significant chi-square probabilities or fit residual SDs. Disordered thresholds were observed for all items

except 8, 9 and 16 (Additional file 1). There were 15 misfitting persons (out of 183 responses) and none of the items demonstrated DIF for any of the person factors. In order to achieve model fit, a number of modifications were made. Items 2, 4, 5, 9, 11, and 14 were rescored (Additional file 1) and this resolved the disordering for all items. Eighteen misfitting persons were removed from the analysis - these persons were not significantly different from the analysed persons with regard to demographics. All items demonstrated ordered thresholds and there was no DIF for any item. There were no residual correlations. The PCA and subsequent paired t-test of the positively and negatively loading items on the Rasch factor were statistically significant indicating the factor was unidimensional. With the item rescoring, the possible total score for this factor is 39. The mean person-item distribution for this factor is 2.35 (Figure 3). The item fit statistics are presented in Table 3.

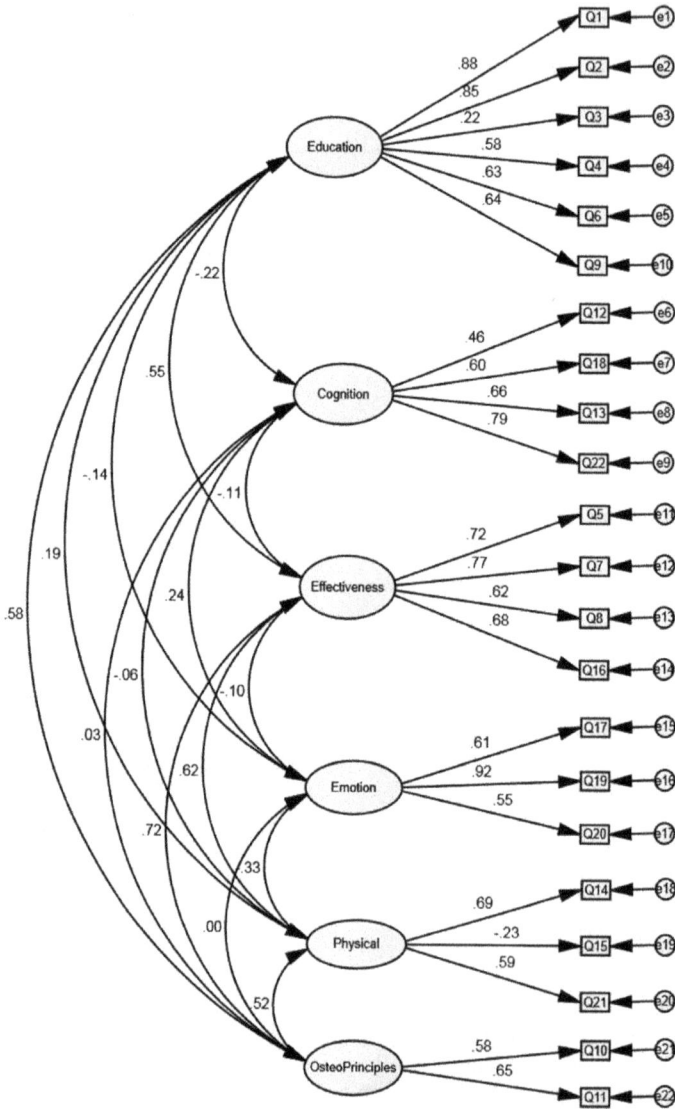

Figure 1 Path diagram for the 22-item Patient Perception Measure - Osteopathy.

Rasch analysis of the cognition & fatigue factor

The Cognition & Fatigue factor fitted the Rasch model ($\chi 2 = 19.37$, df = 12, p = 0.079). The fit residual SDs for both items and person were 1.15 and 0.86 respectively, indicting fit to the Rasch model. Threshold disordering was identified for items 13, 17 and 19 (Additional file 2). Twenty-two misfitting persons, of the 183 analysed, were also identified and subsequently removed from the analysis. The PSI was 0.659 indicating average internal consistency of the factor. DIF was not observed for any of the person factors. Two separate analyses were undertaken in order to achieve fit to the Rasch model. Fit to the Rasch model was achieved ($\chi 2 = 15.82$, df = 8, p = 0.045)

by removing items 17 and 19 and 13 misfitting persons - these persons were not significantly different from the analysed persons with regard to demographics. Rescoring of item 13 resolved the threshold disordering (Additional file 2). The PSI was 0.611 and the fit residual SDs were 1.18 for items and 0.88 for persons. The items and scoring structure for the revised factor are presented in Additional file 3 with the item fit statistics at Table 3. There was no DIF for any person factor nor were there any residual correlations. The paired t-test between the positively and negatively loaded items on the Rasch factor in the PCA was significantly different indicating a unidimensional subscale. All items on this factor require rescoring prior to

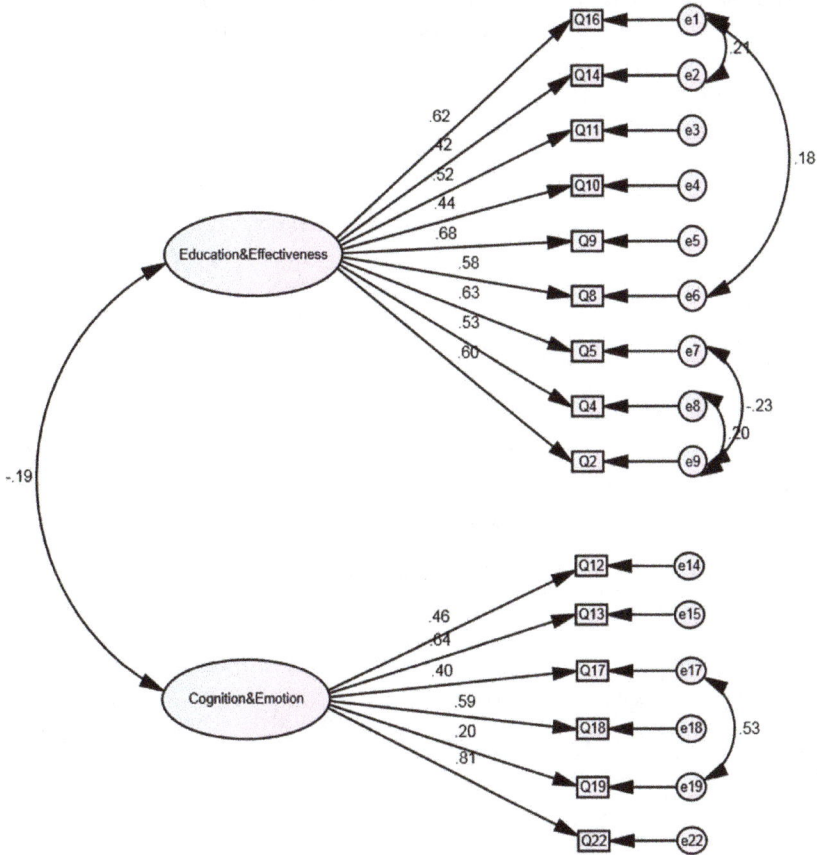

Figure 2 Path diagram for the 2-factor, 15-item Patient Perception Measure -Osteopathy.

summing the total score. The total score for this factor is 19. The person-item distribution has a mean of –1.336 reflecting the negatively worded items on this factor (Figure 4).

The lack of DIF for any of the person factors on both subscales supports the construct validity of the 13-item PPM-O [21].

Confirming the structure of the two-factor, 13-item PPM-O

The Rasch analysed two-factor PPM-O was then analysed with a CFA. The path diagram for the revised 13-item PPM-O is presented in Figure 5 and the model fit statistics are presented in Table 1. The negative association between the two factors (–0.17) supports the fact

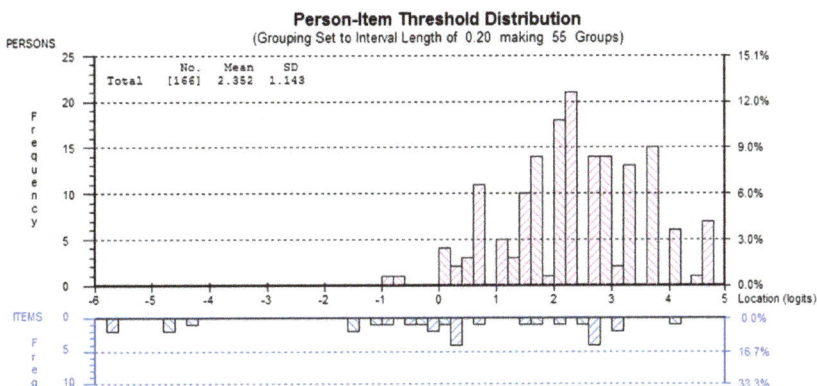

Figure 3 Person-item map for the Education & Effectiveness factor.

Table 3 Item fit statistics for the 2-factor, 13-item Patient Perception Measure – Osteopathy (PPM-O13)

	Response options	Location	Fit residual	Chi-square	Probability
Education & effectiveness					
1. The way my osteopath answers all of my questions is	Poor, fair, good, very good, excellent	−1.307	−1.157	9.672	0.007
2. The instructions my osteopath gives me regarding my home exercise program are	Poor, fair, good, very good, excellent	0.581	0.776	3.696	0.157
3. Osteopathic treatment has helped my condition	Never, rarely, sometimes, mostly, always	−1.050	−0.071	3.230	0.198
4. As a result of osteopathic treatment, my general health is	Poor, fair, good, very good, excellent	−0.136	−0.091	0.300	0.860
5. During my treatment, the questions my osteopath asked were	Poor, fair, good, very good, excellent	−1.024	−0.608	7.443	0.024
6. After my osteopathic treatment I felt like my whole body was treated rather than just one area	Never, rarely, sometimes, mostly, always	0.495	1.029	4.701	0.095
7. Osteopaths at this clinic talk about the body's ability to heal itself	Never, rarely, sometimes, mostly, always	1.828	0.863	0.485	0.784
8. I feel calmer after my osteopathic treatment	Never, rarely, sometimes, mostly, always	0.917	0.853	4.371	0.112
9. How helpful is osteopathic treatment in managing your condition	Poor, fair, good, very good, excellent	−0.303	−0.269	2.031	0.362
Cognition & Fatigue					
10. Osteopathic treatment makes me feel vague	Never, rarely, sometimes, mostly, always	−0.146	0.913	3.192	0.202
11. I cannot focus on tasks after my osteopathic treatment	Never, rarely, sometimes, mostly, always	−0.355	−1.429	2.966	0.226
12. I feel tired after osteopathic treatment	Never, rarely, sometimes, mostly, always	−0.872	1.225	3.126	0.209
13. I find it hard to concentrate after my osteopathic treatment	Never, rarely, sometimes, mostly, always	1.373	−0.745	2.536	0.281

Note: negatively phrased items are in italics and require rescoring prior to analysis.
Legend – response option scoring.
Poor (1), fair (2), good (3), very good (4), excellent (5).
Never (1), rarely (2), sometimes (3), mostly (4), always (5).
NB these scores are reversed for negatively phrased items.

the PPM-O is multidimensional and that a total score for PPM-O should not be calculated. Rather a score for each of the factors should be calculated.

Discussion

The purpose of the present study was to investigate the construct validity of the Patient Perception Measure – Osteopathy. The study used both classical test theory (CTT) and modern test theory (MTT) to investigate the properties of the questionnaire. The focus of the discussion is the CTT and MTT results rather than the descriptive statistics derived from the completed questionnaires.

Psychometrics

The initial phase of the current research involved the analysis of the data set using confirmatory factor analysis

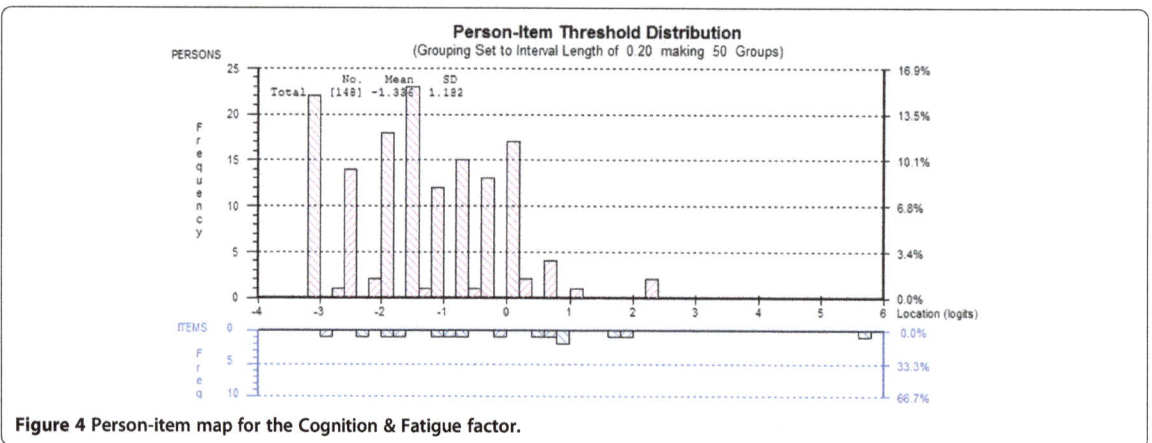

Figure 4 Person-item map for the Cognition & Fatigue factor.

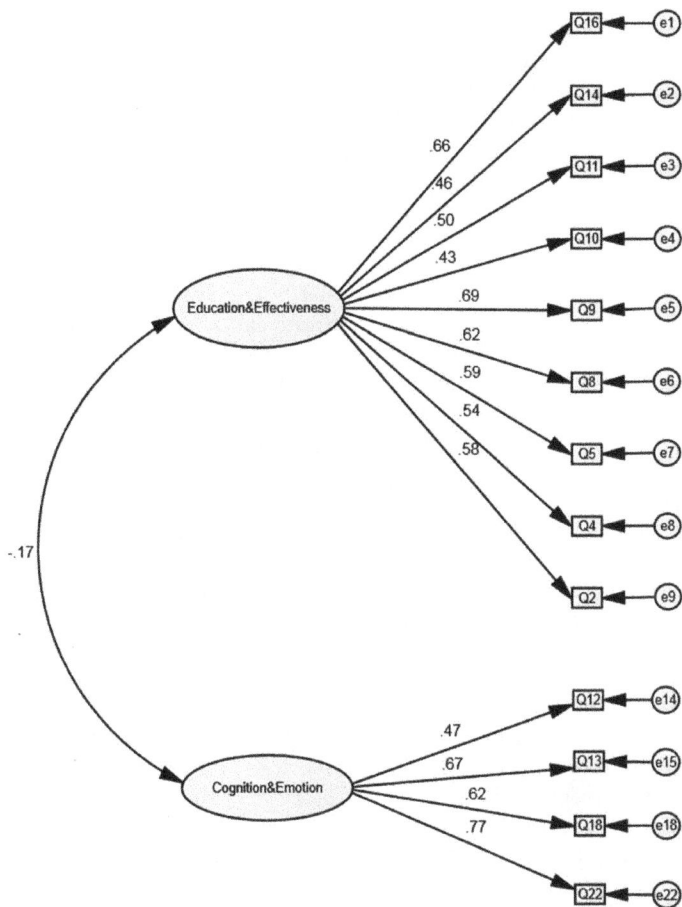

Figure 5 Confirmatory factor analysis path diagram for the 2-factor, 13-item Patient Perception Measure -Osteopathy.

(CFA). CFA is appropriate given that the *a-priori* domain structure of the PPM-O had previously been hypothesised by Mulcahy et al. [13]. The results of the CFA suggest that the domain structure proposed by these authors does not fit the data in the present study. Such a result would suggest that another subscale structure is more appropriate. Subsequent analysis using the Rasch model indicated substantial issues with a range of items and a multidimensional structure. The MTT and CTT results challenged the construct validity of the 22-item PPM-O suggesting further analysis was required.

Drawing on the results from the first CFA, modifications were made to the 22-item PPM-O in order to develop a subscale structure that fitted the data obtained in the present study. A two-factor, 15 item measure was produced and Rasch-analysed. To ensure that as many items as possible were retained to capture the patient experience with osteopathic treatment, both the Education & Effectiveness and Cognition & Fatigue subscales were Rasch-analysed separately. In essence, this produced two unidimensional subscales within the PPM-O. Following these Rasch analysis, a 2-factor, 13-item questionnaire was developed. It is important to note that given both subscales are unidimensional, they cannot be added together to form a single score for the PPM-O. This result is also supported by the CFA of the 13-item questionnaire where the data fitted the model and the correlation between the factors was negative. Support for the construct validity of the 13-item PPM-O is demonstrated by the lack of DIF for any of the items, that is, the response to an individual item was not affected by gender, age, satisfaction with life and meaningful daily activity.

The 13-item PPM-O measures two dimensions of the patients' experiences of osteopathic treatment: information, education and effectiveness of treatment; and cognitive changes and fatigue experienced post-osteopathic treatment.

Education & effectiveness factor

In the physical and manual therapy research, patients' perceptions and experiences of treatment, information and education are often associated with favourable patient treatment outcomes [29-31] and meeting the patient's expectations [11]. These aspects are also strongly represented in the patient satisfaction literature in physical therapy [3,6,32,33]. Given the literature identified here, the fact that information, education and effectiveness of treatment are contained in one dimension of the PPM-O in the current study is not surprising. Of note however is that previous measures have not included (i) Information, (ii) Education and (iii) Effectiveness into one dimension as has been demonstrated in the 13-item PPM-O. The items within this factor provide the practitioner with an overview of the effectiveness of their treatment, and suggest that there is a strong relationship between these three aspects of the patients' perception of their treatment. Patient responses to the individual items in the Education & Effectiveness factor may assist practitioners in their future treatment and management of individual patients - if an individual patient's ratings on a specific aspect of osteopathic care was not rated as being adequate or satisfactory by the patient, these aspects of care may be addressed by the clinician in future treatment.

To the authors' knowledge, the PPM-O is the first self-report measure to evaluate the patients' perception of the influence of the osteopathic principles on their treatment. Items 6 and 7 capture two of these principles [34]: 1) The human being is a dynamic unit of function (item 6), and 2) The body possesses self-regulatory mechanisms that are self-healing in nature. Cotton [35] contends that without using the principles "...osteopathy ceases to exist as a distinctive form of healthcare." The presence of the two PPM-O items related to the osteopathic principles may assist in ascertaining whether the patient perceives osteopathy to be a "...distinctive form of healthcare".

Cognition & fatigue factor
Perceived change in cognitive function and fatigue associated with osteopathic treatment are captured in the PPM-O. Clinicians do not routinely assess cognitive effects of manual therapy, and there are no valid and reliable measures to assess these treatment outcomes. However, the PPM-O Cognition & Fatigue factor provides an avenue to explore these aspects of osteopathic treatment. The concept of assessing fatigue in the PPM-O is supported by its presence in the SF-36 [36]. The PPM-O may be used, albeit with caution at this stage, to assess osteopathic patients' perceived effect of their treatments on cognitive functioning. Changes in cognitive function have been demonstrated in intensive care [37,38] and anaesthesia settings [39] however there is no support in the manual therapy literature for these post-treatment responses. This may be of some interest as

the factor relates to the ability of patients to focus on tasks, concentrate, and feeling vague post osteopathic treatment, and could be the focus of subsequent studies. If patients frequently experience these cognitive responses to osteopathic treatment, clinicians should consider them when treating and managing their patients. In particular care should be taken to ensure that a patient is sufficiently alert and capable of performing their daily activities post-treatment. Consequently testing of cognitive responses to osteopathic treatment is required. To further explore cognitive responses to osteopathic treatment, future research may also include a pre- and post- treatment testing of visual or auditory attention, problem solving, or short-term memory [38].

Future opportunities
From a practical standpoint, the PPM-O is a brief 13-item measure and would take less than five minutes for patients to complete. Clinicians and educators can score and analyse the measure in less than five minutes. Subsequently the implementation of the questionnaire in both research and clinical practice settings is feasible. Users of the PPM-O should be aware that it is not designed to have a total questionnaire score calculated. Rather, the total score for each factor should be calculated separately using the questionnaire interpretation provided in Additional file 3.

Prior to using the PPM-O in practice or research settings, the concurrent validity of the items in the Education & Effectiveness factor needs to be assessed against other patient satisfaction measures such as the measure developed by Hawthorne et al. [9]. Assessment of the concurrent validity of the Cognition & Fatigue factor items may prove more challenging, and may require a range of measures of cognitive functioning to be employed. Identifying the presence of depression, anxiety or other conditions that may affect vitality and energy is also recommended.

Limitations
A limitation of the study is the population who participated in the study. These patients were attending Australian osteopathy university-based teaching clinics and may not necessarily be representative of the population who attend for private osteopathic care [40]. Further work is required to investigate the validity of the PPM-O in a private osteopathic patient population. In addition, the removal of approximately 18% of the questionnaires from the data set to be analysed in the CFA may have introduced bias into the results. No analysis of the questionnaires that were removed prior to the analysis was undertaken therefore it is not possible to comment on how the responses to these questionnaires may have impacted upon the results. The decision to remove

incomplete questionnaires was made *a priori* as it was felt this would be more efficient for the CFA. The characteristics of the patients who did not complete all items on the PPM-O and the demographic questionnaire were analysed to ascertain whether this population differed from those who completed all items. There were no differences between these groups, however there was no record of the number of questionnaires provided to patients and therefore a count of those potentially not returned for analysis was not possible. Further, no data were collected as to why any patients chose not to complete the PPM-O and this may have introduced some bias into the study.

Conclusions

The present study has modified a measure of patients' perception of their osteopathic treatment (the PPM-O) and, in part, established the construct validity of the modified measure through the use of both CTT and MTT. The use of both of these statistical approaches has developed a measure with strong psychometric properties across the two factors in the PPM-O13. Currently the PPM-O provides a measure of the patient-therapist interaction, including information, education and effectiveness, as well as a potential measure of cognitive functioning and fatigue experienced during, and after, osteopathic treatment. The items in the Education & Effectiveness factor are consistent with previous literature, however the inclusion of items that relate to the osteopathic principles in a PROM is described in the literature for the first time. The patients' perception of osteopathy principles has not previously been explored and provides an interesting avenue for future research. The cognitive and fatigue aspects related to treatment outcomes has received little attention in the manual and physical therapy literature, and on the basis of the observations made in this study warrants further investigation.

Additional files

Additional file 1: PPM-O Education & Effectiveness Factor – Category Probability Curves.

Additional file 2: PPM-O Cognition & Fatigue Factor – Category Probability Curves.

Additional file 3: PPM-O scoring guide.

Competing interests
The authors declare that they have no competing interests.

Authors' contributions
Both authors conceived and designed the study. Both authors undertook the literature, data collection, data analysis and write-up. Both authors approved the final version of the manuscript.

Authors' information
Brett Vaughan is a lecturer in the College of Health & Biomedicine, Victoria University, Melbourne, Australia and a Professional Fellow in the School of Health & Human Sciences at Southern Cross University, Lismore, New South Wales, Australia. His interests are competency and fitness-to-practice assessments and evaluation, clinical education in allied health, and musculoskeletal rehabilitation.
Jane Mulcahy is a lecturer in the College of Health & Biomedicine at Victoria University, Melbourne, Australia. Her interests include scale development, health psychology, chronic illness and population health.

Acknowledgements
The authors wish to thank Dr Sandra Grace, Dr Keri Moore, Bridget Easdon, Amy Lawton and Courtney Lyons for their assistance with the data collection. Thanks are also extended to Tracy Morrison for her comments on the manuscript.

Author details
[1]Centre for Chronic Disease Prevention & Management, College of Health & Biomedicine, Victoria University, Melbourne, Australia. [2]Institute of Sport, Exercise & Active Living, Victoria University, Melbourne, Australia. [3]School of Health & Human Sciences, Southern Cross University, Lismore, Australia.

References
1. Kosteniuk JG, Dickinson HD. Tracing the social gradient in the health of Canadians: primary and secondary determinants. Soc Sci Med. 2003;57(2):263–76.
2. Australian Institute of Health and Welfare. Australia's health 2012. Australia's health series no.13. Cat. no. AUS 156. Canberra; 2012.
3. Beattie P, Pinto M, Nelson M, Nelson R. Patient satisfaction with outpatient physical therapy: instrument validation. Phys Ther. 2002;82(6):557–64.
4. Cross V, Leach CMJ, Fawkes CA, Moore AP. Patients' expectations of osteopathic care: a qualitative study. Health Expect. 2013. doi:10.1111/hex.12084.
5. Strutt R, Shaw Q, Leach J. Patients' perceptions and satisfaction with treatment in a UK osteopathic training clinic. Man Ther. 2008;13(5):456–67.
6. Hush JM, Cameron K, Mackey M. Patient satisfaction with musculoskeletal physical therapy care: a systematic review. Phys Ther. 2011;91(1):25–36.
7. Hall AM, Ferreira PH, Maher CG, Latimer J, Ferreira ML. The influence of the therapist-patient relationship on treatment outcome in physical rehabilitation: a systematic review. Phys Ther. 2010. doi:10.2522/ptj.20090245.
8. Rajendran D, Bright P, Bettles S, Carnes D, Mullinger B. What puts the adverse in 'adverse events'? Patients' perceptions of post-treatment experiences in osteopathy - a qualitative study using focus groups. Man Ther. 2012;17:305–11.
9. Hawthorne G, Sansoni J, Hayes L, Marosszeky N, Sansoni E. Measuring patient satisfaction with health care treatment using the short assessment of patient satisfaction measure delivered superior and robust satisfaction estimates. J Clin Epidemiol. 2014;67(5):527–37.
10. Dworkin RH, Jensen MP, Gould E, Jones BA, Xiang Q, Galer BS, et al. Treatment satisfaction in osteoarthritis and chronic low back pain: the role of pain, physical and emotional functioning, sleep, and adverse events. J Pain. 2011;12(4):416–24.
11. Leach CMJ, Mandy A, Hankins M, Bottomley LM, Cross V, Fawkes CA, et al. Patients' expectations of private osteopathic care in the UK: a national survey of patients. BMC Complement Altern Med. 2013;13:122.
12. Mulcahy J, Vaughan B. Sensations experienced and patients' perceptions of osteopathy in the cranial field treatment. J Evid Based Complement Altern Med. 2014;19(4):235–46.
13. Mulcahy J, Vaughan B, Boadle J, Klas D, Rickson C, Woodman L. Item development for a questionnaire investigating patient self reported perception, satisfaction and outcomes of a single Osteopathy in the Cranial Field (OCF) treatment. Int J Osteopath Med. 2013;16(2):81–98.
14. Hurley AE, Scandura TA, Schriesheim CA, Brannick MT, Seers A, Vandenberg RJ, et al. Exploratory and confirmatory factor analysis: guidelines, issues, and alternatives. J Org Behav. 1997;18(6):667–83.
15. DiStefano C, Hess B. Using confirmatory factor analysis for construct validation: an empirical review. J Psychoeduc Assess. 2005;23(3):225–41.
16. Jackson DL, Gillaspy Jr JA, Purc-Stephenson R. Reporting practices in confirmatory factor analysis: an overview and some recommendations. Psychol Methods. 2009;14(1):6–23.
17. Brown TA. Confirmatory factor analysis for applied research. New York, USA: Guilford Press; 2006.

18. Schreiber JB, Nora A, Stage FK, Barlow EA, King J. Reporting structural equation modeling and confirmatory factor analysis results: a review. J Educ Res. 2006;99(6):323–38.

19. Rasch G. Studies in mathematical psychology: I. Probabilistic models for some intelligence and attainment tests. 1960.

20. Tavakol M, Dennick R. Psychometric evaluation of a knowledge based examination using rasch analysis: an illustrative guide: AMEE Guide No. 72. Med Teach. 2013;35(1):e838–48.

21. Pallant JF, Tennant A. An introduction to the rasch measurement model: an example using the Hospital Anxiety and Depression Scale (HADS). Br J Clin Psychol. 2007;46(1):1–18.

22. Tor E, Steketee C. Rasch analysis on OSCE data: an illustrative example. Australas Med J. 2011;4(6):339.

23. Retief L, Potgieter M, Lutz M. The usefulness of the rasch model for the refinement of likert scale questionnaires. Afr J Res Math Sci Technol Educ. 2013;17(1–2):126–38.

24. Pallant JF, Miller RL, Tennant A. Evaluation of the Edinburgh post natal depression scale using rasch analysis. BMC Psychiatry. 2006;6(1):28.

25. Mulcahy JC. Meaningful daily activity and chronic pain. Melbourne, Australia: Victoria University; 2011.

26. Edelen MO, Reeve BB. Applying Item Response Theory (IRT) modeling to questionnaire development, evaluation, and refinement. Qual Life Res. 2007;16(1):5–18.

27. Tennant A, Conaghan PG. The rasch measurement model in rheumatology: what is it and why use it? When should it be applied, and what should one look for in a rasch paper? Arthritis Care Res. 2007;57(8):1358–62.

28. Andrich D, Sheridan B, Luo G. Rasch models for measurement: RUMM2030. Perth, Western Australia: RUMM Laboratory Pty Ltd; 2010.

29. Licciardone JC, Gamber R, Cardarelli K. Patient satisfaction and clinical outcomes associated with osteopathic manipulative treatment. J Am Osteopath Assoc. 2002;102(1):13–20.

30. Licciardone JC, Herron KM. Characteristics, satisfaction and perceptions of patients receiving ambulatory healthcare from osteopathic physicians: a comparative national survey. J Am Osteopath Assoc. 2001;101(7):374–86.

31. Medina-Mirapeix F, Jimeno-Serrano FJ, Escolar-Reina P, Del Bano-Aledo ME. Is patient satisfaction and perceived service quality with musculoskeletal rehabilitation determined by patient experiences? Clin Rehabil. 2012;27(6):1–10.

32. Monnin D, Perneger TV. Scale to measure patient satisfaction with physical therapy. Phys Ther. 2002;82(7):682–91.

33. Beattie P, Turner C, Dowda M, Mirchener L, Nelson R. The MedRisk instrument for measuring patient satisfaction with physical therapy care: a psychometric analysis. J Orthop Sports Phys Ther. 2005;35(1):24–32.

34. Ward RC, Hruby RJ, Jerome JA, Jones JM, Kappler RE, Kuchera ML, et al. Foundations for osteopathic medicine. Baltimore, USA: Lippincott Williams & Wilkins; 2002.

35. Cotton A. Osteopathic principles in the modern world. Int J Osteopath Med. 2013;16(1):17–24.

36. Ware JE, Sherbourne CD. The MOS 36-Item Short-Form Health Survey (SF-36): I. conceptual framework and item selection. Med Care. 1992;30(6):473–83.

37. Wolters AE, Slooter AJ, van der Kooi AW, van Dijk D. Cognitive impairment after intensive care unit admission: a systematic review. Intensive Care Med. 2013;39(3):376–86.

38. Torgersen J, Hole JF, KvÅLe R, Wentzel-Larsen T, Flaatten H. Cognitive impairments after critical illness. Acta Anaesthesiol Scand. 2011;55(9):1044–51.

39. Nadelson M, Sanders R, Avidan M. Perioperative cognitive trajectory in adults. Br J Anaesth. 2014. doi:10.1093/bja/aet420.

40. Burke SR, Myers R, Zhang AL. A profile of osteopathic practice in Australia 2010–2011: a cross sectional survey. BMC Musculoskel Disord. 2013;14(1):1–10.

2

Change in lumbar lordosis during prone lying knee flexion test in subjects with and without low back pain

Amir M Arab[1*], Ailin Talimkhani[2], Noureddin Karimi[2] and Fetemeh Ehsani[2]

Abstract

Background: Prone lying knee flexion (PLKF) is one of the clinical tests used for assessment of the lumbo-pelvic movement pattern. Considerable increase in lumbar lordosis during this test has been considered as impairment of movement patterns in lumbar-pelvic region. However, no study has directly evaluated the change in lordosis during active PLKF test in subjects with low back pain (LBP). The purpose of this study was to investigate the change of lumbar lordosis in PLKF test in subjects with and without LBP.

Methods: A convenience sample of 80 subjects participated in the study. Subjects were categorized into two groups: those with chronic non-specific LBP (N = 40, mean age: 40.84 ± 17.59) and with no history of LBP (N = 40, mean age: 23.57 ± 10.61). Lumbar lordosis was measured with flexible ruler, first in prone position and then on active PKF test in both subjects with and without LBP. Data was analyzed by using statistical methods such as, independent t-test and paired t-test.

Results: There were statistically significant differences in lumbar lordosis between prone position and after active PLKF in both subjects with and without LBP (P < 0.0001). The amount of change in lordosis during PLKF test was not significant between the two groups (P = 0.65). However these changes were greater among patients with LBP.

Conclusion: Increase in lumbar lordosis during this test may be due to excessive flexibility of movement of the lumbar spine in the direction of extension and abnormal movement patterns in the individuals with LBP.

Keywords: Low back pain, Lumbar lordosis, Movement pattern, Prone knee flexion, Flexible ruler

Background

Low back pain (LBP) is a world-wide health problem and the most common and costly musculoskeletal disorder in the today's societies [1,2]. The prevalence of LBP is estimated to be between 10% and 80% depending on the population [3,4]. Despite its high prevalence and detrimental effects on subjects' activities, the exact causes of mechanical LBP have not yet been fully understood. However, during the past decades the approach in evaluation and management of LBP has been changed from strengthening or stretching of the lumbo-pelvic muscles toward modification of the motor system and movement pattern [5].

A balanced motor system is obtained from coordinated activity of synergist and antagonist muscles. Normal functioning of the trunk depends not only on passive joint mobility, but also on normal muscular activity and central nervous system regulation. Muscles produce and control the movement and stabilize the spine, protecting if from excessive load during functional activities [6,7].

With regard to this point of view, repetitive movements and long-term faulty postures and movements can change muscle tissue characteristics and can lead to muscle dysfunction, altered movement pattern, pain and finally movement disorders [5]. Hence, the main emphasis has been recently placed on assessment of the altered movement pattern in patients with musculoskeletal pain and disorders such as LBP and on the important of achieving normal pattern of the movement for the prevention and treatment of LBP [6-11].

* Correspondence: arabloo_masoud@hotmail.com
[1]Department of Physical Therapy, University of Social Welfare and Rehabilitation Sciences, Velenjak, Tehran, Iran
Full list of author information is available at the end of the article

Several studies have demonstrated that LBP is associated with muscle imbalance and altered activation pattern of the lumbo-pelvic muscles during different tasks [12-15]. Some clinical tests have been used to assess the altered movement pattern in subjects with musculoskeletal disorders. Prone lying knee flexion (PLKF) is an accepted test for assessment and treatment of the lumbo-pelvic movement patterns [5]. In this test, a patient lays prone and actively flexes his or her dominant knee as far as possible. Muscle imbalance and altered activation of the lumbo-pelvic muscles has been reported during PLKF test in patients with chronic LBP [5]. Excessive anterior pelvic tilt, lumbar rotation, lumbar hyperextension, increased lumbar lordosis and decreased knee flexion during the PLKF has been considered as abnormal movement patterns during PLKF [5]. Coordination between muscles in the lumbo-pelvic region is thought to balance the position of the pelvis in normal posture and during the lower limb or trunk movement. It has been assumed that during PLKF, lack of sufficient stiffness in the abdominal and anterior supporting structures of the lumbar spine produces anterior tilt in the pelvic and increased lumbar lordosis specially in person with lower cross syndrome [5].

However, to our knowledge, no study has investigated the change in lumbar lordosis during PLKF in patients with chronic LBP. The purpose of this study was to investigate the change in the degree of lumbar lordosis during PLKF in subjects with and without chronic LBP and to determine if this change varies between two groups.

Methods

Subjects

The quasi-experimental study design with repeated measurements was used to investigate the lumbar lordosis changes during PLKF in two groups: subjects with chronic non-specific LBP (N = 40, average age: 40.84 [SD = 17.59] years old, average height: 165.0 [SD = 9.0] cm, average weight: 70.31 [SD = 16.06] kg, body mass index (BMI): 25.55 [SD = 3.99] kg/m^2) and subjects with no history of LBP (N = 40, average age: 23.57 [SD = 10.61] years old, average height: 162.0 [SD = 7.0] cm, average weight: 55.62 [SD = 6.55] kg, BMI: 21.05 [SD = 2.26] kg/m^2).

Power analysis was used to determine the sample size for test. Type I error (α) was set at 0.05 and power of the test was 0.80. Considering this, the calculated sample size showed that sample size in this study was appropriate to test the hypothesis and the results derived from the study are meaningful.

The subject population in this study was a sample of convenience. The LBP patients were referred by orthopedic specialist and physiotherapy clinics. The patients were included if they had a history of non-specific LBP for more than six weeks duration before the study date. They were also included if had intermittent (on and off) LBP

with at least three previous episodes each lasting more than one week, during the year before the study [16].

The control group was evaluated and found to have no complaint of any pain or dysfunction in their low back, pelvis, thoracic and lower extremities. The healthy subjects were recruited from the university students.

The exclusion criteria in both groups were pregnancy, history of dyspnea, history of hip pain, dislocation or fracture, history of lumbar spine surgeries, history of anterior knee ligament injury or rupture, history of anterior knee pain, inability to perform active PLKF without pain, history of lower extremity injury in the past 3 months, shortness of hip flexors, positive neurological symptoms and cardiopulmonary disorders. Each eligible subject was enrolled after signing an informed consent form approved by the human subjects committee at the University of Social Welfare and Rehabilitation Sciences. Ethical approval for this study was granted from the internal ethics committee at the University of Social Welfare and Rehabilitation Sciences (Date: 2013.03.09).

Procedures

The subject was on the examining table in the prone position. The lumbar lordosis was measured first in prone position. Then the subject was asked to perform knee flexion (PLKF) and then the lumbar lordosis was measured after PLKF test in both subjects with and without LBP. The dominant leg was chosen for investigation.

Measuring lumbar lordosis

A standard flexible ruler was used to measure the degree of lumbar lordosis in prone position before and after active knee flexion (Figure 1). For this purpose, the subject's position was prone lying on a treatment table with the arms along the sides and head face was down. The base of sacrum and spinous process of L1 was located by palpation and marked with removable stickers.

A standard flexible ruler was fitted on subject's lumbar curve, over the lumbar spinous processes of L1 – S1. The curve of the flexible ruler, resembling the size of subject's lumbar curvature, was graphed on a paper, noting where the two reference points for L1 and S1 were located. The method explained by others was used to quantify the degree of lumbar lordosis [16-20].

Two points on the curve, representing L1 and S1, were connected by a line (L). A perpendicular line (H), representing the height of the lumbar curve, bisected line L. The length of each line was calculated in millimeters, and the values were used in the following formula to calculate the degree of lumbar lordosis.

$$\theta = 4 \left[\text{Arc tan} \left(2H/L \right) \right]$$

A very high correlation (r = 0.92) has been found between degrees of lumbar lordosis measured by a flexible

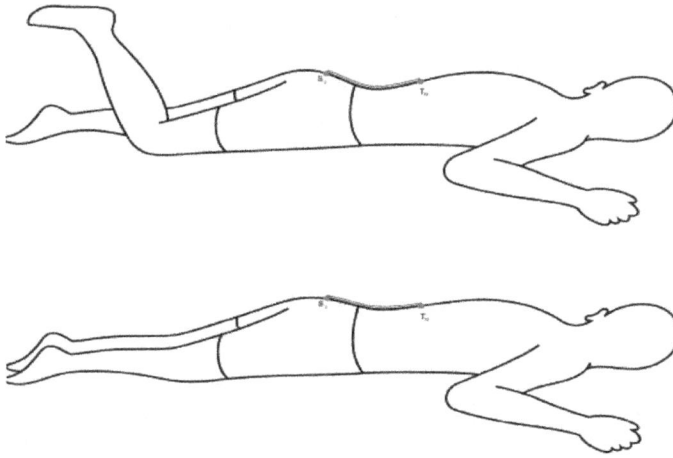

Figure 1 Measurement of lumbar lordosis with flexible ruler in prone position and active PLKF.

ruler and from lumbar X-rays [21-23]. The reliability of flexible curve for measurement of lumbar lordosis has been previously established [24].

Data analysis
Statistical analysis was performed using SPSS version 16.0.

A paired t-test was used to demonstrate changes in lumbar lordosis before and after PLKF test in both subjects with and without LBP.

An independent t-test was used to compare changes in lumbar lordosis during PLKF between subjects with and without LBP and also to compare demographic data between subjects with and without LBP. Statistical significance was attributed to P value less than 0.05.

Ethical approval
This research was reviewed and was approved by the Human Subject Committee at University of Social Welfare and Rehabilitation Sciences.

Results
The demographic data for the subjects are presented in Table 1. No statistical significance was found in the height between groups. However, there was a statistically

significant difference in subjects' age, weight and BMI between the two groups (P = 0.000).

There was no significant difference in lumbar lordosis at the baseline in prone relaxed position between two groups (P = 0.21, %95 CI: 1.77-7.44). There was a statistically significant difference in lumbar lordosis between prone position and after PLKF in subjects without LBP (P = 0.000) and subjects with LBP (P = 0.000) (Table 2, Figure 2). Overall, the lumbar lordosis was significantly greater in the PLKF compared to prone-relaxed position in both subjects with and without LBP. The mean difference in lumbar lordosis between positions was 6.47 and 5.65 for subjects with LBP and without LBP respectively.

There was no statistically significant difference in the changes of lumbar lordosis after performing PLKF between subjects with and without LBP (P = 0.65) (Table 3). However, the changes in lumbar lordosis were greater among patients with LBP compared to those without LBP.

Discussion
The current study shows changes in lumbar lordosis during active PLKF test in subjects with and without LBP. The results of this study demonstrated that there were statistically significant differences in lumbar lordosis between prone position and after PLKF in both subjects with and without LBP (P < 0.0001). But the amount of changes in lordosis during PLKF test was not significant between two

Table 1 Demographic data of the subjects in each group

Variables	With no LBP (n = 40)	With LBP (n = 40)
Age (years)	23.57 (10.61)	40.84 (17.59)
Weight (kg)	55.62 (6.55)	70.31 (16.06)
Height (cm)	162.0 (7.0)	165.0 (9.0)
BMI (kg/m^2)	21.05 (2.26)	25.55 (3.99)

Continuous data: Mean (Standard Deviation).
LBP = Low Back Pain, BMI = Body Mass Index.

Table 2 Lumbar lordosis in both groups

Variables	Before PLKF	After PLKF	P-value
With no LBP	35.02 (9.25)	40.67 (13.09)	**0.000**
With LBP	32.35 (12.43)	38.82 (14.43)	**0.000**

Continuous data: Mean (Standard Deviation). Bold p-values indicate statistical significance.
LBP = Low Back Pain, PLKF = Prone Lying Knee Flexion.

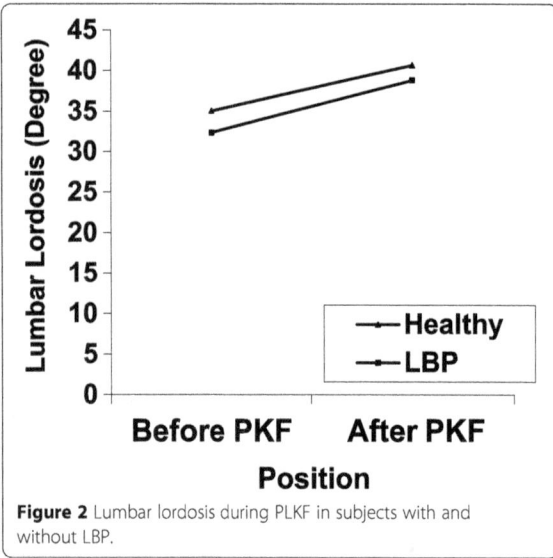

Figure 2 Lumbar lordosis during PLKF in subjects with and without LBP.

groups (P = 0.65). These changes were greater among patients with LBP compared to subjects without LBP.

In this study, the subjects had no pain during the test and none of the subjects reported that pain was a limiting factor to perform PLKF test, so, direct effects of pain on the measurement can be minimized.

Lumbar extension and anterior rotation of the pelvis are often observed during the PLKF test. Increase in the degree of lumbar lordosis during PLKF test found in both groups can be attributed to the accompanied lumbar extension during flexion of the knee. In theory, it is proposed that excessive anterior pelvic tilt, lumbar hyperextension and increased lumbar lordosis during the PLKF are commonly seen as abnormal movement patterns in patients with chronic LBP [5]. Investigators attributed these to muscle imbalance and altered activation of the lumbo-pelvic muscles [5].

Previous investigators attributed excessive lumbar extension and hyper lordosis during PLKF to a deficiency in controlling anterior pelvic rotation during PLKF because of muscular dysfunction in the lumbo-pelvic region [5,25]. Sahrmann [5] proposed the concept of "relative flexibility or stiffness" that has been linked to uncontrolled movement, pain and pathology by causing direction related stress and strain during various functional movements in the patients with LBP. Sahrmann

[5] suggested that increased stiffness of the anterior supporting structures of the thigh, hip, knee and lumbar spine can result in compensatory exaggerated anterior pelvic tilt with lumbar extension motion during prone knee flexion or hip extension. In this study, stiffness in thigh and anterior supporting structures of the lumbar spine was not measured, just measured the change in lumbar lordosis during PLKF.

Scholtes et al. [26] found that during knee flexion and hip lateral rotation in prone lying, subjects with LBP demonstrated a greater maximal lumbar-pelvic rotation angle compared to those without LBP, as the lumbar-pelvic region may move more frequently during the early ranges of lower limb movement in daily activities.

In this study, lumbar lordosis was significantly higher during PLKF compared to prone relaxed position in both subjects with and without LBP. However, this change in lumbar lordosis during PLKF was not significant between two groups. The reason for this may be due to the healthy subjects being recruited from university students and staff used to performing sustained postures and repeated movements in their daily activities.

It has been thought that, if the lumbar-pelvic motion occurs more during a limb movement, then the frequency of lumbar-pelvic motion may be increased through the day. The increased frequency of the movements in lumbar-pelvic region can contribute to increased mechanical stress and strain on lumbar-pelvic region. This can also change the characteristics of muscular tissue, in turn, leading to abnormal movement patterns in lumbar-pelvic region [26,27]. Previous studies supported increased mobility of the lumbar-pelvic region in LBP patients which can be associated with degeneration of lumbar-pelvic region tissues [28,29].

In this study, compensatory lumbar extension motion during active PLKF test may be due to instability in lumbar-pelvic region and also, excessive flexibility of movement of the lumbar spine in the direction of extension. This hypothesis has been supported by findings which suggest active limb movements which contribute to accumulation of tissue stress can affect decrease in spinal stability in patients with LBP [30]. However, more studies are needed to resolve the existing ambiguities in this field.

Limitations

We acknowledge some limitations. In this study the patients with chronic non-specific LBP were examined and other LBP patients (acute or specific LBP) were not examined. Another limitation of this study was that LBP subjects were not categorized based on movement system impairment-based categories for LBP as described by Sahrmann [5].

Table 3 Changes in lumbar lordosis between two groups

Variable	With no LBP (n = 40)	With LBP (n = 40)	P-value
Changes in lumbar lordosis during PLKF	5.65 (10.13)	6.47 (6.67)	0.65

Continuous data: Mean (Standard Deviation).
LBP = Low Back Pain, PLKF = Prone Lying Knee Flexion.

It has been suggested investigating the lumbar lordosis change in LBP patients with different movement system impairment-based categories. Again in this study, we did not measure lumbar -pelvic kinematics and electromyography (EMG) activity of the stabilizing and prime mover muscles during PLKF to find the pattern of muscles recruitment.

The fact that the healthy subjects were recruited from university students and staff performing sustained postures and repeated movements in their daily activities may be used to question the results showing no significant difference in lumbar lordosis change during PLKF between two groups.

Considering the non statistically different but measurable changes in lumbar lodosis during PLKF between subjects with and without LBP, we suggest that PLKF can be used as an evaluation tool of lumbar-pelvic movement patterns in the individuals with LBP and even healthy individuals with poor postural alignment and poor movement habits.

Conclusion

This study investigated the chansge in lumbar lordosis during PLKF test between subjects with and without LBP. The results of this study indicate an increase in the degree of lumbar lordosis during PLKF compared to prone-relaxed position in subjects with and without LBP. However, greater change in lumbar lordosis was found in the subjects with LBP compared to healthy subjects. More studies are needed to resolve the existing ambiguities in this field.

Competing interests
The authors declare that they have no competing interests.

Authors' contributions
AMA contributed to conception, design, analysis, interpretation of data and drafting the manuscript. AT carried out the data collection and drafting the manuscript. NK participated in design and interpretation of data. FE participated in analysis and helped to draft the manuscript. All authors read and approved the final manuscript.

Author details
[1]Department of Physical Therapy, University of Social Welfare and Rehabilitation Sciences, Velenjak, Tehran, Iran. [2]University of Social Welfare and Rehabilitation Sciences, Velenjak, Tehran, Iran.

References
1. Marras WS, Allread WG, Burr DL, Fathallah FA. Prospective validation of a low-back disorder risk model and an assessment of ergonomic interventions associated with manual materials handling tasks. Ergonomics. 2000;43:1866–86.
2. Lahiri S, Markkanen P, Levenstein C. The cost-effectiveness of occupational health interventions: preventing occupational back pain. Am J Ind Med. 2005;48(6):515–29.
3. Verhaak PF, Kerssens JJ, Dekker J, Sorbi MJ, Bensing JM. Prevalence of chronic benign pain disorder among adults: a review of the literature. Pain. 1998;77(3):231–9.
4. Gilgil E, Kacar C, Butun B, Tuncer T, Urhan S, Yildirim C, et al. Prevalence of low back pain in a developing urban setting. Spine. 2005;30:1093–8.
5. Sahrmann S. Diagnosis and treatment of movement impairment syndromes. 1. Missouri: Mosby. Inc; 2002. p. 121–92.
6. Jull GA, Janda V. Muscles and motor control in low back pain: Assessment and management. In: Twomey LT, Taylor JR, editors. Physical Therapy of the Low Back. Chuchill Livingstone: New York; 1987. p. 253–78.
7. Norris CM. Spinal stabilisation: an exercise programme to enhance lumbar stabilistion. Phys Ther. 1995;81(3):13–39.
8. Cholewicki J, Van Dieen JH, Arsenault AB. Muscle function and dysfunction in the spine. J Electromyoger Kinesiol. 2003;13(4):303–4.
9. Janda V. On the concept of postural muscles and posture in man. Aust J Physiother. 1983;29:83–4.
10. Janda V. Pain in the locomotor system-A broad approach. Aspects of manipulative therapy. Melbourne: Churchill Livingstone; 1985. p. 148–51.
11. O'Sullivan P, Phyty D, Twomey L, Allison GT. Evaluation of specific stabilizing exercise in the treatment of chronic low back pain with radiologic diagnosis of spondylolysis or spondylolisthesis. Spine. 1997;22(24):2959–67.
12. Hodges P, Moseley G. Pain and motor control of the lumbopelvic region: effect and possible mechanisms. J Electromyogr Kinesiol. 2003;13:361–70.
13. Hungerford B, Gilleard W, Hodges P. Evidence of altered lumbopelvic muscle recruitment in the presence of sacroiliac joint pain. Spine. 2003;28:1593–600.
14. Leinonen V, Kankaanpaa M, Airaksinen O, Hanninen O. Back and hip extensor activities during trunk flexion/extension: Effects of low back pain and rehabilitation. Arch Phys Med Rehabil. 2000;81:32–7.
15. Newcomer K, Jacobson T, Gabriel D, Larson DR, Brey RH, An KN. Muscle activation patterns in subjects with and without low back pain. Arch Phys Med Rehabil. 2002;83:816–21.
16. Nourbakhsh MR, Arab AM. Relationship between mechanical factors and incidence of low back pain. J Orthop Sports PhysTher. 2002;32:447–60.
17. Link CN, Nicholson GG, Shaddeau SA, Birch R, Gossman MR. Lumbar curvature in standing and sitting in two types of chairs: relationship of hamstring and hip flexor muscle length. PhysTher. 1990;70:611–8.
18. Nourbakhsh MR, Arab AM, Salavati M. The relationship between pelvic cross syndrome and chronic low back pain. J Back Musculoskeletal Rehabil. 2006;19:119–28.
19. Youdas JW, Garrett TR, Harmsen SS. Lumbar lordosis and pelvic inclination of asymptomatic adults. Phys Ther. 1996;76:1066–81.
20. Youdas JW, Garrett TR, Egan KS, Therneau TM. Lumbar lordosis and pelvic inclination in adults with chronic low back pain. Phys Ther. 2000;80:261–75.
21. Seidi F, Rajabi R, Ebrahimi TJ, Tavanai AR, Moussavi SJ. The Iranian flexible ruler reliability and validity in lumbar lordosis measurments. Sport Sci. 2009;2(2):95–9.
22. Hart DL, Rose SJ. Reliability of a noninvasive method for measuring the lumbar curve. Orthop Sports Phys Ther. 1986;8(4):180–4.
23. Youdas JW, Vj S, Garrett TR. Reliability of measurments of lumbar spine sagittal mobility obtained with the flexible curve. Orthop Sports Phys Ther. 1995;21(1):13–20.
24. Nourbakhsh MR, Moussavi SJ, Salavati M. Effects of lifestyle and work-related physical activity on the degree of lumbar lordosis and chronic low back pain in a Middle East population. Spinal Disord. 2001;14:283–92.
25. Jae-Seop O. Effects of Peforming an abdominal drwing-in maneuver during prone hip extension exercises on hip and back extensormuscle activity and amount of anterior pelvic tilt. J OrthopSports Phys Ther. 2007;37(6):320–4.
26. Scholtes SA, Gombatto SP, Van Dillen LR. Differences in lumbopelvic motion between people with and people without low back pain during two lower limb movement tests. Clin Biomech. 2009;24(1):7–12.
27. Van Dillen LR, Sahrmann SA, Norton BJ, Caldwell CA, Fleming D, McDonnell MK, et al. Effect of active limb movements on symptoms in patients with low back pain. J Orthop Sports Phys Ther. 2001;31:402–18.
28. Leone A, Guglielmi G, Cassar-Pullicino VN, Bonomo L. Lumbar intervertebral instability: a review. Radiology. 2007;245(1):62–77.
29. Singer KP, Fitzgerald D, Milne N. Neck retraction exercises and cervical disk disease. In: Singer KP, editor. Proceeding of the Biennial manipulative physiotherapist conference. Australia: Perth; 1993. p. 88–93.
30. Scholtes SA, Van Dillen LR. Gender-related differences in prevalence of lumbopelvic region movement impairments in people with low back pain. J Orthop Sports Phys Ther. 2007;37:744–53.

3

Do MRI findings identify patients with chronic low back pain and Modic changes who respond best to rest or exercise: a subgroup analysis of a randomised controlled trial

Rikke K. Jensen[1]*, Peter Kent[1,2] and Mark Hancock[3]

Abstract

Background: No previous clinical trials have investigated MRI findings as effect modifiers for conservative treatment of low back pain. This hypothesis-setting study investigated if MRI findings modified response to rest compared with exercise in patients with chronic low back pain and Modic changes.

Methods: This study is a secondary analysis of a randomised controlled trial comparing rest with exercise. Patients were recruited from a specialised outpatient spine clinic and included in a clinical trial if they had chronic low back pain and an MRI showing Modic changes. All patients received conservative treatment while participating in the trial. Five baseline MRI findings were investigated as effect modifiers: Modic changes Type 1 (any size), large Modic changes (any type), large Modic changes Type 1, severe disc degeneration and large disc herniation. The outcome measure was change in low back pain intensity measured on a 0–10 point numerical rating scale at 14-month follow-up ($n = 96$). An interaction $\geq$ 1.0 point (0–10 scale) between treatment group and MRI findings in linear regression was considered clinically important.

Results: The interactions for Modic Type 1, with large Modic changes or with large Modic changes Type 1 were all potentially important in size (−0.99 (95 % CI −3.28 to 1.29), −1.49 (−3.73 to 0.75), −1.49 (−3.57 to 0.58), respectively) but the direction of the effect was the opposite to what we had hypothesized—that people with these findings would benefit more from rest than from exercise. The interactions for severe disc degeneration (0.74 (−1.40 to 2.88)) and large disc herniation (−0.92 (3.15 to 1.31)) were less than the 1.0-point threshold for clinical importance. As expected, because of the lack of statistical power, no interaction term for any of the MRI findings was statistically significant.

Conclusions: Three of the five MRI predictors showed potentially important effect modification, although the direction of the effect was surprising and confidence intervals were wide so very cautious interpretation is required. Further studies with adequate power are warranted to study these and additional MRI findings as potential effect modifiers for common interventions.

Background

In most patients with low back pain (LBP), the cause of pain cannot be definitively attributed to a specific pathology and patients are therefore labelled as having 'non-specific LBP'. Non-specific LBP is estimated to be approximately 85 % of LBP in primary care [1]; however,

* Correspondence: rikke.kruger.jensen@rsyd.dk
[1]Research Department, Spine Centre of Southern Denmark, Hospital Lillebaelt, Institute of Regional Health Research, University of Southern Denmark, Oestre Hougvej 55, 5500 Middelfart, Denmark
Full list of author information is available at the end of the article

most clinicians believe that it is not one condition but consists instead of several different subgroups. They also treat non-specific LBP differently depending on patterns of signs and symptoms [2] and preliminary results suggest that targeting treatment to LBP subgroups might be more effective than generic 'one-size-fits all' approaches [3].

There are many ways to potentially classify non-specific LBP into treatment-relevant subgroups, one of which is to use pathoanatomic findings seen on Magnetic Resonance Imaging (MRI). Although there is little evidence for the clinical relevance of most MRI findings, some, such as

Modic changes, have been shown to be associated with LBP. A systematic review in 2008 [4] that investigated this relationship found positive associations between the presence of Modic changes and LBP in seven of 10 studies, with odds ratios ranging from 2 to 20. In addition, a stronger association with pain for Modic changes Type 1 than for other types was shown by Thompson et al. [5], who reported a higher positive predictive value for pain generation during discography for Modic changes Type 1 (0.81) than for Type 2 (0.64) or Type 3 (0.57).

Exercise therapy is a management strategy for non-specific LBP that is guideline-recommended and widely used [6]. As patients' pathoanatomical source of pain is most likely diverse, it may be that MRI findings can identify subgroups of patients with chronic non-specific LBP who benefit more from exercise therapy than others. For example, on theoretical grounds, patients with chronic LBP and Modic changes could be a subgroup of patients that would be less likely to benefit from exercise, as the histology of Modic changes has shown fissured and disrupted endplates [7] that might indicate less tolerance of additional, exercise-induced, loading of the spine.

Based on the hypothesis that rest and reduction of spinal load would lead to better healing of the bone and subsequent reduction in pain, a two-group randomised controlled trial (RCT) investigated if rest was more effective than exercise [8] for people with Modic changes. The results showed no difference between the two treatment outcomes on pain, disability, quality of life or any other outcome measures immediately post-treatment (10 weeks) and at 14-month follow-up. A limitation of those results was that all patients had some type of Modic change, so it was not possible to determine if the presence of any Modic change acted as an effect modifier. However, we also collected information on the type and size of Modic changes as well as the presence or absence of other MRI findings such as disc herniation and disc degeneration. These data now provide the unique opportunity to investigate if the type or size of Modic changes, or the presence or absence of other MRI findings, acted as effect modifiers. To our knowledge, MRI findings have not previously been tested as effect modifiers for response to conservative interventions in an RCT, which seems a major gap in our knowledge.

Therefore, the purpose of this hypothesis-setting, secondary analysis was to investigate if MRI findings modified the treatment response to rest or exercise in patients with chronic LBP and Modic changes.

Method

Study design
This secondary analysis was performed using data from a (two-group) RCT that investigated the effect of rest compared with exercise in patients with chronic LBP and Modic changes. To increase the validity of this subgroup analysis, it was performed using the approach recommended by Sun et al. [9] which included pre-specification of both the direction of subgroup effects and the hypotheses underlying them, and the investigation of only a limited number of subgroups.

Study population
Patients were recruited from a specialised outpatient spine clinic, the Spine Centre of Southern Denmark, where they had been referred by medical practitioners and chiropractors in primary care for investigation of non-response to conservative care. From August 2007 to December 2008, MRI was routinely performed on all patients meeting the following criteria: (i) no contraindications for MRI, (ii) LBP or leg pain of at least 3 on a 0–10 point Numerical Rating Scale (NRS), (iii) duration of current symptoms from 2 to 12 months, and (iv) age above 18 years.

Patients with an MRI showing Modic changes (Type 1, 2 or 3) that extended beyond the endplate into the vertebral body underwent a clinical examination and were invited to participate in the study unless they met any of the following exclusion criteria: (i) unable to participate in the project because of other physical or mental conditions, (ii) had symptoms and clinical signs of lumbar nerve root compression (e.g. leg pain dominating over back pain, positive straight-leg-raise test or neurological deficit), or (iii) had undergone previous spinal surgery with no pain relief after the operation.

Randomisation and intervention
Patients were allocated to one of the two intervention groups (rest or exercise) by means of computerised minimisation software [10]. In total, 100 patients were included and of those, 49 were randomised to the rest group and 51 to the exercise group.

The rest group was instructed to avoid physically demanding activity and to rest twice daily for 1 h, by lying down. The patients participated in a group meeting once every second week to imitate the treatment session structure of the exercise group and thereby, the potential non-specific effect of being in a group. The exercise group received exercises for the stabilising muscles in the low back and abdomen together with dynamic exercises, exercises for postural instability and light physical fitness training. The patients exercised in a group once a week and were instructed to do additional home exercises three times a week. The duration of the interventions was 10 weeks and follow-up data were obtained at the end of this period (post-treatment at 10 weeks) and at 14 months after baseline. At 14 months, follow-up data on 96 participants were available (96 %). For the flow of the trial, see

Fig. 1. Full details of the recruiting procedure and interventions have previously been reported [8].

Outcomes

Current back pain measured on a 0–10 point NRS [11] was the primary outcome in the original trial, collected via self-reported questionnaire. For this secondary analysis, the change in current back pain between baseline and 14-month follow-up was chosen a priori as the treatment outcome, as this enabled the marginal means to be calculated for each subgroup.

Variables of interest

MRIs were obtained at baseline. The MRI system was a 0.2 T (Magnetom Open Viva; Siemens AG, Erlangen, Germany) and a body spine surface coil was used with the patient in the supine position. The imaging protocol consisted of sagittal and axial T1- and T2-weighted sequences. The evaluation of the MRI changes (L1 to S1) was performed by an experienced musculoskeletal radiologist using standardised evaluation protocols [12, 13]. Previous evaluation of the use of these protocols by the same radiologist had shown substantial to almost perfect reproducibility with Kappa values from 0.73 to 1.0 for the Modic change variables [12] and from moderate to almost perfect with values from 0.59 to 0.97 for the disc-related changes [13]. The radiologist was blinded to any patient information except for name, age and sex.

Five potential effect modifiers for treatment with either rest or exercise were chosen from the baseline MRI variables and limited to that number to reduce the risk of type I error. The potential effect modifiers of interest were (i) type of Modic changes (Type 1 compared with not having Type 1 changes), (ii) size of Modic changes (large Modic changes compared with small), (iii) large Modic Type 1 changes (large Modic changes Type 1 compared with not having this finding), (iv) disc degeneration (severe disc degeneration compared with not having this finding) and (v) disc herniation (large disc herniations compared with not having this finding). The rationales for these variables are reported in Table 1.

The definition of a patient being positive for *Modic changes Type 1* was the presence of a Type 1 finding on at least one of the 11 lumbar endplates and regardless of other types present on the same or other segmental levels. A patient was classified as being positive for *large Modic changes* if they had any type of Modic change, of ≥25 % of vertebral height on at least one of the 11 lumbar endplates regardless of other Modic changes present on other segmental levels. *Large Modic changes Type 1* was defined as having at least one Modic change which was both Type 1 and ≥25 % of vertebral height. In the MRI protocol [13], 'disc height' was graded from 0 to 3 and 'disc signal intensity' was graded from 0 to 3 (with higher numbers indicating more severe changes). For the purpose of this study, *severe disc degeneration* was defined as one or more discs with either (i) 'disc height' = grade 3, or (ii) the combination of 'disc height' = grade 2 and 'disc signal intensity' = grade 3 within the same disc. Disc herniations was evaluated according to the same MRI protocol [13], and for the purpose of this study, patients were classified as being positive for *large disc herniation* if they had one or more disc herniations categorised as broad-based protrusion, extrusion or a sequestration independent of the status of the other discs.

Analysis

Data were analysed by linear regression models performed separately for each of the five potential effect modifiers. The dependent variable was change score in pain on a 0–10 point NRS (baseline score minus 14-month follow-up score). Each model included the treatment group variable, the potential effect modifier and the

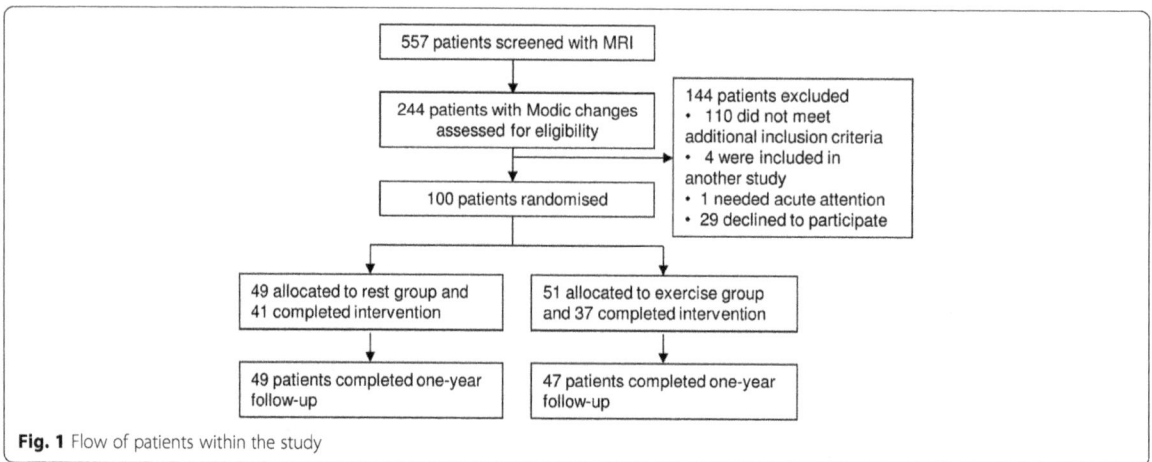

Fig. 1 Flow of patients within the study

Table 1 Rationale for variables

Modic changes Type 1 (compared with not having Type 1)

The histology of Type 1 shows fissured endplates and vascular granulation tissue adjacent to the endplate [7] and could potentially be an early state of bone healing. Therefore, we hypothesised that patients with Modic changes Type 1 would benefit more from rest than from exercise, as rest would facilitate bone healing compared with the compression forces added from exercise.

Large modic changes (compared with small ones)

Kuisma et al. [26] found that extensive Modic changes (≥25 % of vertebral height) were associated with a higher pain score in a working population. Large Modic changes could represent larger disruptions of the endplate and vertebral body and might therefore signal a better outcome from rest than from exercise.

Large modic changes Type 1 (compared with not having this finding)

Based on the hypotheses mentioned above for Modic type and size, we expected that people with large Modic changes Type 1 would benefit more from rest than from exercise.

Severe disc degeneration (compared with not having this finding)

Hancock et al. [27] reported that disc degeneration grade of ≥3 (Pfirrmann grade 1–5) was more than 5 times more likely to be present in patients with acute LBP than in controls without current LBP. Severe disc degeneration and mild disc degeneration could respond differently to conservative treatment. However, the available evidence does not clearly indicate a direction of a potential subgroup effect. Patients with severe disc degeneration could benefit from exercise due to the overall positive effects of physical activity. On the other hand, exercise could lead to increased load on a degenerated joint which could potentially result in a negative outcome.

Large disc herniation (compared with not having this finding)

Patients with LBP and sciatica receiving active conservative treatment [28] who also had broad-based protrusions and extrusions ('large' herniations) had a better outcome in leg pain and physical function than patients with disc bulges or focal protrusions. However, the evidence is sparse and it is possible that 'large' herniations could benefit either from the general effects of exercise or from less load with rest.

interaction term between the two. The interaction term was used to quantify size of the effect modification.

It has been estimated that the detection of a statistically significant subgroup interaction effect in an RCT requires a sample size approximately four times that required to detect a main effect of the same size [14]. Previous authors have suggested secondary analysis of RCTs as an approach to develop hypotheses for potentially important effect modifiers that can then be tested in suitably large trials [15]. As the current hypothesis-setting study was clearly underpowered, our focus was on the estimated effect size rather than statistical significance. If the interaction was greater than the threshold for MCID of 1.0 NRS points identified by Lauridsen et al. [16], we further explored the clinical interpretation by assessing the effect of intervention (rest compared with exercise) separately for those positive for the subgroup and negative for the subgroup, by calculating the marginal means for the subgroups. In addition, the number of patients achieving a MCID >1.0 point on a 0–10 NRS was calculated for those patients who were subgroup negative or positive.

Ethics

This analysis was based on existing data collected for an RCT [8] approved by the Ethics Committee for the Region of Southern Denmark (approval # S-VF-20060111), registered in ClinicalTrials.gov (Identifier # NCT00454792) and performed following the Declaration of Helsinki principles. For all participants in the original RCT signed informed consent was obtained as required by the Ethics Committee for the Region of Southern Denmark. In Denmark, such secondary analysis does not require additional ethics approval (The Act on Processing of Personal Data, December 2012, Section 5.2; Act on Research Ethics Review of Health Research Projects, October 2013, Section 14.2).

Results

Data from 49 patients in the rest group and 47 in the exercise group were available from the original RCT and were used for these analyses. The mean age was 46 years (range 21–60) and 69 % were women.

Participants in both treatment groups had similar sociodemographic and clinical characteristics at baseline, including age, sex, body mass index, type of occupation, sick leave, pain, activity limitation, general health, depression and expectations of treatment effect. Also, the distributions of the MRI variables of interest were similar between the two groups (Table 2). Distribution of the MRI variables per disc level is shown in Additional file 1.

In the regression analyses, the interaction terms for type of Modic changes (Modic Type 1 compared with not having Type 1), size of Modic changes (large changes compared with small ones) and large Modic changes Type 1 (compared with not having this finding) were all greater than or approximated the 1.0-point threshold for clinical importance (Table 3). However, although we hypothesized that patients with these characteristics would benefit more from rest than from exercise, the direction of the effect was the opposite for all three variables. For example, the effect of rest versus exercise was less in participants with

Table 2 Distribution of MRI variables in the treatment groups

		Rest	Exercise	p-value
Modic changes Type 1	Yes	38	36	0.91
	No	11	11	
Large Modic changes (any type)	Yes	34	33	0.93
	No	15	14	
Large Modic changes Type 1	Yes	28	28	0.81
	No	21	19	
Severe disc degeneration	Yes	18	18	0.88
	No	31	29	
Large disc herniation	Yes	13	19	0.15
	No	36	28	

Table 3 Results of linear regression models for change score in pain at 14-month follow-up

	Beta coefficient	p-value	95 % confidence interval
Modic changes Type 1			
Treatment[a]	0.82	0.42	−1.19;2.82
Modic changes Type 1	−1.79	0.03	−3.41; −0.17
Interaction: Modic Type 1 & treatment	−0.99	0.39	−3.28;1.29
Constant	2.09	0.004	0.67;3.51
Large Modic changes (any type)			
Large Modic changes	1.23	0.13	−0.37;2.84
Treatment	1.08	0.26	−0.80;2.95
Interaction: large Modic changes & treatment	−1.49	0.19	−3.73;0.75
Constant	−0.14	0.83	−1.49;1.20
Large Modic changes Type 1			
Large Modic changes Type 1	0.07	0.93	−1.42;1.55
Treatment	0.89	0.27	−0.70;2.47
Interaction: large Modic changes Type 1 & treatment	−1.49	0.16	−3.57;0.58
Constant	0.68	0.24	−0.46;1.83
Severe disc degeneration			
Severe disc degeneration	−0.002	0.998	−1.53;1.52
Treatment	−0.24	0.78	−1.55;1.07
Interaction: severe disc degeneration & treatment	0.74	0.50	−1.40;2.88
Constant	0.72	0.13	−0.22;1.67
Large disc herniation			
Large disc herniation	0.73	0.34	−0.78;2.24
Treatment	0.38	0.56	−0.90;1.66
Interaction: large disc herniation & treatment	−0.92	0.42	−3.15;1.31
Constant	0.43	0.38	−0.53;1.39

[a]Rest compared with exercise

large Modic changes than in those with small Modic changes; the point estimate and 95 % CI for the interaction was −1.49 (−3.73 to 0.75). The interaction terms for disc degeneration and disc herniation did not meet the threshold for clinical importance (Table 3). As expected, none of the interaction terms for any of the MRI findings was statistically significant, most likely due to the small sample size.

As the interaction terms for type of Modic changes, size of Modic changes and large Modic changes Type 1 were larger than or approximated the 1.0-point threshold for clinical importance, therefore we further explored treatment effects for those in the subgroup compared with those not in the subgroup (Table 4). Patients with Modic changes Type 1 were 0.17 points (95 % CI −1.28 to 0.93)

worse with rest than exercise, while those without Modic changes Type 1 were 0.82 points (−1.23 to 2.86) better with rest (Table 4). Patients with large Modic changes were 0.41 (−1.62 to 0.79) points worse with rest, while those without large Modic changes were 1.08 points better with rest (−0.97 to 3.12). Similar findings were identified for patients with large Modic changes Type 1 compared with those without this finding (Table 4). We also present the findings as the number of patients achieving an MCID in the subgroups in Table 5. As an example, of those with Modic changes Type 1, 7 % fewer patients reached the MCID if they received rest compared with exercise, while in those without Modic Type 1 changes, 9 % more reached the MCID if they received rest compared with exercise.

A graphical display of the comparison of outcome in pain for the two treatment groups for the three potential effect modifiers reaching the threshold of 1.0 point, together with treatment effect for those in the subgroup or not in the subgroup (i.e. MRI finding positive vs. MRI finding negative) and interaction effect is shown in Figs. 2, 3 and 4.

Discussion
Statement of principal findings
To our knowledge, this is the first study investigating MRI findings as effect modifiers for response to conservative interventions in a LBP RCT. Although none of the interaction terms for any of the MRI findings tested were statistically significant, Modic changes Type 1, large Modic changes and large Modic changes Type 1 showed tentative evidence of effect modification that was potentially important in size (point estimates ranging from −0.99 to −1.49 on the NRS). Surprisingly, the direction of the effect modification was opposite to those specified in our hypothesis and this is further reason for caution when interpreting the findings. That all three results were consistently in the direction opposite to our hypothesis suggests the notion, that exercise would aggravate physically larger or early stage Modic changes, may have been biologically plausible but overly simplistic. Although this study was underpowered, thereby increasing the risk of the results being due to chance, it suggests which of these potential effect modifiers might be analysed in subsequent studies and provides data suitable for calculating sample sizes for such studies.

Strengths and weaknesses of the study
A strength of the current study is that it was based on data from an RCT, which is the definitive type of data in which to quantify effect modification [17]. In addition, the MRIs were reported using a standardised protocol by a radiologist who had previously demonstrated consistency in evaluating spinal pathologies and was blinded to both the treatment group and the clinical outcome, however, in

Table 4 Change in pain at 14-month follow-up in the two treatment groups

	Rest (mean (95% CI))	Exercise (mean (95% CI))	Treatment effect[a] (mean (95% CI))
Modic changes Type 1	0.13 (−0.62;0.88)	0.31 (−0.47;1.08)	−0.17 (−1.28;0.93)
No Modic changes Type 1	2.91 (1.51;4.31)	2.09 (0.69;3.49)	0.82 (−1.23;2.86)
Modic changes large (≥25 %)	0.68 (−0.18;1.53)	1.09 (0.22;1.96)	−0.41 (−1.62;0.79)
Modic changes small (<25 %)	0.93 (−0.35;2.22)	−0.14 (−1.47;1.19)	1.08 (−0.97;3.12)
Large Modic changes Type 1 (≥25 %)	0.14 (−0.79;1.08)	0.75 (−0.18;1.68)	−0.61 (−1.82;0.61)
No large Modic changes Type 1	1.57 (0.49;2.65)	0.68 (−0.45;1.82)	0.89 (−0.93;2.70)

Change in pain (95 % CI) at 14-month follow-up on a 0–10 point NRS in the two treatment groups for type of Modic changes, size of Modic changes and large Modic changes Type 1
[a]Rest compared with exercise

other settings and with other MRI variables the reliability could vary. Our choice of MRI variables as potential effect modifiers was not exhaustive and other variables could have been potentially important. However, as recommended by Sun et al. [9], we limited the number of variables to cautiously selected potential effect modifiers with, whenever possible, pre-specified assumptions about the direction of the effect. The hypotheses were built on the literature but, as this was often sparse, the likely direction of the effect was not always obvious a priori and we took the pragmatic view that an effect modifier might have potential importance regardless of the direction of the effect. A limitation to the generalisability of the results is that patients in the study population all had some type of Modic changes.

In a study by Bendix et al. [18] investigating Modic changes using low-field MRI (0.3 T) compared with high-field MRI (1.5 T), the authors found a difference in the prevalence rate, with Modic changes Type 1 being detected three times more often using low field MRI, whereas Type 2 was detected two times more often when using high field MRI. As the MRI system used in

the current study was low-field (0.2 T), this may have affected the observed prevalence of Type 1 and 2, but it is unknown whether one MRI approach is more accurate than the other or simply more sensitive and less specific. In addition, using only T1- and T2-weighted sequences to identify the type of Modic change may add to the uncertainty of identifying Modic changes Type 1, as this is optimally visualised using a fluid sensitive (STIR) sequence which was not used in the current study.

The MCID was set to 1 point, which is a small difference that is at the lower end of reported estimates for MCIDs. However, the MCID we used was based on the value estimated from a previous chronic LBP sample from the same hospital department and therefore is likely to be the most appropriate for our study sample [16]. Similarly, the RCT from which the data is used in the current study showed that these patients' pain scores, on average, changed very little over 1 year (0.8 (95 % CI 0.3 to 1.3)) suggesting that their MCID would also likely be low [8].

Meaning of the study and comparison with other studies

To our knowledge, there have been very few RCTs that have formally investigated treatment effect modifiers for exercise therapy [19] and previous attempts to identify subgroups of responders to exercise have used aspects of the clinical presentation. For example, Long et al. [20] found that short-term activity and short-term pain limitation were improved in people with a directional preference, if that exercise was matched to their directional preference rather than being unrelated to that preference. In the current study, we have taken a different approach by focusing on MRI findings rather than aspects of the clinical presentation. Both approaches may yield useful evidence but clearly there is a need to improve the effects of exercise by better targeting [19].

There have also been few previous studies of MRI findings as effect modifiers for LBP or sciatica treatments and, to our knowledge, all have investigated invasive interventions, such as injections and various types of surgery. Two of these studies found evidence of significant treatment

Table 5 Number of patients achieving a Minimal Clinical Important Difference

Subgroup	Rest	Exercise	Treatment effect
Modic changes Type 1	24 % (n = 9)	31 % (n = 11)	7 % fewer patients in the rest group achieved MCID
No Modic changes Type 1	64 % (n = 7)	55 % (n = 6)	9 % more patients in the rest group achieved MCID
Modic changes large (≥25 %)	32 % (n = 11)	39 % (n = 13)	7 % fewer patients in the rest group achieved MCID
Modic changes small (<25 %)	33 % (n = 5)	29 % (n = 4)	4 % more patients in the rest group achieved MCID
Large Modic changes Type 1 ((≥25 %)	25 % (n = 7)	36 % (n = 10)	11 % fewer patients in the rest group achieved MCID
No large Modic changes Type 1	43 % (n = 9)	37 % (n = 7)	6 % more patients in the rest group achieved MCID

Number of patients (in percentage) achieving a Minimal Clinical Important Difference (MCID >1.0-point on a 0–10 point NRS) at 14-month follow-up in the two subgroups

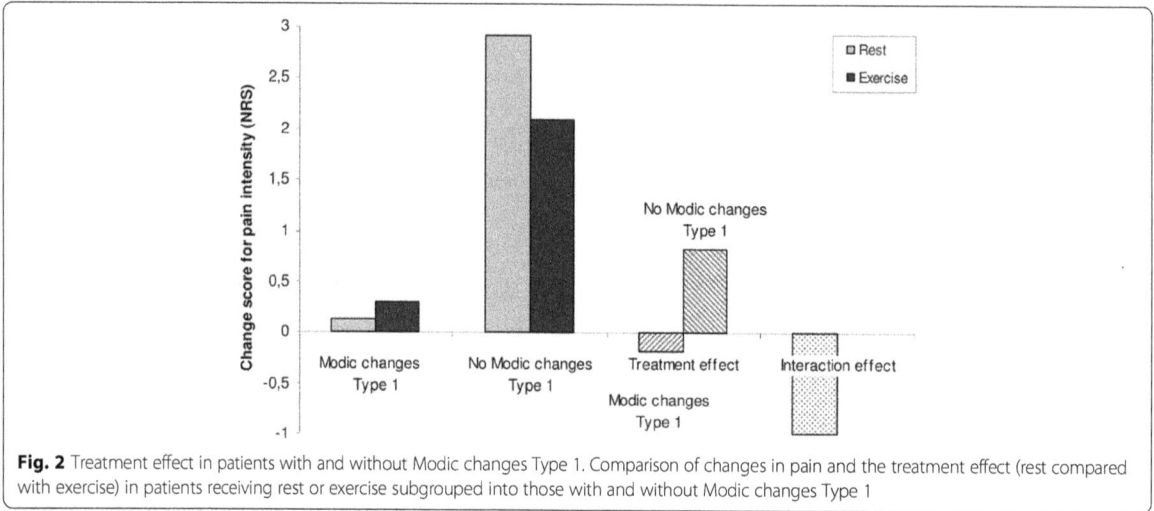

Fig. 2 Treatment effect in patients with and without Modic changes Type 1. Comparison of changes in pain and the treatment effect (rest compared with exercise) in patients receiving rest or exercise subgrouped into those with and without Modic changes Type 1

effect modification (calculations based on data presented in manuscripts) [21, 22]. One study found that people with LBP and Modic changes Type 1 (compared with Modic changes Type 2) had less activity limitation following Disprosan (steroid) injections than if they had saline injections [21]. The other found that sciatica patients with central disc herniation (compared with those without central disc herniation) had less pain following surgery than if they had rehabilitation instead [22]. As early activation and exercise are the most widely recommended treatment for LBP [6], it seems an oversight to not investigate pathoanatomic findings as potential effect modifiers for response to exercise.

Investigation into MRI findings as effect modifiers is complex for a number of reasons. A spinal MRI contains a large amount of anatomical information that requires a detailed protocol to be comprehensively described. When working with a dataset of small sample size, testing for effect modification inevitably leads to data reduction being required and this risks overlooking potentially important information such as location of disc herniation, signal intensity in herniation, location of Modic changes or irregular endplates. Also, numerous MRI findings are present at the same time at a segmental vertebral level and also across all five lumbar segments. For example, vertebral endplate signal changes (Modic changes) and vertebral disc herniation almost always co-exist with other degenerative disc findings, such as reduction of height and signal intensity of the disc [23, 24]. One approach to integrating this multiplicity would be to adjust for the co-existence of other MRI findings in the statistical modelling, but in this study that was not possible due to the lack of power. Alternatively,

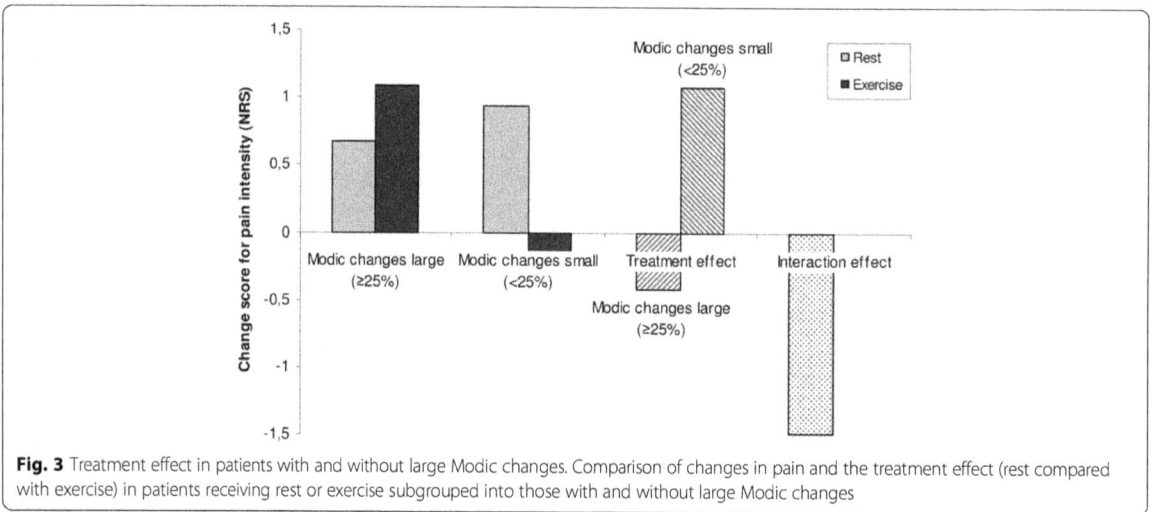

Fig. 3 Treatment effect in patients with and without large Modic changes. Comparison of changes in pain and the treatment effect (rest compared with exercise) in patients receiving rest or exercise subgrouped into those with and without large Modic changes

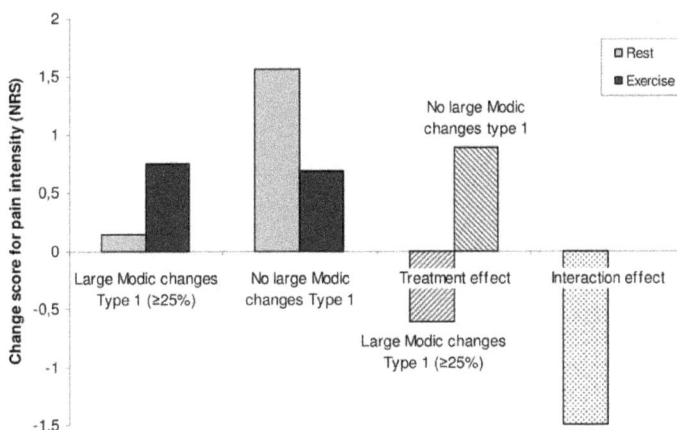

Fig. 4 Treatment effect in patients with and without large Modic changes Type 1. Comparison of changes in pain and the treatment effect (rest compared with exercise) in patients receiving rest or exercise subgrouped into those with and without large Modic changes Type 1

other statistical methods such as Latent Class Analyses could be used to define clusters of MRI findings and those clusters could then be tested as potential effect modifiers, instead of solitary MRI findings [25]. However, those types of analyses using MRI findings are still very novel and require further validation.

Conclusion

In this study, Modic changes Type 1, large Modic changes and large Modic changes Type 1 showed potentially important treatment modification effects by meeting or exceeding our threshold of a 1.0-point difference in pain intensity (0–10 NRS) at 14-month follow-up. Severe disc degeneration and large disc herniations did not reach that threshold. The results need to be interpreted very cautiously as this was a hypothesis-setting study with a relatively small sample, none of the potential effect modifications reached statistical significance, and the effects were in the direction opposite to our hypothesis. Despite this, the findings can be used to indicate some MRI effect modifiers suitable for investigation in subsequent studies of LBP treatment effect and these estimates of effect could be used to adequately power those studies.

Additional file

Additional file 1: Distribution of MRI variables per disc level.
Distribution of type and size of Modic changes per disc level (one disc level = 2 endplates) in 96 patients (1056 endplates) with low back pain and Modic changes. Table B. Distribution of severe disc degeneration and type of herniation per disc level in 96 patients (480 discs) with low back pain and Modic changes. (PDF 35 kb)

Abbreviations

LBP: Low back pain; MRI: Magnetic resonance imaging; RCT: Randomised controlled trial; NRS: Numerical rating scale; MCID: Minimal clinically important difference; CI: Confidence interval; STIR: Short tau inversion recovery.

Competing interests
The authors declare that they have no competing interests.

Authors' contributions
RKJ, PK and MH all participated in conception and design of the project and in interpretation of the data. RKJ performed the analyses and wrote the draft manuscript. PK and MH made substantial contributions to the analyses and revising the manuscript. All authors have given their final approval of the version to be published.

Acknowledgement
RKJ and PMK are partially funded by The Foundation for Chiropractic Research and Postgraduate Education. The authors thank Suzanne Capell, professional English language editor, for editing the manuscript and Joan Solgaard Sorensen, radiologist, for coding the MRI protocols.

Author details
[1]Research Department, Spine Centre of Southern Denmark, Hospital Lillebaelt, Institute of Regional Health Research, University of Southern Denmark, Oestre Hougvej 55, 5500 Middelfart, Denmark. [2]Department of Sports Science and Clinical Biomechanics, University of Southern Denmark, Campusvej 55, 5230 Odense M, Denmark. [3]Faculty of Human Sciences, Macquarie University, Balaclava Rd, North Ryde 2113NSW, Australia.

References
1. Deyo RA, Rainville J, Kent DL. What can the history and physical examination tell us about low back pain? JAMA. 1992;268:760–5. doi:10.1001/jama.1992.03490060092030.
2. Kent P, Keating J. Do primary-care clinicians think that nonspecific low back pain is one condition? Spine (Phila Pa 1976). 2004;29:1022–31.
3. Fersum KV, Dankaerts W, O'Sullivan PB, Maes J, Skouen JS, Bjordal JM, et al. Integration of subclassification strategies in randomised controlled clinical trials evaluating manual therapy treatment and exercise therapy for non-specific chronic low back pain: a systematic review. Br J Sports Med. 2010;44:1054–62. doi:10.1136/bjsm.2009.063289.
4. Jensen TS, Karppinen J, Sorensen JS, Niinimaki J, Leboeuf-Yde C. Vertebral endplate signal changes (Modic change): a systematic literature review of prevalence and association with non-specific low back pain. Eur Spine J. 2008;17:1407–22. doi:10.1007/s00586-008-0770-2.
5. Thompson KJ, Dagher AP, Eckel TS, Clark M, Reinig JW. Modic changes on MR images as studied with provocative diskography: clinical relevance–a retrospective study of 2457 disks. Radiology. 2009;250:849–55.

6. Koes BW, van Tulder M, Lin CW, Macedo LG, McAuley J, Maher C. An updated overview of clinical guidelines for the management of non-specific low back pain in primary care. Eur Spine J. 2010;19:2075–94.
7. Modic MT, Steinberg PM, Ross JS, Masaryk TJ, Carter JR. Degenerative disk disease: assessment of changes in vertebral body marrow with MR imaging. Radiology. 1988;166:193–9.
8. Jensen RK, Leboeuf-Yde C, Wedderkopp N, Sorensen JS, Manniche C. Rest versus exercise as treatment for patients with low back pain and Modic changes. A randomized controlled clinical trial. BMC Med. 2012;10:22. doi:10.1186/1741-7015-10-22.
9. Sun X, Briel M, Walter SD, Guyatt GH. Is a subgroup effect believable? Updating criteria to evaluate the credibility of subgroup analyses. BMJ. 2010;340:c117. doi:10.1136/bmj.c117.
10. 'Minim', an MS-DOS program by Stephen Evans, Patrick Royston and Simon Day. [http://www-users.york.ac.uk/~mb55/guide/minim.htm]. Accessed 8 July 2015.
11. Childs JD, Piva SR, Fritz JM. Responsiveness of the numeric pain rating scale in patients with low back pain. Spine (Phila Pa 1976). 2005;30:1331–4.
12. Jensen TS, Sorensen JS, Kjaer P. Intra- and interobserver reproducibility of vertebral endplate signal (modic) changes in the lumbar spine: the Nordic Modic Consensus Group classification. Acta Radiol. 2007;48:748–54.
13. Solgaard SJ, Kjaer P, Jensen ST, Andersen P. Low-field magnetic resonance imaging of the lumbar spine: reliability of qualitative evaluation of disc and muscle parameters. Acta Radiol. 2006;47:947–53.
14. Brookes ST, Whitely E, Egger M, Smith GD, Mulheran PA, Peters TJ. Subgroup analyses in randomized trials: risks of subgroup-specific analyses; power and sample size for the interaction test. J Clin Epidemiol. 2004;57:229–36.
15. Kamper SJ, Maher CG, Hancock MJ, Koes BW, Croft PR, Hay E. Treatment-based subgroups of low back pain: a guide to appraisal of research studies and a summary of current evidence. Best Pract Res Clin Rheumatol. 2010;24:181–91. doi:10.1016/j.berh.2009.11.003.
16. Lauridsen HH, Hartvigsen J, Manniche C, Korsholm L, Grunnet-Nilsson N. Responsiveness and minimal clinically important difference for pain and disability instruments in low back pain patients. BMC Musculoskelet Disord. 2006;7:82.
17. Kent P, Hancock M, Petersen DH, Mjosund HL. Clinimetrics corner: choosing appropriate study designs for particular questions about treatment subgroups. J Man Manip Ther. 2010;18:147–52. doi:10.1179/106698110X12640740712419.
18. Bendix T, Sorensen JS, Henriksson GA, Bolstad JE, Narvestad EK, Jensen TS. Lumbar modic changes-a comparison between findings at low- and high-field magnetic resonance imaging. Spine (Phila Pa 1976). 2012;37:1756–62.
19. Kent P, Mjosund HL, Petersen DH. Does targeting manual therapy and/or exercise improve patient outcomes in nonspecific low back pain? A systematic review. BMC Med. 2010;8:22. doi:10.1186/1741-7015-8-22.
20. Long A, Donelson R, Fung T. Does it matter which exercise? A randomized control trial of exercise for low back pain. Spine (Phila Pa 1976). 2004;29:2593–602.
21. Cao P, Jiang L, Zhuang C, Yang Y, Zhang Z, Chen W, et al. Intradiscal injection therapy for degenerative chronic discogenic low back pain with end plate Modic changes. Spine J. 2011;11:100–6. doi:10.1016/j.spinee.2010.07.001.
22. Pearson AM, Blood EA, Frymoyer JW, Herkowitz H, Abdu WA, Woodward R, et al. SPORT lumbar intervertebral disk herniation and back pain: does treatment, location, or morphology matter? Spine (Phila Pa 1976). 2008;33:428–35. doi:10.1097/BRS.0b013e31816469de.
23. Schmid G, Witteler A, Willburger R, Kuhnen C, Jergas M, Koester O. Lumbar disk herniation: correlation of histologic findings with marrow signal intensity changes in vertebral endplates at MR imaging. Radiology. 2004;231:352–8.
24. Wang Y, Videman T, Battie MC. ISSLS prize winner: lumbar vertebral endplate lesions: associations with disc degeneration and back pain history. Spine (Phila Pa 1976). 2012;37:1490–6. doi:10.1097/BRS.0b013e3182608ac4.
25. Jensen RK, Jensen TS, Kjaer P, Kent P. Can pathoanatomical pathways of degeneration in lumbar motion segments be identified by clustering MRI findings. BMC Musculoskelet Disord. 2013;14:198. doi:10.1186/1471-2474-14-198.
26. Kuisma M, Karppinen J, Niinimaki J, Ojala R, Haapea M, Heliovaara M, et al. Modic changes in endplates of lumbar vertebral bodies: prevalence and association with low back and sciatic pain among middle-aged male workers. Spine (Phila Pa 1976). 2007;32:1116–22.
27. Hancock M, Maher C, Macaskill P, Latimer J, Kos W, Pik J. MRI findings are more common in selected patients with acute low back pain than controls? Eur Spine J. 2012;21:240–6. doi:10.1007/s00586-011-1955-7.
28. Jensen TS, Albert HB, Sorensen JS, Manniche C, Leboeuf-Yde C. Magnetic resonance imaging findings as predictors of clinical outcome in patients with sciatica receiving active conservative treatment. J Manipulative Physiol Ther. 2007;30:98–108.

4

Chiropractor interaction and treatment equivalence in a pilot randomized controlled trial: an observational analysis of clinical encounter video-recordings

Stacie A Salsbury[1*], James W DeVocht[1], Maria A Hondras[2], Michael B Seidman[1], Clark M Stanford[3] and Christine M Goertz[1]

Abstract

Background: Chiropractic care is a complex health intervention composed of both treatment effects and non-specific, or placebo, effects. While doctor-patient interactions are a component of the non-specific effects of chiropractic, these effects are not evaluated in most clinical trials. This study aimed to: 1) develop an instrument to assess practitioner-patient interactions; 2) determine the equivalence of a chiropractor's verbal interactions and treatment delivery for participants allocated to active or sham chiropractic groups; and 3) describe the perceptions of a treatment-masked evaluator and study participants regarding treatment group assignment.

Methods: We conducted an observational analysis of digital video-recordings derived from study visits conducted during a pilot randomized trial of conservative therapies for temporomandibular pain. A theory-based, iterative process developed the 13-item *Chiropractor Interaction and Treatment Equivalence Instrument*. A trained evaluator masked to treatment assignment coded video-recordings of clinical encounters between one chiropractor and multiple visits of 26 participants allocated to active or sham chiropractic treatment groups. Non-parametric statistics were calculated.

Results: The trial ran from January 2010 to October 2011. We analyzed 111 complete video-recordings (54 active, 57 sham). Chiropractor interactions differed between the treatment groups in 7 categories. Active participants received more interactions with clinical information (8 vs. 4) or explanations (3.5 vs. 1) than sham participants within the therapeutic domain. Active participants received more directions (63 vs. 58) and adjusting instrument thrusts (41.5 vs. 23) in the procedural domain and more optimistic (2.5 vs. 0) or neutral (7.5 vs. 5) outcome statements in the treatment effectiveness domain. Active participants recorded longer visit durations (13.5 vs. 10 minutes). The evaluator correctly identified 61% of active care video-recordings as active treatments but categorized only 31% of the sham treatments correctly. Following the first treatment, 82% of active and 11% of sham participants correctly identified their treatment group. At 2-months, 93% of active and 42% of sham participants correctly identified their group assignment.

Conclusions: Our findings show the feasibility of evaluating doctor-patient interactions in chiropractic clinical trials using video-recordings and standardized instrumentation. Clinical trial design and clinician training protocols should improve and assess the equivalence of doctor-patient interactions between treatment groups.

(Continued on next page)

* Correspondence: stacie.salsbury@palmer.edu
[1]Palmer College of Chiropractic, Palmer Center for Chiropractic Research, 741 Brady Street, Davenport, IA 52803, USA
Full list of author information is available at the end of the article

(Continued from previous page)

Trial registration: This trial was registered in ClinicalTrials.gov as NCT01021306 on 24 November 2009.

Keywords: Chiropractic, Musculoskeletal manipulations, Observational study, Physician-patient relations, Placebo effect, Randomized controlled trials, Sham treatment, Verbal behavior, Video recording

Background

Chiropractic care is a complex health intervention. Complex health interventions are those healthcare therapies constructed from multiple independent and interacting components rather than composed of a single active ingredient, such as a medication [1-3]. With chiropractic care, these interacting components may include the biomechanical characteristics of spinal or joint manipulation, the therapeutic components of chiropractic care, and the non-specific effects of health interventions in general. The biomechanical characteristics of spinal manipulation [4-8] are commonly described in terms of force-time profile (e.g., loading rates, peak and pre-load forces) [8-10] or the thrust characteristics of location, direction and duration [9,11]. Therapeutic components of chiropractic care may include the underlying theoretical paradigm (i.e., subluxation, biomechanical, or somatic dysfunction) [12-15], specific techniques applied [16-19], and treatment frequency or dose [20]. The non-specific or contextual effects of health interventions are often termed 'placebo effects' [3,21,22]. Placebo effects are physiological responses to an intervention that vary by individual and in extent due to the nature of an intervention, its invasiveness, and the patient's expectations for cure or relief and which may have an impact on patient-reported outcomes, such as pain [23-26]. Placebo effects of a health intervention may include such diverse facets as treatment credibility [3,27], therapeutic ritual [28-30], patient response to clinical observation [28], patient and provider expectations [21,27,31-34], classical conditioning [32,34], the biological pathways involved in pain perception [22,31,32], and patient-practitioner interactions [21,27,31,35].

In clinical trials of chiropractic, manual therapy, acupuncture, medical or surgical interventions, or complementary and alternative medicine (CAM), the notion of the placebo effect may be conflated with the placebo treatment, that is, the comparative or control group [22,23,28,34]. These placebo treatments often are termed 'sham' treatments [36,37]. An ideal sham intervention is a procedure that mimics the active treatment in every way except for the absence of the therapeutic component under investigation [23]. Thus, when conducting a randomized controlled trial (RCT) that involves a placebo or sham treatment group, it is not sufficient to provide a sham that is both credible and non-therapeutic [3,21,38,39]. In order to accurately determine the effectiveness of an active treatment, investigators must ensure

that non-specific treatment effects (e.g., doctor-patient interactions, time demands, touch or other contact) are the same for participants in the sham group as for the therapeutic group [3,21,23,38,39].

While clinical trials of chiropractic care and other complex health interventions may examine the effects of a treatment on patient-centered outcomes, such as pain or disability [40-42], few trials have considered how placebo effects associated with these therapies may impact patient outcomes [3,21,22,27,43]. One reason researchers have not evaluated placebo effects in clinical trials of chiropractic is the lack of research instruments or data collection processes to quantify these effects. The overall purpose of this observational study was to assess the feasibility of quantifying doctor-patient interactions in sham-controlled chiropractic clinical trials. We also compared these findings to participant perceptions of their treatment group assignment from that same trial. Thus, our specific aims were fourfold. First, we developed a theory-derived data collection tool, the *Chiropractor Interactions and Treatment Equivalence Instrument* (CITE-I), to assess video-recordings of clinical encounters between doctors of chiropractic (DCs) and chiropractic patients. Secondly, we evaluated the equivalence of one chiropractor's verbal interactions and treatment delivery for participants randomized to the active treatment and sham-controlled chiropractic care groups in an expertise-based, pilot RCT of Activator Methods Chiropractic Technique (AMCT) for temporomandibular disorder (TMD) [44]. Next, we described the video evaluator's masked assessment of participant treatment assignment with the RCT participants' beliefs about their treatment group assignment. Finally, we described participants' perceptions of their treatment group assignment after the first treatment visit and following 2 months of treatment.

Methods

We conducted an observational analysis of digital video-recordings derived from study visits with participants who received an active or sham chiropractic treatment during a pilot RCT of 4 conservative therapies for TMD-related jaw pain. A theory-based, iterative process developed the 5-domain, 13-variable, *Chiropractor Interaction and Treatment Equivalence Instrument*. In these methods, we describe the design of the pilot RCT, video-recording procedures, the instrument development process, and data collection and analysis procedures.

Pilot RCT design

The institutional review boards of the Palmer College of Chiropractic, Davenport, Iowa (Approval Number 2009D121), and The University of Iowa, Iowa City, Iowa (Approval Number 200808726) approved the study protocol and human research participant protections for the pilot RCT. This trial was registered in ClinicalTrials. gov as NCT01021306 on 24 November 2009. The trial began January 2010, with data collection completed October 2011. The methods and results of the pilot RCT were described elsewhere [44]. Participants had at least a 6-month history of jaw pain consistent with chronic myofascial TMD. Eighty participants were randomly allocated to one of four treatment groups: active AMCT (n = 20), sham AMCT (n = 19), dental reversible interocclusal splint therapy (RIST) (n = 20), or self-care only (n = 21). Participants in all four groups received a basic self-care training module of relaxation, stretching and self-awareness pain modulation therapy. The self-care treatment group received this module, alone. Participants signed a written informed consent. The informed consent document instructed participants that they may be randomized to a "placebo treatment group" with treatments similar in appearance to AMCT and that the investigators did not expect the TMD condition of participants assigned to this group to worsen over the course of the study [23,38]. The consent document informed participants that study visits would be video-recorded to evaluate the doctor's interactions with participants and that these recordings would not be destroyed.

One DC with over 20 years of experience using the AMCT protocol provided the intervention to all participants in both the active and sham AMCT groups. The DC delivered both treatments with a hand-held, spring-loaded device – the Activator Adjusting Instrument (AAI) (Activator IV, Activator Methods International Ltd., Phoenix, AZ) instead of a manual thrust common to many forms of chiropractic spinal manipulation [17,45]. The DC mimicked the active AMCT protocol for the sham group by using a detuned AAI that made just a sound (like the active AAI), but delivered no thrust. The DC delivered the AMCT protocol, including treatment to the full spine, extremities, and temporomandibular joints for participants in both groups [44]. The DC also performed a gentle occipital stretching procedure following delivery of the standard AMCT treatment. Training on the study protocol emphasized the DC should offer the same type of verbal communication and spend a similar amount of time with patients in each treatment group, including in self-care instruction, examination and testing procedures, and treatment delivery [44].

All participants randomized to the AMCT groups were to receive 12 study visits over 2 months [44]. Primary outcomes included an 11-point numerical rating scale for TMD-related pain [46] and the 14-item Oral Health Impact Profile (OHIP-14) [47] to assess quality of life at 2 months and 6 months. Participant ratings of treatment believability were gathered for all 4 treatment groups following the first and twelfth study visits [19]. Participants also answered the following statement on a 5-item scale ('strongly believe' to 'do not know'): "There are two types of treatments in this research study: active and inactive (placebo). Please indicate which type of treatment you believe you are receiving". Participant responses for 'strongly believe' and 'somewhat believe' for active treatment and 'strongly believe' and 'somewhat believe' for inactive (placebo) treatment were combined in this analysis.

Video recording and handling process

The study protocol included video recordings of each chiropractic study visit. Thus, our study sample was the video-recorded observations of participant study visits, and not the participants themselves. A digital video-camera (Panasonic model HDC-H520; Newark, NJ, USA) was set up on a tripod in a corner of the treatment room before the participant entered. A card with the participant identification (ID) number and current date was placed in front of the video-camera and recorded for a few seconds. The video-camera was to be positioned to visualize the participant's entire body lying on the treatment table (from crown of head to feet), as well as the DC as he moved around the table delivering the study treatment. The clinic receptionist used a remote control unit to begin the video-recording process as the participant entered the treatment room and to stop the recording when the participant left the treatment room. The video files were copied from the camera to an external hard drive and named with the participant ID number and recording date. No other identifying information was recorded to maintain participant confidentiality. A study co-leader (JWD) copied the video files from the external hard drive in the chiropractic clinic to a second external hard drive for data transfer to the research center. The HD video-recordings were converted from *. m2ts to *.mp4 files using Roxio Toast Titanium 10 software (Corel Corporation, Ottawa, Ontario, Canada). This version of the video-recordings was stored at the research center on a password-protected computer for long-term back-up and data analysis.

Instrument development process

Four team members developed the assessment instrument and data collection process to codify the doctor-patient interactions during the chiropractic visits (see Author Information for respective contributions). Team members remained blinded to participants' treatment assignment throughout the instrument development, data collection and analysis processes. The instrument development process went through 3 primary stages as described below.

Stage 1: Preliminary video-recordings review and research question

Two researchers (JWD, SAS) jointly reviewed several video-recordings to examine various aspects of the doctor-patient interactions such as verbal communications (i.e., clinician utterances, participant replies), non-verbal behaviors, and contextual effects (e.g., social interactions, humor, or use of touch) as well as factors related to the recording process to identify the initial coding framework and the strengths and limitations of these video-recordings as data sources. For example, most of the video-recordings did not visualize the participant during pre-treatment consultations or post-treatment interactions due to camera position. In addition, the audio-track often did not record the participants' side of these conversations clearly. The treatment table muffled participants' voices when lying prone during much of the AMCT-protocol. Similarly, the camera position for many video-recordings did not allow complete visualization of the non-verbal behaviors (e.g., facial expressions, body position, treatment delivery, AAI positioning) of the DC when his back was to the camera, nor could participants observe these doctor behaviors when they were lying prone. Further, the participants' ideal body position (i.e., from the crown of the head to the feet) was captured in only about 25% of the videos recorded.

Based on such contextual factors, the investigators (SAS, JWD, MAH) concluded that an analysis of doctor-patient interactions could neither focus on the non-verbal communications of the DC nor emphasize participants' verbal responses. However, we noted the recordings captured most of the chiropractor's verbal utterances as well as the "clicking" sounds produced by the thrust of the active and detuned AAIs. A previous study using AAI as a placebo treatment noted this clicking sound supported patients' assessments of treatment credibility [37]. The team then focused the research question and instrument development process on quantification of the equivalence of the DC's verbal communications and AAI delivery between the active and sham AMCT groups.

Stage 2: Construct identification and instrument development

Literature reviews identified published instruments available for the assessment of doctor-patient interactions in medical encounters [48-50]. Among these, the Roter Interaction Analysis System (RIAS) was identified as the most widely used method of analyzing patient-provider interactions during healthcare encounters [49], and served as the theoretical framework from which our instrument was derived. The RIAS classifies medical communications into two conceptual categories - the socioemotional and task dimensions [49]. While the RIAS has excellent

psychometric properties [49], a major limitation of this instrument for an analysis of patient-provider communications within the context of clinical research is that conversational styles of communication in RCTs differ from those in naturally-occurring medical encounters [30,35,51]. In routine clinical practice, physicians may tailor patient education, advice and support to the individual needs of the patient [27]. In contrast, the communications from the research clinician to the research participant within an RCT is a protocol-driven, or scripted, conversation to minimize its influence on treatment outcomes [28,35,43]. In addition, while research participants are masked to their treatment assignment at the start of a RCT, clinician behavior may lead them to identify whether they are receiving an active or placebo/sham treatment [27,30,35,37,43,51,52]. Thus, the clinician's verbal communications and treatment delivery should not unmask participants to treatment assignment [43]. Finally, the research clinicians' verbal interactions may directly impact outcomes assessments in an RCT should the doctor communicate any observed or perceived changes in health status, such as an improvement or decline, to participants [43,51,53].

At this stage, the team first focused instrument development on two theoretical categories of the RIAS: socio-emotional, or 'care-oriented', communications and instrumental, or 'cure-oriented', communications [49,54] to assure these key features of doctor-patient interactions were identified. Video-recordings were viewed over several team meetings to identify how these thematic constructs were expressed by the clinician during treatment. Each member coded the video-recordings using a paper copy of the current assessment form. Video reviewers placed a hash mark in the appropriate cell for each utterance from the clinician and any clicks from the AAI thrust. An utterance was defined as any verbalization that expressed a single idea to a participant. Thus, a sentence in which the DC directed the participant to "turn your head to the right, and to the center, and to the left" would equate 3 unique utterances. Team members stopped the video-recording frequently to discuss how each had categorized the various utterances, the rationale for such categorization, and sought consensus on each classification.

The team reviewed 2–4 video-recordings per session, determined categorical or definitional revisions, and identified form changes. For instance, clinician utterances on participants' health status (i.e., need for more or fewer adjustments since the last visit) required an added domain for "treatment effectiveness" with optimistic, pessimistic and neutral statements on patient outcomes constituting key variables. This category was of particular importance within a sham-controlled trial where verbal indications of treatment effectiveness may increase participant expectancies for future response [31], serve as a conditioning protocol [31], and impact patient outcome measures [31]. We included a variable for the duration of the study visit to assess whether the clinician spent an equivalent amount time with participants in each group. We also added a tally of AAI clicks (an auditory stimulus that may condition the participant and increase the placebo response [31]) as a rough indicator of the 'dose' delivered of active or sham AMCT.

Stage 3: Process pre-testing, evaluator training and instrument refinement

SAS and JWD evaluated video-recordings until the team members achieved consensus on the instrument domains, variables, examples and data collection format as no new categories were identified with additional video-recording reviews. MAH confirmed the completeness of initial data collection form. While the team did not assess inter-rater agreement using formal statistics, comparison of categorical totals at the end of each data collection session revealed a high level of agreement between reviewers, with most categories tallying within 1 [for categories with low tallies (0–8 hash marks), such as treatment effectiveness] to 3 points [for categories with high tallies (30–50 hash marks) such as directions or AAI clicks] for each evaluator.

During pre-testing, the team also identified treatment duration differences, with the first treatment visit (T1) lasting 10–20 minutes longer than subsequent study visits (T2-T12). During the T1 visit, the DC spent considerable time discussing the participants' past medical history, the study protocol, and follow-up activities. As these visits appeared tailored to the individual participant, and differed considerably in duration and content from the other treatment visits, we decided not to include these visits in the analysis for this study.

The team member (MBS) who served as the video evaluator was trained on the video analysis instrument. As in previous coding rounds, team members coded the recordings as a group and discussed unclear utterances, variable definitions and examples. Early in the training, the video evaluator had categorical inconsistencies (primarily with therapeutic domain variables) that were resolved through these discussions. The instrument was reorganized so the most used variables (*clinical information, directions, Activator clicks*) were placed at the top of the grid. Categorical tallies after each coding round noted few differences between the team members.

The team members reviewed and accepted the Chiropractor Interaction and Treatment Equivalence Instrument (CITE-I) for use in the interaction equivalence study. This version of the CITE-I included 5 domains with 13 variables. The affective domain consisted of 2 socio-emotional variables [49,54] categorizing the clinician's verbal interactions as *social/humor* or *name use*. The

therapeutic domain included 3 instrumental variables [49,54]: *clinical information, explanations*, and *logistics*. The procedural domain consisted of 3 variables addressing treatment implementation and fidelity [55] including adherence, delivery, and dose: *directions, cautions*, and *Activator clicks*, or the sound produced by the adjusting instrument. The treatment effectiveness domain categorized *optimistic, pessimistic* and *neutral* statements about health or treatment outcomes [31]. Lastly, the encounter context domain tabulated the *duration* of the treatment encounter as an additional measure of dose, as well as any *unclear statements* made by the clinician that the video evaluator could not definitively place into another category. The CITE-I also included a field to denote how much of the participant's *body position* was on the video and a *notes field* to record additional details of the interaction context, blinding issues, etc. The final item on the CITE-I asks the video evaluator to denote which study treatment he believed the participant to have received (active, placebo/sham or not sure). Figure 1 presents the CITE-I instrument including variable definitions and examples.

Data collection

One team member (MBS) evaluated the video-recordings of the chiropractic visits using the CITE-I. A flash drive of video-recordings included mixed participants from discontinuous study visits to assure the evaluator did not view an entire treatment series sequentially. The evaluator viewed the recordings while wearing headphones to minimize external distractions. When necessary, portions of the video-recordings were replayed to enhance the accuracy of data collection. This process was repeated until all video recordings were evaluated.

Data management and data analysis

Completed CITE-I forms were submitted to the Office of Data Management for double key entry into an electronic spreadsheet once all video-recordings in an analytic set were evaluated. Tally marks were counted twice and entered as a total for each category by the evaluator, with these sums double checked by data entry personnel. Data were organized by participant ID number, treatment date, and treatment visit number. Participant treatment believability items were data entered at the time of the pilot RCT. Data were analyzed using the SAS statistical analysis software package (Version 9.2, SAS Institute Inc., Cary, North Carolina, USA). We report simple descriptive statistics (median, interquartile ranges [IQR], and/or number and percentage) to characterize our sample of video-recordings. Formal statistical tests of significance were not appropriate at this stage of instrument development as our primary aim was to assess whether video-recordings were a feasible means of evaluating

PTID:_____   Tx Date (mm/dd/yy):___/____/____   Tx Duration: ___:___ ___:___ ___   **Chiropractor Interaction and Treatment Equivalence Instrument (CITE-I)**

Variable	Definition	Examples	5	10	15	20	25	30	35	40	45	50	Total
Clinical Info Seeking	Questions/comments to obtain clinical or health information	How are you feeling?											
		How are you feeling?											
Directions or Instructions	Instructions given to participant related to treatment protocol	Place your arm... Lift your head. Relax.											
		Place your arm... Lift your head. Relax.											
	If two or move body movements are instructed in one sentence, count each movement separately.	Place your arm... Lift your head. Relax.											
Activator Clicks	Sounds produced by Activator Adjusting Instrument	Click!											
		Click!											
Optimistic Health Statement	Positive statement on health improvement / treatment success	Leg check is even. Good. Very nice.											
Pessimistic Health Statement	Negative statements on health decline / treatment nonsuccess	Much worse... Need adjustments											
Neutral Statement	Neutral statements about health or noncommittal sounds	Hmmm... I see... OK.											
Social / Humor	Statements or questions about everyday life / attempt at humor	Family, work, hobby, jokes, weather, laugh											
Cannot Make Out	Statement unclear or soft volume	(whispers)											
Explanation or Recommendation	Info given on protocol or actions pt should take to improve health	I do this to... You should do this...											
Cautions	Statements on uncomfortable or startling touch or treatments	This touch might hurt. I am lowering table.											
Study Logistics	Statements on study or schedule	Appointments, call-ins											

Number of times participant's name spoken: [_____]

Participant body position (upper- and lowermost body sections visible, such as head to knee, shoulder to feet, etc):

NOTES (Interaction context, blinding issues, etc.):

In your opinion, which study treatment did this participant receive? ☐₁ Active (Activator) Treatment   ☐₂ Placebo/Sham   ☐₃ Not sure

Evaluator ID: __ __ __ __   Evaluation Date (mm/dd/yy):___/____/____

Figure 1 Chiropractor Interaction and Treatment Equivalence Instrument (CITE-I).

doctor-patient interactions and not to test hypotheses based on those interactions.

Results

Video-recording evaluation flowchart

Figure 2 presents a flowchart of the video-recordings evaluated for this study. Each participant allocated to a chiropractic group (n = 39) was to receive 12 visits to the chiropractor per study protocol (n = 468). An equal number of participants from each group (n = 13) had at least 1 video-recording reviewed for this study. Four participants (3 in active AMCT, 1 in sham AMCT) withdrew from the trial before the first treatment, while 9 participants (5 in active AMCT, 4 in sham AMCT) did not have any video-recordings made during the trial. The mean number of video-recordings completed for all participants was 4.4 (range from 0–11).

For this analysis, we excluded all T1 visits from this analysis due to their longer durations and the more personalized nature of the encounters as compared to the T2-T12 visits. Other video-recordings were either not available or incomplete and not included. Of these, the number of missed appointments (n = 59), missed video-recordings (n = 172), and video-recordings excluded due to incomplete recordings (n = 43), either from video-recordings that began after the visit was in progress or that ended before the visit concluded, were equivalent between groups. In total, we analyzed 24% (111/468) of the planned active and sham AMCT study visits in this pilot RCT. The video evaluator coded 54 video-recordings from 13 active AMCT participants and 57 video-recordings from 13 sham AMCT participants for this analysis.

Chiropractor interactions and treatment equivalence

Table 1 presents results for the video analysis of clinician interaction and treatment equivalence between active and sham AMCT groups. Five categories, *clinical information, explanations, directions, optimistic statements*, and *neutral statements* revealed notable differences in the DC's verbal interactions, while two categories, *Activator clicks* and *encounter duration*, denoted disparities in treatment equivalence between the active and sham AMCT groups.

Within the therapeutic domain, the participants in active AMCT had twice as many verbal interactions where

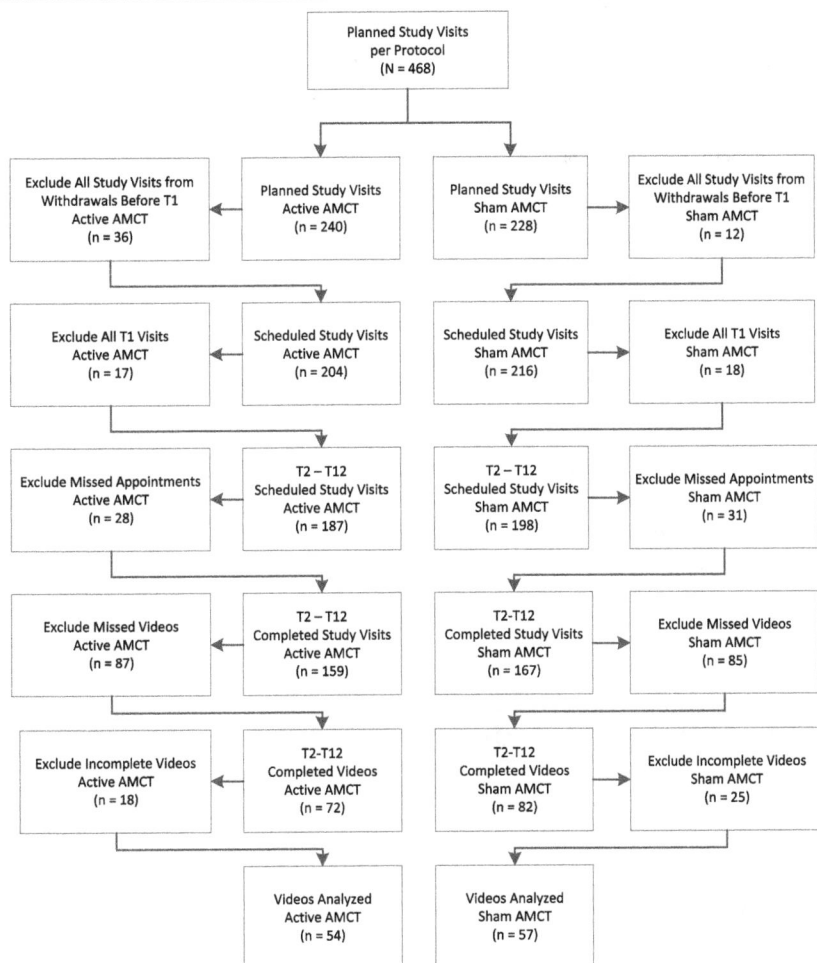

Figure 2 Video-recording flowchart.

the clinician sought *clinical information* than did sham AMCT participants (median 8.0 vs. 4.0 per visit). Active AMCT participants also received more *explanations* on the study protocol or recommendations on actions to take to improve health compared to sham AMCT participants (median 3.5 vs. 1.0 per visit). Statements about study *logistics* favored sham ACMT participants over active AMCT participants (median 2.0 vs. 1.0 per visit).

Within the procedural domain, active AMCT participants received more *directions* from the clinician than did sham AMCT participants (median 63 vs. 58 per visit). Active AMCT participants also received more *Activator clicks* than did sham AMCT participants (median 41.5 clicks vs. 23 clicks per visit). *Cautions* were similar between groups.

Within the treatment effectiveness domain, the DC offered active AMCT participants more *optimistic statements* about health improvements or treatment success than participants in the sham AMCT group (median 2.5 comments vs. 0 comments per visit). Active AMCT participants also received more *neutral statements* about their treatments than did sham AMCT participants (median 7.5 comments vs. 5 comments per visit), while few *pessimistic statements* were offered to participants in either treatment group.

Within the encounter context domain, the mean *encounter duration* was somewhat longer for the active AMCT group than the sham AMCT group (13.5 minutes vs. 10.0 minutes per treatment). More *unclear statements* were recorded for the active AMCT group (median 2.0 versus 1.0). Neither of the affective domain variables (*social/humor* or *name use*) differed appreciably between the treatment groups.

Treatment group assignment evaluation

Table 2 presents the results of the masked assessment of treatment assignment by the video evaluator and compares

Table 1 Video-analysis of chiropractor interaction equivalence between active and sham Activator Methods Chiropractic Technique (AMCT) treatment groups

Domain	Variable	Definition	Active AMCT (n =54)		Sham AMCT (n =57)	
			Median (SD)	IQR	Median (SD)	IQR
Affective	Social/Humor	Statements or questions about everyday life or attempts at humor	9.0 (14.9)	14	8.0 (11.2)	13
	Name Use	Number of times the name of the participant was spoken	2.0 (1.3)	2	2.0 (1.5)	1
Therapeutic	Clinical Information	Questions or comments to obtain clinical or health information	8.0 (5.3)	7	4.0 (3.1)	4
	Explanations	Information on protocol or actions to take to improve health	3.5 (9.2)	8	1.0 (3.6)	3
	Logistics	Statements on study procedures or treatment schedule	1.0 (1.4)	2	2.0 (2.5)	1
Procedural	Directions	Instructions given related to treatment protocol	63.0 (11.6)	15	58.0 (6.7)	8
	Cautions	Statements on uncomfortable or startling touch or treatments	3.0 (1.5)	2	3.0 (1.2)	1
	Activator Clicks	Sounds produced by Activator Adjusting Instrument	41.5 (30.1)	44	23.0 (10.1)	13
Treatment Effectiveness	Optimistic	Positive statement on health improvement or treatment success	2.5 (4.0)	6	0 (1.6)	0
	Pessimistic	Negative statement on health improvement or treatment success	0 (1.1)	1	0 (0.7)	0
	Neutral	Neutral statement about health or noncommittal sounds	7.5 (4.1)	6	5.0 (3.6)	4
Encounter Context	Encounter Duration	Duration of treatment in minutes	13.5 (4.1)	5	10.0 (1.8)	2
	Unclear Statement	Statement unclear or spoken at soft volume	2.0 (2.6)	3	1.0 (2.0)	3

Table 2 Video evaluator assessment of treatment assignment compared to participant treatment believability ratings

Variable	Response	Active AMCT Videos (n =54)		Sham AMCT Videos (n =57)	
		n^	%	n^	%
Video Evaluator Assessment of Treatment Assignment	Active AMCT	33	61	16	28
	Sham AMCT	3	6	18	31
	Not Sure	17	31	22	39
		Active AMCT participants (n =17)		Sham AMCT participants (n =18)	
Variable	Response	n	%	n	%
Participant Believability 1st Treatment Visit	Active Treatment+	14	82	12	66
	Inactive Treatment (Placebo)+	1	6	2	11
	Do Not Know	2	12	4	22
		Active AMCT participants (n =14)		Sham AMCT participants (n =14)	
Variable	Response	n	%	n	%
Participant Believability Month 2	Active Treatment+	13	93	8	58
	Inactive Treatment (Placebo)+	1	7	6	42
	Do Not Know	0	0	0	0

+Strongly believe and somewhat believe were combined for presentation.
^Missing data.

these data to participant's perceptions about their treatment assignment. The video evaluator correctly assigned an assessment of 'active treatment' to 33 (61%) of the active AMCT video-recordings, with most of the remaining (n = 17; 31%) video-recordings receiving a 'not sure' designation. The video evaluator assigned an assessment of 'active treatment' (n = 16; 28%), 'placebo/sham' (n = 18; 31%), and 'not sure' (n = 22; 39%) to the sham AMCT video-recordings.

In contrast to the treatment-masked evaluator, study participants more readily identified their treatment group assignments, particularly those in the active AMCT group. After the first study visit, 82% (n = 14) of active AMCT participants rated their treatment as an 'active treatment', with 6% (n = 1) rating the treatment as inactive or placebo, and 12% (n = 2) stating they did not know which treatment they received. After their first treatment, 66% (n = 12) of sham AMCT participants rated their treatment as active, 11% (n = 2) as inactive or placebo, and 22% (n = 4) as did not know. At the 2-month assessment, participant ratings of 'active treatment' increased to 93% (n = 13) for active AMCT participants. For sham AMCT participants, active treatment ratings dropped to 58% (n = 8), with inactive or placebo ratings increasing to 42% (n = 6). No participant in either group stated they did not know their treatment group at the 2-month evaluation.

Discussion

To our knowledge, this study is the first to assess the equivalence of verbal interactions and treatment delivery for a doctor of chiropractic providing active and sham chiropractic interventions within the context of a randomized controlled trial. Many studies of spinal manipulation or other chiropractic therapies have used sham adjustments as a comparator [36,56], including those using a detuned Activator adjusting instrument as the sham [37,57]. Researchers who conduct sham or placebo-controlled trials of complementary therapies, including chiropractic, have espoused the need for the standardization of the non-specific aspects of treatment, including treatment duration and the interventionists' verbal and non-verbal communications, between study groups [37,52,58]. And yet, most have evaluated only patient perceptions of the believability of the sham or their success in masking treatment assignment [37,52,59-61]. Few studies, if any, of chiropractic interventions have discussed the potential placebo effects derived from the doctor's interpersonal interactions with patients.

This study showed the feasibility of quantifying the verbal interactions and treatment equivalence of chiropractors within a clinical trial using a standardized data collection process. This finding has relevance for future clinical studies. Our data collection tool, the Chiropractor Interaction and Treatment Equivalence Instrument, may be tailored for specific chiropractic techniques, other manual therapies, and complementary and alternative medicine therapies, and perhaps to interventions delivered by other healthcare providers. The CITE-I also may be useful for several stages of the clinical trial development and implementation process [53,55,62,63]. For example, researchers might use the CITE-I to train clinicians in the delivery of the study protocol in an effort to provide participants in each treatment group with equivalent doses of interactions with the treatment provider, and equivalent treatments when more than one clinician delivers the study treatments [63]. This training procedure might be performed via video-recordings that are either reviewed by the investigators or by the clinicians themselves, to identify areas to treatment standardization (e.g., number of adjustments, clinical information queries) before the start of the trial [62]. Once the trial is underway, the same instrument might be used for quality control purposes to minimize drift in treatment delivery over the course of the trial [64]. Finally, once the trial is concluded, the CITE-I might be used to assess treatment fidelity over the course of the study [53,55].

Our study found potentially important discrepancies in the DC's verbal interactions, including in communications related to clinical information, explanations, protocol-related directions, and statements about treatment effectiveness between the active and sham groups. In essence, active AMCT participants may have received an 'augmented interaction' with the DC, similar to that delivered by acupuncturists in an RCT specifically designed to assess various components of the placebo effect in patients with irritable bowel syndrome [28]. In that study, participants allocated to the augmented interaction group received acupuncturists' communications that emphasized 5 behaviors shown to support optimal patient-practitioner relationships: a friendly manner, active listening, empathy, thoughtful silence, and communication of confidence in and positive expectations for treatment [28]. These augmented communication styles were not dissimilar to the added interactions the active AMCT participants received when the DC sought more clinical information, offered treatment explanations or self-care recommendations, or shared optimistic statements about participants' changes in health status. These differences in the practitioner's verbal interactions may explain the higher satisfaction levels of participants in the active AMCT group reported in the pilot RCT, and possibly account for some of the difference in outcomes between the two chiropractic groups [44].

We also reported the video evaluator's perceptions of treatment assignment and the RCT participants' perceptions of treatment believability. The video evaluator correctly attributed 'active treatment' to 61% of the active AMCT videos, while incorrectly ascribing 'placebo/sham' to only 6% of the active AMCT group. This finding suggests a perceptible difference in the DC's interactions between treatment groups that allowed a trained evaluator to correctly identify participants who received active AMCT more often than by chance. Similarly, 82% and 93% of active AMCT participants correctly identified their treatment as an active treatment after the first and final treatments, respectively. In contrast, sham AMCT participants shifted their treatment perceptions as inactive from 11% at first treatment to 42% at the final treatment. The video evaluator's and participants' perceptions of treatment assignment might be based on two notable differences in treatment delivery identified in this analysis: treatment duration and number of audible sounds generated by the adjusting instrument during its thrust. Active AMCT participants received study visits that were three minutes longer in duration and during which almost twice as many instrument-assisted adjustments were delivered. The sounds made by the adjusting instrument were identified in a previous study as evidence of treatment credibility [37]. Future chiropractic trials with sham treatment groups should develop study protocols that maximize equivalence in such components of treatment delivery.

While our analysis focused on the doctor's verbal interactions, the non-verbal communications which were not measured in this study may account for the differences noted in the treatment group assignment perceptions of the video evaluator and study participants. Other researchers have identified the importance of such non-verbal communications as tone of voice, facial expression and eye contact [65], the use of touch [65,66], and provider time spent sitting versus standing during clinical encounters [67] on patient satisfaction and health outcomes. Future studies may more closely examine the contributions of non-verbal communication to the placebo effects of chiropractic care although those may be more difficult to adequately record and quantify than were verbal interactions.

Our study has several strengths. Our method of video-recording doctor-patient interactions during chiropractic care is similar to other studies using video-recordings to assess the clinical or communication skills of health professionals [68]. The advantages of video-recordings for this type of research are numerous [69,70]. First, a video-recording is a permanent account of human interactions that are complex, fleeting, and difficult to detail or verify using standard documentation techniques for observational data (e.g., field notes, memos) [69]. As we did during the instrument development process, observers may view video-recorded interactions repeatedly, at different speeds and directions, and with pauses, allowing for thorough and reliable analyses [69,70]. Multiple reviewers also may analyze the same interaction, which may decrease the subjectivity inherent in observational techniques [69,70]. Another strength was the number of recordings analyzed, recorded from multiple participants at different phases of

the treatment protocol. In addition, team members were blinded to the treatment assignment of participants throughout the instrument development process as well as during video-recording analysis. These procedures enhance the validity of the study findings [69].

This study had its limitations, including the challenges inherent in the video-recording process [68-71]. Mechanical limitations, such as camera malfunctions, static camera positions, or muffled audio mechanisms, are known issues in research using video-recordings [69-71]. Future studies might position the video-camera on the ceiling, employ two cameras, or use cameras that automatically follow movement to allow fuller visualization of the doctor-patient interaction, as researchers have done in similar studies conducted in emergency departments, physician consultations, or during surgical procedures [64,71,72].

Another limitation is the potential influence of the video-recoding process on the behaviors of the persons whose interactions are recorded [69,70]. Some studies have shown few differences in camera-related behaviors [73] or doctor-patient interactions during video-recorded clinical encounters [68,74], while others indicate improved performance by physicians whose clinical encounters were video-recorded [75]. The frequency with which such behaviors occurred was not evaluated in this analysis, although some patterns were noted that may suggest clinician discomfort with the video-recording process. For example, the camera often was positioned in such a way that it did not visualize the participants' entire body (most notably the neck and head region) or pick up DC utterances while seated at the head of the treatment table. Future studies should assess clinician comfort with the video-recording process directly.

Another limitation is missing data. We analyzed just 24% of the planned study visits in this pilot RCT. While some missing data-points were from missed appointments, more were from unrecorded treatment visits or incomplete video-recordings. Clinic staff missed or truncated the video-recordings when the office was busy or other clinical demands tasks were prioritized. Similar analyses have reported similar challenges capturing all possible events due to problems with the recording device or human error in initiating the video-recording process [72]. Future studies collecting video-recordings to assess doctor-patient interactions should institute pre-treatment checklists and on-going quality control procedures to assure complete datasets.

In this analysis, we opted not to evaluate the video-recordings for the first treatment visit due to the extended duration and content differences for these visits compared to the T2-T12 study visits. Eight active AMCT participants and 6 sham AMCT participants did not have their T1 study visits video-recorded. Finniss and colleagues note, however, that first treatment encounters may

Chiropractor interaction and treatment equivalence in a pilot randomized controlled trial...

37

be of critical importance in the "development of subsequent robust placebo responses" (p. 688) through a chain of treatment expectancy, conditioning mechanisms, and the perceived effectiveness of the initial interaction [31]. A future study using this or similar datasets might evaluate the doctor-patient interactions using a more discrete data collection system such as the RIAS to assess group differences in medical history taking, rapport building, self-care instructions, and other socio-emotional relationship components during the initial treatment encounter [49]. Such an evaluation also would allow a comparison of the communication strategies of DCs to other healthcare professionals [76-80].

Lastly, this study was a preliminary investigation of doctor-patient interactions with a pilot clinical trial of chiropractic care. We developed the Chiropractic Interaction and Treatment Equivalence Instrument specifically for this preliminary study. While the conceptual framework for the instrument seems logical and our analysis did identify differences in the doctor's interactions between treatment groups, the CITE-I requires further refinement, including formal instrument testing to establish its reliability and validity. Item analysis may identify different domains than those presented here, as well as individual items that are redundant or that might be omitted. Psychometric evaluations of the CITE-I should occur before its use in other clinical studies of chiropractic care or in other manual therapy trials.

Conclusion
Our findings show the feasibility of evaluating doctor-patient verbal interactions and treatment equivalence in chiropractic clinical trials using video-recordings of doctor-patient encounters and a standardized data collection tool, the Chiropractor Interaction and Treatment Equivalence Instrument. The results of our study indicated that doctor-patient interactions in randomized controlled trials of chiropractic therapies may vary between the active care and sham-controlled treatment groups. It is not known how much effect such variation in doctor-patient interaction has on clinical outcomes. However, to accurately compare the clinical value of one form of treatment to that of another, clinical trial design and training protocols of clinicians who deliver study interventions should include steps to minimize the variation of doctor-patient interactions between treatment groups. Future studies to establish the psychometric properties of the CITE-I are needed.

Abbreviations
AAI: Activator adjusting instrument; AMCT: Activator methods chiropractic technique; CAM: Complementary and alternative medicine; CITE-I: Chiropractor interaction and treatment equivalence instrument; DC: Doctor of chiropractic; ID: Identification number; RCT: Randomized controlled trial; RIAS: Roter interaction analysis system; T: Treatment (number); TMD: Temporomandibular joint disorder.

Competing interests
The authors declare that they have no competing interests.

Authors' contributions
MAH, CMS, JWD, CMG and SAS conceived of this study. SAS, MAH, and JWD designed the study methodology and participated in instrument design. SAS directed instrument development, conducted literature reviews, and coordinated the coder training process. JWD coordinated the video-recording, data management and data analysis processes. MAH was a co-investigator for the pilot RCT and provided oversight throughout this study. MBS participated in instrument refinement and completed data collection. SAS, JWD, and MAH interpreted the data and drafted the manuscript. CMG, CMS and JWD provided leadership on the Center grant and the clinical trial that provided the data used in this study. All authors were involved in manuscript revision and gave final approval of the manuscript.

Acknowledgements
This study was supported by grant U19AT004663 from the National Center for Complementary and Alternative Medicine (NCCAM), National Institutes of Health (NIH), Bethesda, MD, USA. This study was conducted in part in a facility constructed with support of the Research Facilities Improvement Program grant C06 RR15433 from the National Center for Research Resources (NCRR), NIH. The contents of this manuscript are solely the responsibility of the authors and do not necessarily represent the official views of NCCAM, NCRR, or NIH.
The results of this study were presented at the 2012 International Research Congress on Integrative Medicine and Health in Portland, OR, USA.
The authors thank Activator Methods International, Phoenix, AZ, for providing the Activator IV instruments used in the pilot study.
The authors thank the study participants for their important contributions to this research. We thank the doctor of chiropractic and office staff for their involvement in the clinical trial. We acknowledge research staff members for their project and data management contributions. We are grateful to Robert D. Vining, DC for his many valuable and thoughtful insights on the nature of doctor-patient relationships.

Author details
[1]Palmer College of Chiropractic, Palmer Center for Chiropractic Research, 741 Brady Street, Davenport, IA 52803, USA. [2]Institute of Sports Science and Clinical Biomechanics, University of Southern Denmark, Odense, Denmark. [3]The University of Illinois, 801 South Paulina Street, 102c (MC621), Chicago, IL 60612, USA.

References
1. Campbell NC, Murray E, Darbyshire J, Emery J, Farmer A, Griffiths F, Guthrie B, Lester H, Wilson P, Kinmonth AL: Designing and evaluating complex interventions to improve health care. BMJ 2007, 334(7591):455–459.
2. Craig P, Dieppe P, Macintyre S, Michie S, Nazareth I, Petticrew M: Developing and evaluating complex interventions: the new Medical Research Council guidance. BMJ 2008, 337:a1655.
3. Paterson C, Dieppe P: Characteristic and incidental (placebo) effects in complex interventions such as acupuncture. BMJ 2005, 330(7501):1202–1205.
4. Jones CH: The spectrum of therapeutic influences and integrative health care: classifying health care practices by mode of therapeutic action. J Altern Complement Med 2005, 11(5):937–944.
5. Herzog W: The biomechanics of spinal manipulation. J Bodywork Mov Ther 2010, 14(3):280–286.
6. Graham BA, Clausen P, Bolton PS: A descriptive study of the force and displacement profiles of the toggle-recoil spinal manipulative procedure (adjustment) as performed by chiropractors. Man Ther 2010, 15(1):74–79.
7. Bronfort G, Haas M, Evans R, Kawchuk G, Dagenais S: Evidence-informed management of chronic low back pain with spinal manipulation and mobilization. Spine J 2008, 8(1):213–225.
8. Downie AS, Vemulpad S, Bull PW: Quantifying the high-velocity, low-amplitude spinal manipulative thrust: a systematic review. J Manipulative Physiol Ther 2010, 33(7):542–553.

9. Kawchuk GN, Herzog W: Biomechanical characterization (fingerprinting) of five novel methods of cervical spine manipulation. *J Manipulative Physiol Ther* 1992, **16**(9):573–577.

10. DeVocht JW, Owens EF, Gudavalli MR, Strazewski J, Bhogal R, Xia T: Force-time profile differences in the delivery of simulated toggle-recoil spinal manipulation by students, instructors, and field doctors of chiropractic. *J Manipulative Physiol Ther* 2013, **36**(6):342–348.

11. Nambi SG, Inbasekaran D, Khuman R, Devi S, Satani K: Clinical effects of short and long lever spinal thrust manipulation in non-specific chronic low back pain: a biomechanical perspective. *Int J Health Allied Sci* 2013, **2**(4):230–236.

12. McGregor M, Puhl A, Reinhart C, Injeyan H, Soave D: Differentiating intraprofessional attitudes toward paradigms in health care delivery among chiropractic factions: results from a randomly sampled survey. *BMC Complement Altern Med* 2014, **14**(1):51.

13. Smith M, Carber LA: Survey of US chiropractor attitudes and behaviors about subluxation. *J Chiropr Human* 2008, **15**:19–26.

14. Murphy DR, Schneider MJ, Seaman DR, Perle SM, Nelson CF: How can chiropractic become a respected mainstream profession? The example of podiatry. *Chiropr Osteop* 2008, **16**:10.

15. Gleberzon B, Stuber K: Frequency of use of diagnostic and manual therapeutic procedures of the spine currently taught at the Canadian Memorial Chiropractic College: a preliminary survey of Ontario chiropractors. Part 2 – procedure usage rates. *J Can Chiropr Assoc* 2013, **57**(2):165–175.

16. Mykietiuk C, Wambolt M, Pillipow T, Mallay C, Gleberzon BJ: Technique Systems used by post-1980 graduates of the Canadian Memorial Chiropractic College practicing in five Canadian provinces: a preliminary survey. *J Can Chiropr Assoc* 2009, **53**(1):32–39.

17. Huggins T, Boras AL, Gleberzon BJ, Popescu M, Bahry LA: Clinical effectiveness of the activator adjusting instrument in the management of musculoskeletal disorders: a systematic review of the literature. *J Can Chiropr Assoc* 2012, **56**(1):49–57.

18. Gleberzon BJ: Chiropractic "name techniques": a review of the literature. *J Can Chiropr Assoc* 2001, **45**(2):86–99.

19. Christensen MG, Kollasch MW, Hyland JK: *Practice Analysis of Chiropractic 2010: A Project Report, Survey Analysis, and Summary of Chiropractic Practice in the United States.* Greeley, CO: National Board of Chiropractic Examiners; 2010.

20. Haas M, Spegman A, Peterson D, Aickin M, Vavrek D: Dose response and efficacy of spinal manipulation for chronic cervicogenic headache: a pilot randomized controlled trial. *Spine J* 2010, **10**(2):117–128.

21. Witt CM, Schützler L: The gap between results from sham-controlled trials and trials using other controls in acupuncture research: the influence of context. *Complement Ther Med* 2013, **21**(2):112–114.

22. Gay C, Bishop M: Research on placebo analgesia is relevant to clinical practice. *Chiropr Man Therap* 2014, **22**(1):6.

23. Brim RL, Miller FG: The potential benefit of the placebo effect in sham-controlled trials: implications for risk-benefit assessments and informed consent. *J Med Ethics* 2013, **39**(11):703–707.

24. Hróbjartsson A, Gøtzsche PC: Placebo interventions for all clinical conditions. *Cochrane Database Syst Rev* 2010, 1:CD003974.

25. Puhl AA, Reinhart CJ, Rok ER, Injeyan HS: An examination of the observed placebo effect associated with the treatment of low back pain: a systematic review. *Pain Res Manag* 2011, **16**(1):45–52.

26. Krogsbll LT, Hróbjartsson A, Gøtzsche PC: Spontaneous improvement in randomised clinical trials: meta-analysis of three-armed trials comparing no treatment, placebo and active intervention. *BMC Med Res Methodol* 2009, **9**(1):1.

27. Licciardone JC, Russo DP: Blinding protocols, treatment credibility, and expectancy: methodologic issues in clinical trials of osteopathic manipulative treatment. *J Am Osteopath Assoc* 2006, **106**(8):457–463.

28. Kaptchuk TJ, Kelley JM, Conboy LA, Davis RB, Kerr CE, Jacobson EE, Kirsch I, Schyner RN, Nam BH, Nguyen LT: Components of placebo effect: randomised controlled trial in patients with irritable bowel syndrome. *BMJ* 2008, **336**(7651):999–1003.

29. Kaptchuk TJ: The placebo effect in alternative medicine: can the performance of a healing ritual have clinical significance? *Ann Intern Med* 2002, **136**(11):817–825.

30. Kaptchuk TJ, Shaw J, Kerr CE, Conboy LA, Kelley JM, Csordas TJ, Lembo AJ, Jacobson EE: "Maybe I made up the whole thing": placebos and patients' experiences in a randomized controlled trial. *Cult Med Psychiatry* 2009, **33**(3):382–411.

31. Finniss DG, Kaptchuk TJ, Miller F, Benedetti F: Biological, clinical, and ethical advances of placebo effects. *Lancet* 2010, **375**(9715):686–695.

32. Price DD, Finniss DG, Benedetti F: A comprehensive review of the placebo effect: recent advances and current thought. *Annu Rev Psychol* 2008, **59**:565–590.

33. Bialosky JE, Bishop MD, Robinson ME, Barabas JA, George SZ: The influence of expectation on spinal manipulation induced hypoalgesia: an experimental study in normal subjects. *BMC Musculoskelet Disord* 2008, **9**:19.

34. Bensing JM, Verheul W: The silent healer: the role of communication in placebo effects. *Patient Educ Couns* 2010, **80**(3):293–299.

35. Paterson C, Zheng Z, Xue C, Wang Y: "Playing their parts": the experiences of participants in a randomized sham-controlled acupuncture trial. *J Altern Complement Med* 2008, **14**(2):199–208.

36. Ernst E, Harkness E: Spinal manipulation: a systematic review of sham-controlled, double-blind, randomized clinical trials. *J Pain Symptom Manag* 2001, **22**(4):879–889.

37. Hawk C, Azad A, Phongphua C, Long CR: Preliminary study of the effects of a placebo chiropractic treatment with sham adjustments. *J Manipulative Physiol Ther* 1999, **22**(7):436–443.

38. Miller FG, Emanuel EJ, Rosenstein DL, Straus SE: Ethical issues concerning research in complementary and alternative medicine. *JAMA* 2004, **291**(5):599–604.

39. Margolin A, Avants SK, Kleber HD: Investigating alternative medicine therapies in randomized controlled trials. *JAMA* 1998, **280**(18):1626–1628.

40. Schulz KF, Altman DG, Moher D, CONSORT Group: CONSORT 2010 statement: updated guidelines for reporting parallel group randomised trials. *BMC Med* 2010, **8**(1):18.

41. Goertz CM, Pohlman KA, Vining RD, Brantingham JW, Long CR: Patient-centered outcomes of high-velocity, low-amplitude spinal manipulation for low back pain: a systematic review. *J Electromyogr Kinesiol* 2012, **22**(5):670–691.

42. Khorsan R, Coulter ID, Hawk C, Choate CG: Measures in chiropractic research: choosing patient-based outcome assessments. *J Manipulative Physiol Ther* 2008, **31**(5):355–375.

43. Sikorskii A, Wyatt G, Victorson D, Faulkner G, Rahbar MH: Methodological issues in trials of complementary and alternative medicine interventions. *Nurs Res* 2009, **58**(6):444–451.

44. DeVocht JW, Goertz CM, Hondras MA, Long CR, Schaeffer W, Thomann L, Spector M, Stanford CM: A pilot study of a chiropractic intervention for management of chronic myofascial temporomandibular disorder. *J Am Dent Assoc* 2013, **144**(10):1154–1163.

45. Fuhr AW, Menke JM: Status of activator methods chiropractic technique, theory, and practice. *J Manipulative Physiol Ther* 2005, **28**(2):e1–e20.

46. Farrar JT, Young JP Jr, LaMoreaux L, Werth JL, Poole RM: Clinical importance of changes in chronic pain intensity measured on an 11-point numerical pain rating scale. *Pain* 2001, **94**(2):149–158.

47. Locker D, Allen PF: Developing short-form measures of oral health-related quality of life. *J Public Health Dent* 2002, **62**(1):13–20.

48. Epstein RM, Franks P, Fiscella K, Shields CG, Meldrum SC, Kravitz RL, Duberstein PR: Measuring patient-centered communication in patient–physician consultations: theoretical and practical issues. *Soc Sci Med* 2005, **61**(7):1516–1528.

49. Roter D, Larson S: The Roter interaction analysis system (RIAS): utility and flexibility for analysis of medical interactions. *Patient Educ Couns* 2002, **46**(4):243–251.

50. Ong L, De Haes J, Hoos A, Lammes FB: Doctor-patient communication: a review of the literature. *Soc Sci Med* 1995, **40**(7):903–918.

51. Barlow F, Scott C, Coghlan B, Lee P, White P, Lewith GT, Bishop FL: How the psychosocial context of clinical trials differs from usual care: A qualitative study of acupuncture patients. *BMC Med Res Methodol* 2011, **11**(1):79.

52. White AR, Filshie J, Cummings TM: Clinical trials of acupuncture: consensus recommendations for optimal treatment, sham controls and blinding. *Complement Ther Med* 2001, **9**(4):237–245.

53. Sidani S, Braden CJ: *Evaluating Nursing Interventions: A Theory-Driven Approach.* Thousand Oaks, CA: SAGE Publications; 1998.

54. Desjarlais-deKlerk K, Wallace J: Instrumental and socioemotional communications in doctor-patient interactions in urban and rural clinics. *BMC Health Serv Res* 2013, **13**(1):261.

55. Carroll C, Patterson M, Wood S, Booth A, Rick J, Balain S: **A conceptual framework for implementation fidelity.** *Implement Sci* 2007, **2**(40):1–9.

56. Scholten-Peeters GG, Thoomes E, Konings S, Beijer M, Verkerk K, Koes BW, Verhagen AP: **Is manipulative therapy more effective than sham manipulation in adults? A systematic review and meta-analysis.** *Chiropr Man Therap* 2013, **21**(1):34.

57. Reed WR, Beavers S, Reddy SK, Kern G: **Chiropractic management of primary nocturnal enuresis.** *J Manipulative Physiol Ther* 1994, **17**(9):596–600.

58. Sawyer CE, Evans RL, Boline PD, Branson R, Spicer A: **A feasibility study of chiropractic spinal manipulation versus sham spinal manipulation for chronic otitis media with effusion in children.** *J Manipulative Physiol Ther* 1999, **22**(5):292–298.

59. Vernon H, MacAdam K, Marshall V, Pion M, Sadowska M: **Validation of a sham manipulative procedure for the cervical spine for use in clinical trials.** *J Manipulative Physiol Ther* 2005, **28**(9):662–666.

60. Brose SW, Jennings DC, Kwok J, Stuart CL, O'Connell SM, Pauli HA, Liu B: **Sham manual medicine protocol for cervical strain-counterstrain research.** *PM&R* 2013, **5**(5):400–407.

61. Vernon HT, Triano JJ, Ross JK, Tran SK, Soave DM, Dinulos MD: **Validation of a novel sham cervical manipulation procedure.** *Spine J* 2012, **12**(11):1021–1028.

62. Ozcakar N, Mevsim V, Guldal D, Gunvar T, Yildirim E, Sisli Z, Semin I: **Is the use of videotape recording superior to verbal feedback alone in the teaching of clinical skills?** *BMC Public Health* 2009, **9**(1):474.

63. Kihlgren M, Kuremyr D, Norberg A, Brane G, Karlson I, Engstrom B, Melin E: **Nurse-patient interaction after training in integrity promoting care at a long-term ward: analysis of video-recorded morning care sessions.** *Int J Nurs Stud* 1993, **30**(1):1–13.

64. Mackenzie CF, Xiao Y: **Video techniques and data compared with observation in emergency trauma care.** *Qual Saf Health Care* 2003, **12**(suppl 2):ii51–ii57.

65. Marcinowicz L, Konstantynowicz J, Godlewski C: **Patients' perceptions of GP non-verbal communication: a qualitative study.** *Br J Gen Pract* 2010, **60**(571):83–87.

66. Cocksedge S, George B, Renwick S, Chew-Graham CA: **Touch in primary care consultations: qualitative investigation of doctors' and patients' perceptions.** *Br J Gen Pract* 2013, **63**(609):e283–e290.

67. Swayden KJ, Anderson KK, Connelly LM, Moran JS, McMahon JK, Arnold PM: **Effect of sitting vs. standing on perception of provider time at bedside: a pilot study.** *Patient Educ Couns* 2012, **86**(2):166–171.

68. Coleman T: **Using video-recorded consultations for research in primary care: advantages and limitations.** *Fam Pract* 2000, **17**(5):422–427.

69. Latvala E, Vuokila-Oikkonen P, Janhonen S: **Videotaped recording as a method of participant observation in psychiatric nursing research.** *J Adv Nurs* 2000, **31**(5):1252–1257.

70. Caldwell K, Atwal A: **Non-participant observation: using video tapes to collect data in nursing research.** *Nurse Res* 2005, **13**(2):42–54.

71. Ram P, Grol R, Rethans JJ, Schouten B, van der Vleuten C, Kester A: **Assessment of general practitioners by video observation of communicative and medical performance in daily practice: issues of validity, reliability and feasibility.** *Med Educ* 1999, **33**(6):447–454.

72. Oakley E, Stocker S, Staubli G, Young S: **Using video recording to identify management errors in pediatric trauma resuscitation.** *Pediatrics* 2006, **117**(3):658–664.

73. Penner LA, Orom H, Albrecht TL, Franks MM, Foster TS, Ruckdeschel JC: **Camera-related behaviors during video recorded medical interactions.** *J Nonverbal Behav* 2007, **31**(2):99–117.

74. Pringle M, Stewart-Evans C: **Does awareness of being video recorded affect doctors' consultation behaviour?** *Br J Gen Pract* 1990, **40**(340):455–458.

75. Rex DK, Hewett DG, Raghavendra M, Chalasani N: **The impact of videorecording on the quality of colonoscopy performance: a pilot study.** *Am J Gastroenterol* 2010, **105**(11):2312–2317.

76. Innes M, Skelton J, Greenfield S: **A profile of communication in primary care physician telephone consultations: application of the Roter Interaction Analysis System.** *Br J Gen Pract* 2006, **56**(526):363–368.

77. Paasche-Orlow M, Roter D: **The communication patterns of internal medicine and family practice physicians.** *J Am Board Fam Prac* 2003, **16**(6):485–493.

78. Bensing JM, Roter DL, Hulsman RL: **Communication patterns of primary care physicians in the United States and The Netherlands.** *J Gen Internal Med* 2003, **18**(5):335–342.

79. Shaw JR, Adams CL, Bonnett BN, Larson S, Roter DL: **Use of the Roter interaction analysis system to analyze veterinarian-client-patient communication in companion animal practice.** *J Am Vet Med Assoc* 2004, **225**(2):222–229.

80. Ong LM, Visser MR, Kruyver IP, Bensing JM, Brink-Muinen A, Stouthard JM, Lammes FB, de Haes JC: **The Roter Interaction Analysis System (RIAS) in oncological consultations: psychometric properties.** *Psychooncology* 1998, **7**(5):387–401.

5

Public health engagement: detection of suspicious skin lesions, screening and referral behaviour of UK based chiropractors

Sara Glithro[1*], David Newell[2], Lorna Burrows[3^], Adrian Hunnisett[1] and Christina Cunliffe[1]

Abstract

Background: UK morbidity and mortality rates from skin cancer are increasing despite existing preventative strategies involving education and early detection. Manual therapists are ideally placed to support these goals as they see greater quantities of exposed patient skin more often than most other healthcare professionals. The purpose of this study therefore was to ascertain the ability of manual therapists to detect, screen and refer suspicious skin lesions.

Method: A web-based questionnaire and quiz was used in a sample of UK chiropractic student clinicians and registered chiropractors to gather data during 2011 concerning skin screening and referral behaviors for suspicious skin lesions.

Results: A total of 120 questionnaires were included. Eighty one percent of participants agreed that screening for suspicious skin lesions was part of their clinical role, with nearly all (94%) assessing their patients for lesions during examination. Over 90% of the participants reported regularly having the opportunity for skin examination; with nearly all (98%) agreeing they would refer patients with suspicious skin lesions to a medical practitioner. A third of respondents had referred a total of 80 suspicious lesions within the last 12 months with 67% warranting further investigation.

Conclusions: Nearly all respondents agreed that screening patients for suspicious skin lesions was part of their clinical role, with a significant number already referring patients with lesions.

Keywords: Skin lesion, Skin cancer, Screening, Referral behaviour, Prevention, Detection, Dermatology, Chiropractor, Manual therapist

Background

Malignant melanoma incidence rates have increased more than fivefold since the mid-1970s and continue to rise [1]. In 2002, the UK paid over £240 million in total costs associated with skin cancer; of which 42% were direct costs to the NHS [2]. Of the various forms of skin cancer, melanoma treatment was directly responsible for 63% of this total. Early detection of pre-cancerous and cancerous lesions not only improves patient mortality rates [3-5] it also substantially reduces this economic burden by enabling faster, cheaper and less-invasive interventions as out-patients in comparison to the otherwise high costs associated with in-patient care required to treat advanced lesions. Yet, in a study of US patients, 75% reported having

never been advised by their medical practitioner or any other medical professional in their medical practice, to examine their skin for growths or changes in spots or moles. Furthermore, most participants (58% and 83% respectively) reported that their medical practitioner 'never' or 'rarely' looked at the skin on their back or on the backs of their legs [6].

However, in the UK, in addition to medical practitioners, a diverse group of clinical practitioners are in a position to detect, screen and refer suspicious skin lesions [6-10]. Of these, a smaller number regularly see patients unclothed and particularly see areas of the body inaccessible to visual inspection by the patient themselves. Of those that do, manual therapists such as masseurs, osteopaths and chiropractors are ideally placed to regularly screen the skin for suspicious lesions. Chiropractic practice is concerned with the diagnosis and treatment of musculoskeletal syndromes, including low back, neck pain,

* Correspondence: sglithro@bournemouth.ac.uk

^Deceased

[1]McTimoney College of Chiropractic, Abingdon, UK

Full list of author information is available at the end of the article

headaches and peripheral joint problems [11]. Despite 42% of chiropractors regularly examining patients who were in their underwear [12], little if any research exists that has attempted to determine whether chiropractors in the field take advantage of this opportunity to perform basic skin screening. Of that research already carried out, this was restricted to a student population only and recommended that further research should test the ability of chiropractors to identify pathological moles on a broader, evaluative basis [13]. In view of this we investigated the accuracy with which chiropractic student clinicians and registered chiropractors were able to recognise as suspicious or benign, a variety of common skin lesions from images chosen by a dermatologist. More generally we also examined attitudes towards skin screening and the screening and referral patterns within this sample. For the purpose of this article the term 'chiropractic student clinicians' has been adopted to describe chiropractic students or interns in their final year of clinical study.

Methods
Dissemination
A web based, self-administered questionnaire was emailed to the chiropractic student clinicians of both participating UK colleges. These participants were in their final clinical year of study when the survey was distributed in 2011 (n = 154). The questionnaire was also emailed to a sample of 250 practising UK registered chiropractors who were randomly selected by the McTimoney Chiropractic Association from their members list. Finally, a link to the questionnaire was published in the United Chiropractic Association's regular members' e-newsletter. The questionnaire contained closed questions and images designed to gather descriptive information on the participants' frequency and accuracy of detecting suspicious skin lesions.

Inclusion/exclusion criteria
Students were those in their final clinical year of chiropractic study at a UK college or university which on completion of their course, allowed registration with the General Chiropractic Council (GCC). The chiropractors were all registered with the GCC at the time the questionnaire was issued. For inclusion within the data analysis, respondents must have confirmed whether they were either a student or a registered chiropractor. In addition, they had to provide a response to the question concerning whether or not they considered screening patients for suspicious skin lesions to be part of their role as a chiropractor. Only subjects that responded either 'Yes' or 'No' were included as failure to answer this question meant the subject had exited the questionnaire without answering any further questions. Questionnaire completion was advised and taken as consent.

Questionnaire design
The questionnaire had four sections: 1) Participant demographics, 2) Willingness and attitudes towards examination of patients for skin lesions, 3) Skills associated with lesion detection and 4) Identification of training needs associated with lesion detection.

Likert scales were used to evaluate participants' knowledge of risk factors involved with and identification of, suspicious skin lesions. The second part of the questionnaire established participants' skills in identifying lesions. A dermatologist advised on and approved a set of images of commonly occurring skin lesions, including some where early detection could have substantial impact on prognosis and decrease costs to health services. In an attempt to prevent participants from searching for the images online prior to answering questions; a statement encouraging the participants to resist using any reference material was displayed at the beginning of the questionnaire; image references were only revealed to the participants on questionnaire completion and an on-demand document providing all the images, references and correct diagnoses was also provided to participants on questionnaire completion. Face validity and piloting of the questionnaire took place prior to finalising the questionnaire design. Anonymous responses were accepted for a period of four weeks, with emailed reminders sent at pre-identified points during this period.

Sampling
The aim was to capture responses from a sample group reflective of the UK chiropractic profession and a final year pre-registration student chiropractic population. Invitations to take part were made to the four UK chiropractic associations; British Chiropractic Association (BCA), McTimoney Chiropractic Association (MCA), Scottish Chiropractic Association (SCA), United Chiropractic Association (UCA) and all three UK chiropractic colleges; Anglo-European College of Chiropractic (AECC), McTimoney College of Chiropractic (MCC) and the Welsh Institute of Chiropractic (WIOC).

The final sample included 62 UK based registered chiropractors who were members of the MCA and 58 final year students from two UK teaching institutions. Of these, 34 (58%) were from AECC and 25 (42%) were from the MCC.

Analysis
Questionnaire data was analysed using a descriptive approach. Continuous variables where normally distributed were described using means and standard deviations, while non-parametric distributions were described with medians and percentiles. Categorical variables were described using proportions.

Ethics

Ethical approval was granted by the McTimoney College Research Ethics Committee on the 21st of November 2010, prior to commencement of the study.

Results

From the 404 questionnaires that were issued, a total of 139 questionnaires were returned. Nineteen failed to meet the inclusion criteria, leaving 120 included in the analysis and giving a successful response rate of 30%. Eighty (67%) participants were female and 40 (33%) were male. Sixty two (52%) were registered chiropractors and the remaining 58 (48%) were chiropractic students. In the registered chiropractor group, the mean number of years qualified was 5.8 years (SD ± 8.0) and the mean number of patients treated per month was 89 (SD ± 70.3) (Table 1).

Table 1 Demographic characteristics of sample

Variable		n	%	Mean (SD)	Range
Gender	Female	80	67		
Age (years)	21-30	36	30		
	31-40	27	23		
	41-50	31	26		
	51-60	16	13		
	>60	10	8		
Practicing category	Chiropractic student clinician	58	48		
	Registered Chiropractor	62	52		
Years qualified				5.8 (8)	0-35
	Not yet qualified	58	48		
	Less than 5 years	14	12		
	5-9 years	15	13		
	10-14 years	15	13		
	15-19 years	7	6		
	20-24 years	6	5		
	25-35 years	5	4		
New patients per month				12.8 (13)	0-108
	1-4	50	42		
	5-9	18	15		
	10-19	25	21		
	20-39	21	18		
	Over 40	5	4		
Repeat patients per month				76.1 (65)	13-347
	1-49	58	48		
	50-99	28	23		
	100-199	27	23		
	200-799	7	6		

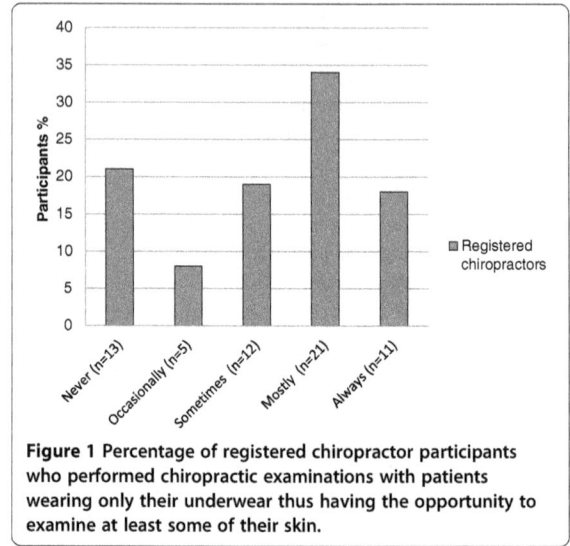

Figure 1 Percentage of registered chiropractor participants who performed chiropractic examinations with patients wearing only their underwear thus having the opportunity to examine at least some of their skin.

As the chiropractic student clinicians approach to examination of patients was likely to be dictated by their college policy on patient gowning, skin exposure analysis was evaluated from the data provided by participating registered chiropractors. Figure 1 shows the degree of patient skin exposure during the examination and treatment by the registered chiropractor. Fifty two percent (n = 32) agreed they 'always' or 'mostly' examined patients in their underwear during the examination. In another question, over half, (71%, n = 44) indicated that their patients were 'never' or 'occassionally' fully clothed during the examination, implying regular opportunities to examine at least some of their patients' skin.

Most chiropractic student clinician and registered chiropractor participants (81%, n = 97) agreed that screening patients for skin lesions was part of their clinical role (Table 2). Of these, 94% (n = 91) indicated they screened each new patient, 53% (n = 51) screened existing patients

Table 2 Screening attitude and behaviours of participants

Question posed		Answered 'Yes'	
		%	n
Do you consider screening patients for suspicious skin lesions to be part of your role as a chiropractor?		81	97
If 'Yes', is this part of your normal patient assessment for...	New patients?	94	91
	Repeat patients at every visit?	53	51
	Repeat patients during regular assessments?	73	71

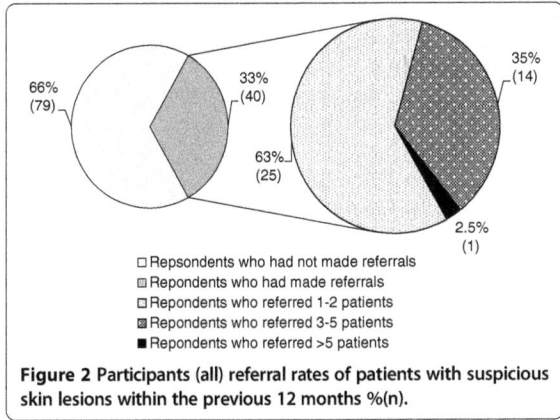

Figure 2 Participants (all) referral rates of patients with suspicious skin lesions within the previous 12 months %(n).

at every visit and 73% (n = 71) at visits scheduled specifically for patient re-assessments.

Registered chiropractors and final year chiropractic students already identify and refer patients with suspicious skin lesions. Within the previous 12 months, 33% (n = 40) of the participants had referred a total of 104 patients with skin lesions they felt warranted further investigation (Figure 2).

Of the 104 referrals made, referrers declared they were aware of 80 outcomes via feedback from their patients or medical practitioners. Over two-thirds of the 80 outcomes known (67%, n = 54), warranted further secondary healthcare investigation by a medical professional. Of these 80 outcomes; 29% (n = 23), were diagnosed as Basal Cell Carcinoma, Malignant Melanoma or Squamous Cell Carcinoma. A further 17% (n = 9) of patients

were still awaiting the outcome and 9% (n = 5) were diagnosed with other conditions requiring medical care. Almost a third (31%, n = 17) of those referred required no further treatment following examination by their medical practitioner (Figure 3).

The participants generally demonstrated a good understanding of the risk factors associated with developing skin cancers, although some frequently occurring features were less understood (Table 3). Few respondents identified having blue/green eyes (10%, n = 12), red hair/freckles (37%, n = 36) or an unprotected balding head (45%, n = 53) as risk factors for developing skin cancer. Yet over 88% recognised an increased risk with having an outdoor occupation, repeated sunburn as a child or history of using UV tanning beds. When assessing whether a lesion should be considered suspicious, over 90% agreed or strongly agreed the importance of a change in the appearance or behavior of a lesion. Furthermore, over 70% agreed or strongly agreed that the recent appearance, an uneven colour or lesion asymmetry should also be looked out for. Additionally, 55% deemed a raised surface to be important although this is not a major feature for all suspicious lesions. The majority practiced a proactive approach in the detection and referral of lesions however, less than 40% advised their patients on preventative strategies in avoiding or reducing risk.

Figures 4a to d document the responses to questions asked about the ten images of skin lesions shown to the subjects. As is shown, with reference to identification of suspicious lesions, over 75% of participants correctly labeled examples of malignant melanoma and squamous cell carcinoma. However, less than 45% did so for superficial basal cell carcinoma and actinic keratosis. Interestingly,

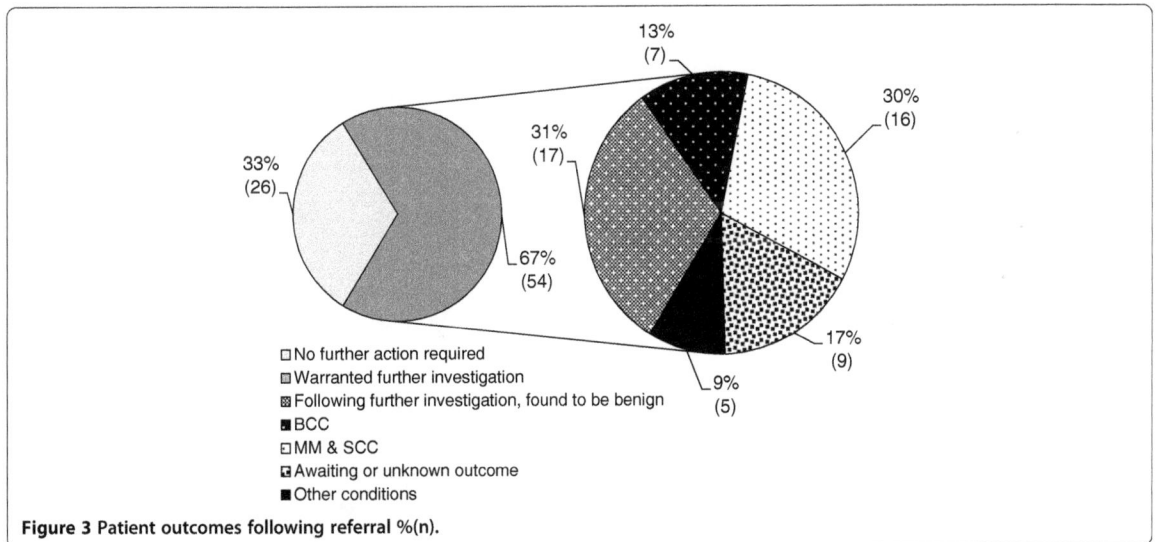

Figure 3 Patient outcomes following referral %(n).

Table 3 Respondents knowledge of the risk factors associated with developing skin cancer and the advice they offer patients

	%	n
The risk of developing skin cancer increases with...'		
An outdoor occupation		
Strongly agree/agree	76	89
Neutral	20	23
Disagree/strongly disagree	4	5
An indoor occupation and holidays in the sun once or twice a year (beach, skiing, outdoor etc.)		
Strongly agree/agree	71	82
Neutral	21	24
Disagree/strongly disagree	8	9
Repeated incidents of having sunburn as a child		
Strongly agree/agree	88	104
Neutral	11	13
Disagree/strongly disagree	1	1
A history of using UV tanning beds		
Strongly agree/agree	93	110
Neutral	6	7
Disagree/strongly disagree	1	1
More than 50 moles		
Strongly agree/agree	56	65
Neutral	38	45
Disagree/strongly disagree	6	7
More than 100 moles		
Strongly agree/agree	69	78
Neutral	27	31
Disagree/strongly disagree	4	4
A history of at least one pre-cancerous or cancerous skin lesion		
Strongly agree/agree	92	109
Neutral	6	7
Disagree/strongly disagree	2	2
A first degree relative with a history of at least one pre-cancerous or cancerous skin lesion		
Strongly agree/agree	69	82
Neutral	22	26
Disagree/strongly disagree	8	10
Freckles and/or red hair		
Strongly agree/agree	37	36
Neutral	51	49
Disagree/strongly disagree	12	12
Blue or green eyes		
Strongly agree/agree	10	12
Neutral	65	75
Disagree/strongly disagree	25	29

Table 3 Respondents knowledge of the risk factors associated with developing skin cancer and the advice they offer patients (Continued)

	%	n
Fair skin		
Strongly agree/agree	58	69
Neutral	34	40
Disagree/strongly disagree	8	9
A history of long-term use of drugs with known side-effects of photosensitivity		
Strongly agree/agree	66	77
Neutral	32	37
Disagree/strongly disagree	3	3
Thinning or balding hair		
Strongly agree/agree	45	53
Neutral	42	50
Disagree/strongly disagree	13	15
A skin lesion should be considered 'suspicious' if...	**%**	**n**
It has uneven colour		
Strongly agree/agree	72	84
Neutral	23	27
Disagree/strongly disagree	4	5
It is asymmetrical		
Strongly agree/agree	73	85
Neutral	22	25
Disagree/strongly disagree	5	6
It has changed in size (growing)		
Strongly agree/agree	95	114
Neutral	2	2
Disagree/strongly disagree	3	4
It has changed in shape (irregular border)		
Strongly agree/agree	97	113
Neutral	2	2
Disagree/strongly disagree	1	1
It has changed in colour (including several different colours)		
Strongly agree/agree	93	112
Neutral	4	5
Disagree/strongly disagree	3	3
It has a crusty keratinised surface		
Strongly agree/agree	71	82
Neutral	22	26
Disagree/strongly disagree	7	8
It bleeds		
Strongly agree/agree	95	110
Neutral	3	3
Disagree/strongly disagree	3	3
It appeared recently		
Strongly agree/agree	71	82

Table 3 Respondents knowledge of the risk factors associated with developing skin cancer and the advice they offer patients *(Continued)*

Neutral	24	28
Disagree/strongly disagree	5	6
It has a raised surface		
Strongly agree/agree	55	66
Neutral	32	38
Disagree/strongly disagree	13	15
It itches		
Strongly agree/agree	78	91
Neutral	17	20
Disagree/strongly disagree	4	5
The patient is concerned about it		
Strongly agree/agree	73	85
Neutral	25	29
Disagree/strongly disagree	3	3
Do you advise your patients on...	**%**	**n**
The risks of sun exposure		
Yes	33	39
No	67	78
The risks of using UV sunbeds		
Yes	37	43
No	63	74
Using sunscreen with an SPF of at least 15		
Yes	32	36
No	68	78
Other factors that can increase photosensitivity (E.g. some antibiotics, anti-depressants, anti-malarial medications etc.)		
Yes	14	16
No	86	96
Have you ever been asked for advice on preventing skin cancer by your patients?		
Yes	7	8
No	93	108

whilst confident to label these lesions as suspicious, less than 10% diagnosed the lesions correctly (Figure 4d). Over 60% incorrectly labeled the benign seborrhoeic wart as suspicious, however more participants correctly labeled the haemangioma and junctional naevus as not suspicious. The majority, 75% (n = 90) correctly identified the intradermal naevus as not suspicious.

Participant's referral rates were slightly greater (<11%) than those declaring the corresponding lesion as 'suspicious' (Figure 4b). Whilst not wanting to over-refer, perhaps this degree of caution demonstrates

respondents recognising when to request help beyond their own expertise. Participant's confidence in their ability to diagnose the images correctly mirrored the actual number of correct diagnoses; however both were low at less than 20%.

Participants were asked whether they had completed any skin lesion identification training as part of their undergraduate course and whether they would be interested in receiving more. The majority (68%, n = 81) had received some form of undergraduate training and 75% (n = 90) of all respondents were interested in receiving further training.

Discussion

A position paper decrying the less than main stream position of chiropractic within the wider health care system and using podiatry as a model to describe how a similar profession has navigated a course toward greater acceptance, cited podiatrists traditional dedication to public health issues as one of the major reasons why they became influential members of the healthcare community [14]. They urged the chiropractic profession to '...openly embrace, and become actively involved in public health initiatives'.

In the context of these discussions this study investigated the degree to which chiropractors were engaging in an important key public health issue, namely early detection of skin cancer.

As long ago as 2003, Mahon [15] concluded that given skin cancer remaining as a major public health problem, efforts following those associated with primary prevention, such as sun screen use and judicial reductions in exposure to UV, should also include secondary prevention such as professional skin examinations. This author went on to suggest that nurses have a major role to play in these secondary preventative efforts.

A recent article by Ramcharan et al. [13] using a cross sectional design, reported that over 80% of chiropractic student clinicians thought that recognising skin cancer in their patients was important or very important in their practice, concluding that chiropractic education should emphasize the opportunity to detect and assess atypical moles as a routine part of primary prevention in clinical education.

Similarly in this study, the majority of participants agreed that screening patients was part of their clinical role and felt they already had the skills to recognise suspicious lesions and refer patients for further investigation. Within this small sample (n = 120), 40 practitioners had referred 80 patients for further investigation within the previous 12 months and at least 23 were found to have skin cancer. Extrapolating to the UK registered chiropractic population of approximately 2827,

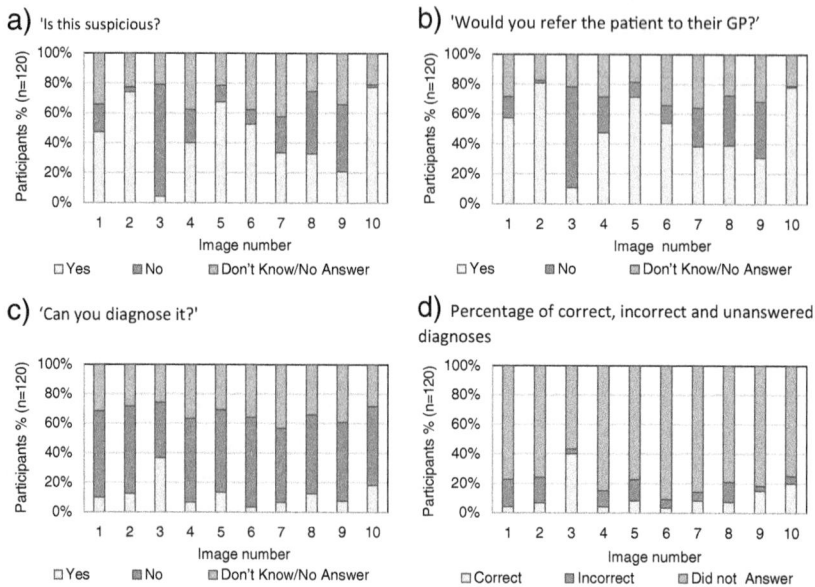

Figure 4 Participants response to questions concerning images. For a) to d): n = 120; Images, 1: Superficial Basal Cell Carcinoma, 2: Squamous Cell Carcinoma, 3: Intradermal Naevus, 4: Actinic Keratosis, 5: Seborrhoeic Wart, 6: Bowen's Disease, 7: Nodular Basal Cell Carcinoma, 8: Haemangioma, 9: Junctional Naevus and 10: Malignant Melanoma. NB: for the purposes of this study, images 1,2,4,6,7 and 10 were considered 'suspicious' by the researchers.

one could estimate that the chiropractic profession might identify and refer 1866 patients annually for further investigation and of these 29% (541) could have skin cancer.

This research indicates that detecting and referring patients with suspicious skin lesions is already taking place, yet patient education in primary prevention by chiropractors is lacking during these consultations. A need and willingness to undertake further training was identified which, if put in place, may improve patient education and contribute to improving outcomes in skin cancer.

Clearly the study has limitations. Firstly, generalizability is limited with the inclusion of participants from only two of the three UK chiropractic educational institutions and only one chiropractic association. This means the results may not be representative of the whole UK chiropractic population, although the one association included does comprise 19% of the UK chiropractic practitioner population. Secondly, whilst every effort was made in the research design to discourage participants, the possibility that reference material was used while completing the questionnaire cannot be overlooked.

Conclusion

Visual screening is an important weapon in the arsenal against the rise of malignant skin lesions and is also highly cost effective [16]. Chiropractors serve to positively contribute to this public health problem and the role of the profession should both be articulated and improved in this respect.

This study has shown that not only do chiropractic student clinicians and registered chiropractors feel this screening to be an important part of their role but it also indicates that significant numbers of patients are referred on to specialist care with the potential to importantly reduce mortality and morbidity together with the substantial costs associated with these lesions.

With focused undergraduate training and further post graduate opportunities, chiropractors may feel more confident in detecting suspicious skin lesions and subsequently prove to be increasingly important advocates in the early detection of skin cancer.

Competing interests
The authors declare that they have no competing interests.

Authors' contributions
SG and DN conceived the study. SG collected data and produced first draft. DN provided statistical advice. LB provided advice and assistance on lesion images. AH reviewed and amended initial draft. All authors read and approved the final manuscript.

Author details
[1]McTimoney College of Chiropractic, Abingdon, UK. [2]Anglo European College of Chiropractic (AECC) and Bournemouth University, Dorset, UK. [3]Salisbury NHS Foundation Trust, Salisbury, UK.

References

1. Cancer Research. Cancer Statistics. http://info.cancerresearchuk.org/ Cancerstats/Types/Skin 2011a; [Accessed 22/09/11].
2. Morris S, Cox B, Bosanquet N. Cost of skin cancer in England. Eur J Health Econ. 2009;10(3):267–73.
3. Karakousis CP, Emrich LJ, Rao U. Tumor thickness and prognosis in clinical stage I malignant melanoma. Cancer. 1989;64(7):1432–6.
4. Mackie R, Bray C, Leman J. Effect of public education aimed at early diagnosis of malignant melanoma: cohort comparison study. BMJ. 2003;326:367.
5. Rossi C, Vecchiato A, Bezze G, Mastrangelo G, Montesco M, Mocellin S, et al. Early detection of melanoma: an educational campaign in Padova, Italy. Melanoma Res. 2000;10:181–7.
6. Weinstock M, Martin R, Risica P, Berwick M, Lasater T, Rakowski W, et al. Thorough skin examination for the early detection of Melanoma. Am J Prev Med. 1999;17(Issue 3):169–75.
7. Boiko P, Colleagues in Skin Cancer Prevention. The family practitioner, pediatrician, internist, gynaecologist, physician assistant and nurse. Clin Dermatol. 1998;16:467–75. Elsevier Science Inc, New York.
8. Cummings SR, Tripp MK, Herrmann NB. Approaches to the prevention and control of skin cancer. Cancer Metastasis Rev. 1997;16(3):309–27.
9. Greenly L. Guide to detecting skin cancer – Part one. Chiropr Tech. 1997.
10. Greenly L. Guide to detecting skin cancer – Part two. Chiropr Tech. 1998.
11. General Chiropractic Council. Code of Practice and Standard of Proficiency. Gen Chiropr Council. 2005.
12. General Chiropractic Council. Consulting the profession: A survey of UK chiropractors. Gen Chiropr Council. 2004.
13. Ramcharan M, Evans MW, Ndetan H, Beddard J. Knowledge, perceptions, and practices of chiropractic interns in the early detection of atypical moles. J Chiropr Med. 2011;10:77–85.
14. Murphy D, Schneider M, Seaman D, Perle S, Nelson C. How can chiropractic become a respected mainstream profession? The example of podiatry. Chiropr Osteopat. 2008;16:10.
15. Mahon S. Skin cancer prevention: education and public health issues. Semin Oncol Nurs. 2003;19(1):52–61.
16. Losina E, Walensky RP, Geller A, Beddingfield FC, Wolf LL, Gilchrest BA, et al. Visual screening for malignant melanoma: a cost-effective analysis. Arch Dermatol. 2007;143(1):21–8.

6

Treatment preferences amongst physical therapists and chiropractors for the management of neck pain: results of an international survey

Lisa C Carlesso[1*], Joy C MacDermid[2,3], Anita R Gross[2], David M Walton[4] and P Lina Santaguida[5]

Abstract

Background: Clinical practice guidelines on the management of neck pain make recommendations to help practitioners optimize patient care. By examining the practice patterns of practitioners, adherence to CPGs or lack thereof, is demonstrated. Understanding utilization of various treatments by practitioners and comparing these patterns to that of recommended guidelines is important to identify gaps for knowledge translation and improve treatment regimens.

Aim: To describe the utilization of interventions in patients with neck pain by clinicians.

Methods: A cross-sectional international survey was conducted from February 2012 to March 2013 to determine physical medicine, complementary and alternative medicine utilization amongst 360 clinicians treating patients with neck pain.

Results: The survey was international (19 countries) with Canada having the largest response (38%). Results were analyzed by usage amongst physical therapists (38%) and chiropractors (31%) as they were the predominant respondents. Within these professions, respondents were male (41-66%) working in private practice (69-95%). Exercise and manual therapies were consistently (98-99%) used by both professions but tests of subgroup differences determined that physical therapists used exercise, orthoses and 'other' interventions more, while chiropractors used phototherapeutics more. However, phototherapeutics (65%), Orthoses/supportive devices (57%), mechanical traction (55%) and sonic therapies (54%) were *not* used by the majority of respondents. Thermal applications (73%) and acupuncture (46%) were the modalities used most commonly. Analysis of differences across the subtypes of neck pain indicated that respondents utilize treatments more often for chronic neck pain and whiplash conditions, followed by radiculopathy, acute neck pain and whiplash conditions, and facet joint dysfunction by diagnostic block. The higher rates of usage of some interventions were consistent with supporting evidence (e.g. manual therapy). However, there was moderate usage of a number of interventions that have limited support or conflicting evidence (e.g. ergonomics).

Conclusions: This survey indicates that exercise and manual therapy are core treatments provided by chiropractors and physical therapists. Future research should address gaps in evidence associated with variable practice patterns and knowledge translation to reduce usage of some interventions that have been shown to be ineffective.

Keywords: Survey, Neck pain, Treatment, Practice patterns, Complementary and alternative medicine

* Correspondence: lccarlesso@gmail.com
[1]Toronto Western Research Institute, University Health Network, 399 Bathurst Street - MP11-328, Toronto, Ontario M5T 2S8, Canada
Full list of author information is available at the end of the article

Background

Clinical practice guidelines (CPG) are developed to provide statements and recommendations with the intention of helping practitioners optimize patient care [1]. By examining the practice patterns of practitioners, adherence to CPGs or lack thereof, is demonstrated. Recommendations for practice can then be formed. Understanding existing practice patterns provides insight into how current evidence impacts on practice and can identify where greater efforts in knowledge translation are needed. Clinical practice will vary dependent on a number of factors such as location, resources available, patient population, and professional background. Several CPGs from varying professionals who treat patients with neck pain exist [2-5]. To our knowledge no examination of practice patterns across health care professionals who treat patients with neck pain has been published.

Neck pain is a common problem with an episodic course that affects a large proportion of the population. Estimates for the prevalence of neck pain vary from 0.4% to 86.8% (mean 23.1%) in the general population, whereas the range for the one year incidence is reported to be smaller (10.4% to 21.3%) [6]. Risk factors for new onset neck pain include being female, between the ages of 35 to 49 years and having a previous episode of neck pain [6-8]. Estimated expenditures on spine related care in the United States have almost doubled in the last decade [7,9]. The number of emergency room visits related to motor vehicle accidents (MVA) has been steadily increasing in the last three decades [10]. Direct healthcare costs may only be a small piece of this burden, while the indirect costs of work absenteeism and disability are much greater [6,11].

Over the past decade the evidence base guiding the choice of effective treatments for reducing symptoms and increasing function has evolved. The association between severity and disability of neck pain has been established by numerous studies [12-15]. There are numerous health care practitioners that treat patients with neck pain with a variety of interventions such as physical medicine, manual therapies, exercise, electrotherapeutic agents, and ergonomics [16]. Manual therapies in combination with exercise may provide optimal treatment effects [17]. Outcomes such as better pain reduction, better patient satisfaction, improved function, increased range of motion and increased strength in people with neck pain have been reported in patients who received manual therapy alone or in combination with other modalities [16,18-22]. While evidence exists for other interventions, the number of studies is few with conflicting results leading to less confidence in their effectiveness [16,23-25].

Our recent reviews of reviews [26,27] provide some guidance for practitioners. There is moderate evidence for specific modalities such as laser and acupuncture for pain reduction while there is evidence of no benefit for the use of collars, ergonomic or physical environment changes in the workplace. Ideally, providers make treatment choices based on their experience, the available evidence, and the clinical presentation of their patient.

In reality however, provider choices of care may be influenced by factors such as scope of practice, patient preferences, types of providers the patient chooses to see or insurance coverage, thereby influencing the types of treatments received and by their interaction with providers. Even within the same profession, providers' choices of care may vary depending upon the degree to which they are aware of current evidence on treatment effectiveness and the degree to which they choose to incorporate the evidence into their practice. For example, care provided by a physical therapist will differ, in some ways from care provided by a physician or from another physical therapist. Patient centered care and the shared decision making model have incorporated patient preferences into treatment planning. This denotes the importance of flexibility in the way that health professionals structure the decision-making process so that individual patient differences can be respected [28]. The incorporation of patient preferences has the potential to shift 'ideal' choices to more practical ones based on preferences of each individual. For example, a patient treated previously for a different problem and presenting with a new problem may have had a successful outcome using an evidence based intervention. However applying the same intervention to a different area may not be supported. Given the favourable outcome, the patient may request that the same intervention be used. The practitioner is therefore faced with making treatment decisions that incorporate patient expectation and it has been suggested that doing so may improve adherence and satisfaction with care [29]. The end result is more varied care and a modification of the 'ideal' treatment allowing incorporation of patient preferences and expectations but straying slightly from recommended guidelines.

There is little evidence in the literature about guideline adherence in patients with neck pain. A study by Oostendorp et al. (2013) used quality indicators of treatment based on guideline recommendations for patients with non specific neck pain [30]. The study by Oostendorp et al. used a sample of 38 physiotherapists and 96 patients in the Netherlands. Adherence to the identified treatment quality indicators ranged from weak (34%) to adequate (59%). These findings provide some initial insight into the potential variability in care that may exist for this patient population and practitioner group but does not provide details about the types of interventions or the frequency with which they were used.

The International Collaboration on Neck Pain (ICON) project is a collaborative project amongst internationally recognized experts in the field of neck pain. The goal of ICON is to establish clear, actionable messages in the areas of diagnosis, prognosis, interventions and outcomes measurement. To establish such data, ICON has implemented an international multidisciplinary survey of clinical practice patterns that will help shape evidence based recommendations.

The purposes of this study were 1. To describe the utilization of interventions in patients with neck pain by clinicians and 2. Where appropriate, to examine whether utilization varies by profession or subgroup of disorder.

Methods

A cross sectional survey to determine practice patterns of clinicians who provide care to patients with neck pain was conducted from February 2012 to March 2013. The survey was approved by the McMaster University Research Ethics Board (REB#11-025).

Survey development and validation

The survey was designed to acquire information in four principle content areas. These four areas included examination/diagnostic procedures, prognostic indicators, interventions (including adverse events), and outcome measures. Two additional content areas determined the demographic and caseload information of respondents.

The survey was developed using Streiner and Norman (2008) [31] methods in three distinct and iterative steps – item generation using literature review, consultation with clinicians which included clinical observation, and ICON content experts - before fielding the questionnaire. 1) The initial core set of items was generated from systematic reviews on conservative treatments for neck pain. 2) This set was then sent to expert clinicians identified within and external to ICON for review of usability, technical functionality of the electronic questionnaire and identification of issues/gaps. 3) The next set was tested using the ICON expert panel of interdisciplinary professionals; this included physicians, psychologists, physiotherapists, massage therapists, chiropractors, and other rehabilitative professions. Additional items created by these experts aimed to address areas missing from the initial item generation to ensure they were designed to be appropriate for administration across different health care professionals commonly treating people with neck pain.

This content area being sufficiently large was divided into the following two separate surveys: 1. Physical medicine or CAM interventions; and 2. Pharmacological and psychological interventions. Items in the physical medicine and CAM survey covered exercise, manual therapies, modalities, mechanical traction, orthoses/supportive devices, ergonomic and work related interventions. An 'other' response option was included where appropriate within each category and allowed respondents to add any interventions that may have been missed. Broadly, items asked about utilization of each treatment category (yes, no, outside scope of practice). The questions progressed in the following sequence. If a respondent indicated 'yes' to the initial utilization question, then inquiry of frequency of use (commonly, occasionally, never) followed. If respondents indicated 'common' or 'occasional' use of an intervention, then use of that intervention (commonly, occasionally, never, not applicable) among the following common subgroups of neck pain disorders was also inquired about:

1. Acute nonspecific neck pain,
2. Chronic nonspecific neck pain,
3. Facet joint dysfunction (as diagnosed by diagnostic block),
4. Acute whiplash associated disorder (WAD),
5. Chronic WAD and
6. Radiculopathy/WADIII.

For the modalities category, respondents were also asked about indications for use. Routing questions were sequentially designed to reduce respondent burden allowing avoidance of categories not relevant to respondents.

Face and content validity of the survey were addressed in an iterative process involving multiple revisions and content experts. In the first round, there was a focus on accuracy of item content and clarity in the wording of each item and response. In the second round, there was a focus on the organizational structure of the survey so as to have logical grouping, sequencing of items and routing questions. In the third round, responses were piloted within the electronic survey format to evaluate presentation and routing. Finally, the ICON working group (n = 38) that had representation from all the disciplines included in our target audience was used for field-testing. These experts reviewed the survey for accuracy, clarity, completeness and burden. After each round of revisions, editing occurred for clarity. This resulted in minor changes to items and a few additions. The finalized version was mounted using LimeSurvey[a], a software program for web-based survey administration.

Sampling frame

Our sampling frame was all health care professional groups identified as having a major role in the management of neck pain, relying on both our reviews and clinical experience to identify these groups. This included physicians (general practitioners, physiatrists, psychiatrists) physiotherapists, chiropractors, massage therapists, occupational therapists, psychologists and complementary medicine specialists. We wanted to include an international perspective. Given the number of national associations and a general lack of willingness for professional associations to burden their members with survey requests we relied on Snowball sampling strategies.

This method allowed clinician experts identified by ICON within each of the professions. Invitations were sent to the contact person identified for each association and requested they assist with sending out links to our survey to their professional links and colleagues. If the association responded and agreed to send out the link on our behalf, it was done so at their discretion. In total 37 groups were contacted, 19 of which did not respond. Survey invitations were distributed via e-mail blast to members, and electronic postings (e.g., e-newsletter, website, Facebook or Twitter pages) by national and international professional groups for chiropractors (Danish Chiropractors' Association; European Academy of Chiropractic; Netherlands Chiropractic Association; New Zealand Chiropractors' Association; Ontario Chiropractic Association); manual therapists (Canadian Academy of Manipulative Physical Therapy; Dutch Association for Manual Therapy; Finnish Association for Orthopedic Manual Therapy; German Manual Therapy Journal; International Federation of Orthopaedic Manipulative Physical Therapists); massage therapists (Massage Therapists' Association of British Columbia); physicians (North American Spine Society; University of British Columbia Department of Family Medicine); physiotherapists (American Physical Therapy Association – Orthopedic Section; Canadian Physiotherapy Association – Pain Sciences Division; Hong Kong Physiotherapy Association; Musculoskeletal Physiotherapy Australia; Physiopedia); and other health care professionals (Osteopathic Society of New Zealand). The method of recruitment meant we were unable to determine how many people received our requests for participation. We were unaware if the associations sent the survey link to all members or only those who agreed to receive it.

Survey administration

The survey was administered through the International Collaboration on Neck (ICON) group and was estimated to take 15-20 minutes to answer. An e-mail including information about the survey, and a registration link were provided. No incentives were offered. Public registration was required to participate in the survey and individuals who volunteered to receive the survey link were considered "registrants". Once respondents registered, an email containing the link to participate in this survey was sent out immediately. Respondents remained anonymous by storing the identification tokens (name and e-mail address) that provided access to the survey on a secure separate database. Registrants were notified that clicking the survey link indicated that they were electronically consenting to participate. Weekly reminders were sent to registrants until they completed the survey, opted out, or received a maximum of four reminders. Response rates amongst registrants were calculated based on the number of registrants who completed at least part of the survey.

Analysis

Data quality was assessed by randomly sampling 10% of the dataset to check for errors. Discrepant entries ($< 1\%$) were resolved through this process. Descriptive statistics were used to summarize participants and their responses to each question. Chi-squared analyses were used to test for differences in the frequency of use of various treatment interventions based on profession. Rank order was used to assess frequency of use of interventions amongst subtypes of neck pain.

Results

There were 360 respondents (332 full and 28 partial) spanning 17 countries. Respondents were mainly physical therapists (38%) or chiropractors (31%) and largely male (41-66%). Due to lack of adequate representation from professions other than physical therapists and chiropractors, we focused the analyses on these two groups. Based on the relevant physiotherapy and chiropractic professional associations' membership information that we were able to ascertain, as many as 17773 individuals were invited to respond to our survey. This is likely a high estimate as more detailed information from a few organizations indicates that variation existed due to inactive emails, unsent links (one international body represents 22 countries) and membership number fluctuations throughout the year. Using this very conservative total, results in a response rate of approximately two percent. Table 1 provides the characteristics for the whole sample and physical therapists and chiropractors only. Within the two professions, there was an average of 15 years of clinical experience, and 34% had obtained a Master's degree. The majority (80%) worked in private practice, with reimbursement through private insurance (79%) in a fee for service private payment model (64%). Over half of the respondents indicated that patients with neck pain made up at least one quarter of their caseload. The largest subset of respondents was from Canada (38%). The gender distribution of this subset of respondents is representative of both professions (males 41% physical therapists; 66% chiropractors) [32,33].

Table 2 demonstrates the frequency of use ('Yes') of the various physical medicine and CAM treatment interventions along with their subtypes. Exercise prescription was used at least by 98% of respondents, as were manual therapies. Ergonomic advice (83%), work related interventions (73%) and thermal agents (73%) rounded out

Table 1 Demographics

Demographics	Respondents (n = 360)	Respondents (n = 251)	
		Chiropractor (n = 113)	Physical therapist (n = 138)
Years in practice since graduation (mean (sd))	16 (12)	16 (12)	16 (12)
Gender	44% female, 48% male	35% female, 66% male	59% female, 41% male
Profession			
Physical therapist (Manual therapist)	38% (13%)	-	55%
Chiropractor	31%	45%	-
Massage therapist	9%	-	-
Physician	5%	-	-
Other	14%	-	-
Country			
Canada	38%	56%	23%
United Kingdom	10%	3%	19%
United States of America	10%	1%	12%
Denmark	9%	26%	-
New Zealand	9%	1%	11%
Netherlands	6%	3%	9%
Other (Australia, Belgium, Brazil, Finland, Germany, Hong Kong, Italy, Norway, Portugal, South Africa, Sweden,)	18%	13%	25%
Practice setting			
Private clinic	72%	95%	69%
General hospital	7%	1%	14%
Teaching hospital	7%	3%	10%
Outpatient rehab facility	7%	6%	9%
Private consultant	6%	3%	7%
Other	9%	4%	12%
% of caseload with neck pain			
<5	3%	0%	3%
6-20	21%	14%	34%
21-50	47%	60%	49%
>50	24%	26%	15%
Health care reimbursement system			
Private insurance	72%	83%	75%
Public health insurance	45%	40%	51%
Workers compensation	36%	40%	36%
Salary reimbursement scheme			
Salary - Fixed	27%	17%	46%
Fee for service – Public	22%	27%	12%
Fee for service – Private	61%	75%	55%
Education - Highest level obtained			
Diploma	9%	4%	5%
Bachelor's degree	19%	6%	33%
Masters degree	29%	*	41%
Doctor of medicine	4%	3%	1%
Doctorate/PhD	16%	27%	15%
Other	14%	35%	4%
		(Doctor of chiropractic)	

*This value for chiropractors is not reported as it overlaps with the 'Other' category.

Table 2 Provision of treatment interventions

Interventions	Yes %	Yes commonly %	Yes occasionally %	Yes never %	No %	Outside scope of practice
Exercise	98				2	0
Stretch neck/upper thorax		79	17	2		
Stretch other body part		47	43	8		
Strengthen neck/upper thorax		77	19	3		
Strengthen other body parts		51	41	7		
Local muscle endurance		63	26	9		
Postural control		84	13	2		
Exercises related to motor control		40	41	18		
Static/dynamic stabilization		55	32	12		
Cardiovascular retraining		25	51	23		
Other:		17	53	29		
Mechanical Traction	28				55	12
Modalities						
Electrotherapeutics	43				47	9
TENS		12	27	4		
EMG biofeedback		1	9	26		
Short wave diathermy		0	5	31		
Muscle stimulation		5	13	19		
Thermal agents	73				22	5
Heat or cold application		55	13	0		
Phototherapeutics	10				65	23
Laser therapy		5	4	1		
Sonic therapies	29				54	17
Ultrasound		11	13	0		
Shock wave		0	2	21		
Acupuncture	46				29	25
Traditional acupuncture		17	17	7		
Dry needling		18	11	12		
Manual therapies	99				1	0
Mobilization		90	8	1		
Manipulation		56	32	11		
Manual traction		55	37	7		
Massage/soft tissue work		79	19	1		
Orthoses/supportive devices	30				57	11
Collars		0	24	5		
Pillows		8	20	3		
Taping		4	16	10		
Adaptive equipment		0	5	25		
Other		0	1	28		
Ergonomic interventions	83				15	8
Work related interventions	73				22	9
Work hardening		8	35	29		
Work site modification		33	36	3		
Communication with employer		16	43	13		
Work site restrictions		19	47	7		
Other		7	23	42		
Other	13				70	6

the top 5 most frequently endorsed treatment approaches. Respondents indicated that they largely did not provide ('No') 'other' interventions (70%), phototherapeutics (65%), orthoses/supportive devices (57%), mechanical traction (55%), sonic therapies (54%) or electrotherapeutics (47%).

Different types of exercise were more *commonly* used such as those for postural control (84%), stretching of the neck/upper thorax (79%) and strengthening of the neck/upper thorax (77%). The exceptions were motor control (41%) and cardiovascular training (51%), which were used more *occasionally*. The most *commonly* used modalities included hot and cold applications (55%) and acupuncture (traditional 17%, dry needling 18%). A substantial number of respondents rarely or never used short wave diathermy (31%), biofeedback (26%), shock wave sonic therapy (21%) and muscle stimulation (19%). The majority of respondents *commonly* used manual therapies and this was most frequently mobilization (90%) compared to manipulation (56%). Work related interventions such as work hardening, site modification, communication with the employer and site restrictions were used *occasionally* (35-47%).

Table 3 highlights the use of modalities and their indications for use. The only two modalities that the majority of respondents indicated that they used were Thermal applications and TENS. Both were indicated for pain relief, 90% and 71% respectively. For the remaining modalities, for all but ultrasound and muscle stimulation (45% each), the majority of respondents indicated that they 'Do not use/outside scope of practice'.

Subgroup analysis
Provider
Looking across physical therapists and chiropractors, differences in their use of the various interventions were found. Table 4 shows that the two differ in their prescription of exercise, phototherapeutics, orthoses/supportive devices and the category of 'other' interventions. Both

collars and taping are used more often by physical therapists than chiropractors ($p = 0.01$ and $p = 0.03$ respectively). Examples of 'other' interventions used more frequently by physical therapists include pain education, referral to other healthcare professionals, use of McKenzie methods [34], self-management strategies, breathing/relaxation strategies and prolotherapy. Figure 1 depicts the differences in exercise prescription between the two. Significant differences were found in the prescription of some types of exercise (greater by physical therapists $p \leq 0.01$) except stretching of other body parts, strengthening of neck/upper back and other body parts and cardiovascular training where there was no difference. Figure 2 shows the differences in use of modalities. Chiropractors use of laser ($p = 0.00$), and electrical muscular stimulation ($p = 0.01$) was significantly greater than physical therapists. Although there is no significant difference between the two in the overall use of manual therapies, there is a significant difference in the use of thrust manipulation ($p = 0.00$) with chiropractors performing it more often.

Disorder subgroup
Table 5 outlines the use of treatment interventions according to disorder subgroup. Respondents reported using exercises, manual therapy, and ergonomic interventions most frequently in patients with chronic nonspecific neck pain compared to the five other conditions. Differences between chronic nonspecific neck pain and chronic WAD were minimal. The use of orthoses/supportive devices was variable across the 6 subgroup disorders. Respondents indicated that collars were used most frequently for patients with acute WAD (24%), pillows for patients with chronic nonspecific neck (27%), while the use of taping (16%) was split across three subgroups and adaptive equipment (5%) in chronic non specific neck pain. Utilization of three of the four work related interventions was equal in patients with chronic non

Table 3 Indications for use of modalities

	Pain relief	Retrain or strengthen muscle	Enhance tissue healing	Alter tissue prior to MT	Do not use/outside scope of practice
TENS	71%	3%	5%	7%	26%
EMG biofeedback	2%	28%	1%	1%	66%
Short wave diathermy	5%	0%	4%	5%	83%
Muscle stimulation	16%	42%	11%	15%	45%
Heat or cold application	90%	1%	34%	42%	1%
Laser therapy	12%	1%	28%	3%	65%
Ultrasound	25%	1%	40%	18%	45%
Shock wave	1%	1%	8%	1%	86%
Traditional acupuncture	37%	5%	18%	12%	55%
Dry needling	34%	4%	15%	21%	55%

Table 4 Differences in provision of treatment interventions across professions

Interventions	Physical therapy versus chiropractic significance and direction
Exercise	p = 0.01, PT–138 CH–107
Electrotherapeutics	No difference
Thermal agents	No difference
Phototherapeutics	p = 0.00, CH–23 PT–10
Sonic therapeutics	No difference
Acupuncture	No difference
Manual therapies	No difference
Mechanical traction	No difference
Orthoses/support devices	p = 0.05, PT–53 CH–26
Ergonomic interventions	No difference
Work related interventions	No difference
Other	p = 0.00, PT–29 CH–4

PT = Physical therapist, *CH* = Chiropractor.

specific neck pain or chronic WAD (43 to 68%). Respondents indicated that they used mechanical traction most frequently for patients with radiculopathy or WAD III (27%). Rank ordering of interventions within the subgroups from most utilized to least utilized resulted in the following: 1. chronic nonspecific neck pain; 2. chronic WAD; 3. radiculopathy; 4. acute nonspecific neck pain; 5. acute WAD; and 6. facet joint dysfunction by diagnostic block. This would indicate that chronic conditions are being treated with the interventions we inquired about more frequently and that respondents are also utilizing a wider range of interventions.

Discussion
Summary of main findings
Our results from this survey demonstrate that the interventions most commonly used by physical therapists and chiropractors for the treatment of people with neck pain (exercise and manual therapy) are those that also have strong evidence for their effectiveness, [17,35-38] particularly when combined. It is these two interventions that are also recommended by clinical practice guidelines [2,4]. Other treatments do not reflect the best evidence for effective treatment. The results also indicate variable use of interventions with low or very low evidence. Some are being used to a larger degree (ergonomic and work related interventions) [39,40] while others are not being used (mechanical traction, orthoses/supportive devices and modalities) [23,24]. Other treatments may be used more as they address immediate or short term symptom relief but they lack sufficient focus on long-term functioning [17,27].

Exercise
A Cochrane review of exercise interventions for patients with neck pain highlighted that a combination of cervical and scapulothoracic stretching and strengthening improves pain and function and leads to greater patient satisfaction in people with chronic neck pain. Endurance exercises of the cervical and scapulothoracic regions are effective at reducing pain, improving function and global perceived effect for subacute/chronic cervicogenic headache, while neck strengthening is effective at reducing pain in acute cervical radiculopathy. Neither upper extremity stretching, strengthening or a general exercise program is recommended for chronic neck pain [35]. In this study, respondents' reported the greatest utilization

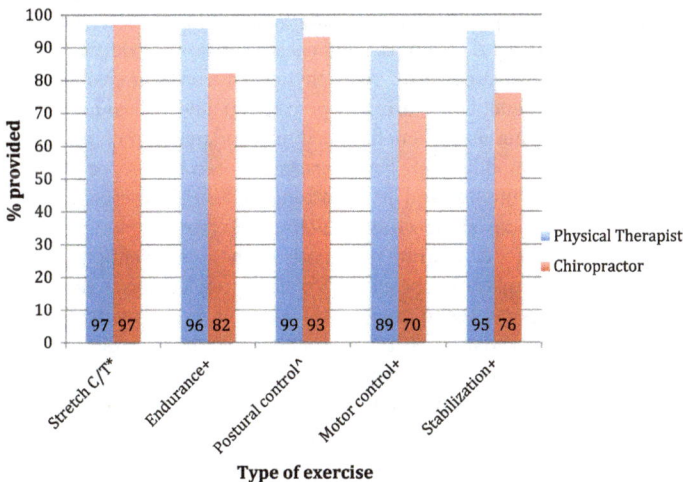

Figure 1 Significant differences between professions in exercise prescription.

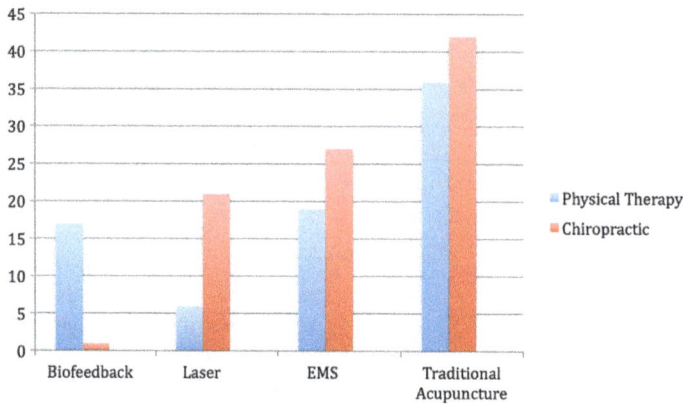

Figure 2 Significant differences between professions in modality use.

of exercise in chronic nonspecific neck pain and WAD conditions demonstrating that current practice patterns are in sync with evidence based recommendations. We did not have a specific category to capture cervicogenic headache so we cannot be certain of how this subgroup was considered. Our response options regarding exercise covered many general concepts ranging from stretching, strengthening, endurance, postural control, motor control and stabilization, but did not allow for details within these categories to be explored. Overall exercise prescription was reported most often in the two chronic neck pain conditions and radiculopathy, which is consistent with the findings of the systematic review.

Manual therapies

Manual therapies are a core skill for the majority of respondents so it is not surprising that they are used as frequently as exercise. Mobilization and massage therapy/soft tissue work were the two most commonly reported of the four techniques. Possible explanations for this lie in our sample representing physical therapists and chiropractors as well as in the evidence base. A Cochrane review has reported the benefit of using mobilization techniques and that no differential benefit for spinal manipulation as opposed to mobilization has been shown for the outcomes of pain, function and patient satisfaction [36]. Using the techniques alone compared to combining them with exercise is mainly of short term benefit on pain only [37]. Regarding the effectiveness of massage therapy/soft tissue techniques, findings of systematic reviews are concordant [41-43]. Evidence indicates some pain reduction and improvement in function for subacute and chronic neck pain immediately post massage therapy/soft tissue treatment but there is inconclusive evidence of any long-term benefit. Despite the lack of clear direction in the literature, the proportion of utilization of massage therapy/soft tissue

techniques was similar between the physical therapists and chiropractors in this survey. Massage/soft tissue techniques may be selected for a variety of reasons including complementary or preparatory effects prior to vertebral mobilization/manipulations [43] and the fact that patients report it being very helpful for neck pain [44,45]. It is possible that there are differences in the type of soft tissue techniques performed by the two different professions, but the nature of survey work does not allow for these distinctions.

Ergonomics, work related interventions and Orthotics/Supportive devices

The association between poor workstation design and awkward work postures with neck pain has been documented [46]. Recent systematic reviews reported limited evidence for decreased neck pain when physical ergonomic interventions were used compared to none at all [39,47]. The following interventions are reported to have no evidence of benefit: ergonomic education (for intervention), workplace physical environment changes (for intervention and primary prevention), and individual worker upper extremity stretching and endurance training program (for intervention, primary and secondary prevention) [26]. In the absence of strong evidence for ergonomic or work related interventions, and considering the difficulties and potential high costs of these interventions it may be that practitioners are less likely to select this treatment approach. Our survey does not allow us to determine why people select different interventions and thus whether it is perceived effectiveness, skills or resources that drive the lower utilization of ergonomic and workplace interventions. The lower rate of utilization of these interventions by respondents, particularly for complex patients like those with chronic WAD may reflect the challenge that practitioners face in addressing interventions for complex patients with limited evidence [48,49].

Table 5 Provision of treatment interventions by subgroups

	Acute non specific NP + %	Chronic non specific NP%	Facet joint dysfunction by diagnostic block %	Acute WAD%	Chronic WAD%	Radiculopathy (WAD III)%
Exercise						
Stretch neck/upper thorax	78	**97**	50	63	92	65
Stretch other body part	69	**86**	42*	63	83	65
Strengthen neck/upper thorax	69	**94**	51	62	92	75
Strengthen other body parts	61	**87**	47	57	86	65
Local muscle endurance	63	**87**	51	59	86	65
Postural control	84	**95**	57	81	92	85
Exercises related to motor control	56	**72**	40*	56	71	59
Static/dynamic stabilization	68	**84**	48	67	83	73
Cardiovascular retraining	29*	**57**	26*	31*	56	38
Manual therapies						
Mobilization (joint or neuromuscular)	95	**97**	61	86	95	89
Manipulation (thrust)	73	**82**	51	51	77	49
Manual traction	82	**83**	51	66	77	79
Massage/soft tissue work	93	**95**	58	85	92	84
Mechanical traction	17	25	15	12	24	**27**
Orthoses/supportive devices						
Collars	21	6*	6*	**24**	8*	20
Pillows	22	**27**	18	23	26	23
Taping	**16**	**16**	10	14	**16**	14
Adaptive equipment	3	**5**	2	3	4	4
Other	2	1	1	2	1	1
Ergonomic interventions	73	**83**	49	70	81	75
Work related interventions						
Work hardening	19*	**43**	21*	21*	**43**	27
Work site modification	56	**68**	37	57	**68**	63
Communication with employer	45	**55**	7*	50	**55**	52
Work site restrictions	59	55	31*	**61**	58	61
Other	21	**22**	13*	20	21	21
Other types of interventions	12	**15**	8*	11	14	12

+NP = Neck Pain.
* = percentage is ≤ to respondents indicating never use/not applicable.
Bolded = highest percentage amongst subgroups.

Overall, respondents provided little endorsement for the use of mechanical traction, and orthoses/supportive devices. However, responses suggest that there may be subgroups where clinicians feel these interventions could be beneficial. For example, mechanical traction was used most frequently in the radiculopathy/WAD III population compared to the other subgroups, despite inconclusive evidence for its use either intermittently or continuously [24]. This may suggest that practitioners expect that a force to unload pressure on the nerve is indicated in nerve root compression. Some evidence does exist for intermittent traction for generalized mechanical neck pain which may be influencing practitioner usage [50] and we have recently found evidence of moderate benefit for intermittent traction for chronic neck pain [27]. We did not ask about intermittent versus continuous application and therefore cannot be certain how this was interpreted.

Cervical pillows were used most commonly in chronic neck pain and WAD conditions while collar use was reported most often in acute non specific neck pain despite evidence of no benefit [51,52] or that collar use is detrimental to recovery [53]. In our concurrent review we found no evidence to support the effectiveness of soft collars in acute neck pain or WAD [26].

Modalities

We did not inquire about modality usage by disorder subgroup but by indications for use. When implemented, the rationale selected by respondents for specific modalities was consistent with their accepted indications. TENS, Heat/cold and acupuncture were used for pain relief and laser therapy for tissue healing. The existing literature base shows moderate evidence supporting the use of these modalities for neck pain [16,23,54] with the exception of heat/cold where little evidence is present. A survey of patients in one state in the USA seeking care for neck pain reported that heat and cold therapy were received by 57% and 48% respectively compared to prescribed exercise (53%), spinal manipulation (37%) or TENS (22%) [55]. A survey of chiropractors in two states in the USA also reported use of thermal and electrical modalities more than exercise [56]. There may be several reasons for these discrepancies between the practice patterns reported in these two American studies versus the current findings. This could include factors such as: patient preferences, time management in busy clinics, clinicians balancing observations of treatment efficacy with the published evidence or perhaps being unaware of the current recommendations for care.

Our concurrent review of reviews indicates that acupuncture (short term pain relief) and low-level laser (short and intermediate term pain relief and function improvement) both have moderate evidence of benefit for chronic neck pain. Evidence of no benefit was found for pulsed ultrasound, or continuous traction [27]. Our data shows that respondents are practicing in line with the evidence in their minimal use of ultrasound and traction and greater use of acupuncture, but deviates from the evidence in their minimal use of low level laser.

Disorder subgroups

Our data indicated some difference in treatment selection across different types of neck pain. Chronic neck pain conditions presented in our survey as non specific and WAD were more likely to be treated with physical medicine and CAM treatment interventions in comparison to radiculopathy/WAD III, (presented in our survey as acute neck conditions and facet joint dysfunction). Although it is tenuous to make assumptions about why respondents selected different interventions from this type of survey, it does appear that the pattern of utilization is consistent with variations in the complexity of the condition. Chronic neck pain conditions, particularly those arising following WAD [13,57] are often more complex, and associated with greater degrees of disability and impairment [57]. Our respondents indicated use of more varied interventions for chronic neck conditions compared to acute conditions, possibly in line with the complexity of the condition. Cervical nerve root pathology leading to upper extremity symptoms is often caused by space occupying lesions such as disc herniation, spondylosis, or osteophytosis that can be resistant to conservative treatment [58]. There is conflicting evidence around the efficacy of manual therapy, exercise, and other modalities for radiculopathy [3,58]. Acute neck pain and WAD if uncomplicated by high levels of pain severity, functional limitation or psychological distress will likely resolve within a reasonable timeframe. Our survey results seem to reflect this as these acute conditions had the lowest frequency of intervention utilization.

There is little published evidence on the effectiveness of conservative treatments for facet joint dysfunction confirmed by diagnostic block. The relative lack of evidence for treatment specific to this syndrome may be why respondents ranked it last of our listed disorders regarding overall frequency of utilization of interventions. Practitioners may suspect facet joint dysfunction after screening but it is likely that few are confirmed by diagnostic block thus making certainty of the diagnosis difficult.

Differences and similarities between professions

Our findings indicate that some differences exist in the utilization of interventions between physical therapists and chiropractors. Although the scope of practice of these two professions is similar, these findings are not unexpected, as differences based on education and clinical paradigms could be expected that may influence their approach to treatment. Practitioner's use of interventions can be shaped by factors other than their entry-level education such as courses taken post professionally, clinical environments, characteristics of the population treated, or use of evidence base medicine. The nature of the survey does not allow us to determine why differences existed between the professional groups. The higher utilization of exercise by physical therapists could reflect the fact that physical therapists have a strong focus on use of therapeutics exercise in their entry-level training or that there is a substantial body of therapeutic exercise evidence developed by physical therapists. We could anticipate that clinicians attend to research that is published within their own professional journals to a greater extent than literature from other disciplines [59-61]. Similarly, innovations in pain education have arisen in physical therapy literature and were cited in the 'other' category by physical therapists [62,63]. The higher use of manipulation by chiropractors (100%) is consistent with this intervention being at the core of chiropractic education. Explanations for the differences in the remaining categories were less dramatic and the reasons for them were less intuitive.

Similarities between the physical therapists and chiropractors were demonstrated in their utilization of electrotherapeutics, thermal agents, sonic agents, acupuncture, manual therapies, mechanical traction, ergonomic and work related interventions. Our review of the evidence has indicated that most of these categories have poor supporting evidence with the exception of manual therapies. The similarity in the use of manual therapies in general is not surprising since they are at the core of entry-level education for both professions. Reasons for their similarity in practice patterns with respect to the remaining interventions can only be speculated. It may be that a combination of factors is contributing to this practice pattern including caseload, patient expectations, infrastructure within the clinics, post-professional training, mentorship and others. For example, patients with neck pain may have a preference for heat applications and in busy private clinics supplementing the treatment sessions with heat may improve patient satisfaction and facilitate other aspects of the treatment program. Although workers compensation accounted for approximately one third of reimbursement in our respondents, it may be that practitioners are seeing patients who are having issues managing their neck pain at work even though the problem may not have directly resulted from a work injury. This along with practitioners implementing primary or secondary prevention strategies could explain the high use of ergonomic and work related interventions.

Overall the practice patterns demonstrated by this data suggest that chiropractors and physical therapists demonstrate strong utilization of interventions widely supported by the literature to manage neck pain. Interventions with limited or conflicting evidence have low to moderate use that is consistent with the uncertainty in the literature. The variability in use of interventions reflects the multimodal practice of practitioners that are commonly used to treat this population. Clinicians faced with applying the evidence-base must customize interventions to the presentation of the individual patient and we know that even within clinical trials response patterns vary across different patients. Therefore, some of the variability in practice patterns reflects this customization. There are multiple patient and practitioner preferences that affect the treatment choices made in clinician and patient interactions around managing neck pain. These can include previous experience, stage of healing, or practitioner type. However understanding the gaps between the evidence base and practice patterns is important for identifying areas needing targeted knowledge translation. Comparing current evidence with our survey results indicates that there are areas for education of chiropractors and physical therapists to increase utilization of interventions with supportive evidence. This includes low level laser and acupuncture therapy that were reported by only 13% and 45% respectively of our respondents. Our results also indicate an even greater need to educate practitioners about their use of interventions with weak supporting evidence such as work related and ergonomic interventions which were utilized by the majority of respondents. A greater understanding of explanatory factors of utilization may require further mixed methods research. As the evidence-based becomes clearer, it might be expected that practice patterns should become less variable.

To our knowledge our practice survey is the first to compare practice patterns of chiropractors and physical therapists for people with neck pain. Previous surveys pertaining to specific professions, reporting more broadly or on specific aspects of treatment have been published making comparison difficult. Within the physical therapy profession, surveys have focused on the utilization of manual therapies with greater attention to spinal (thrust) manipulation for neck pain. Internationally and in Canada, a decrease in manipulative procedures to the neck have been reported [64,65] and there is evidence of them generally being used less often in the neck compared to mobilization techniques [65-68]. Chiropractic surveys report much higher utilization of spinal (thrust) manipulative procedures [56,69,70], and this is not surprising since spinal manipulation is a core intervention within the paradigm of chiropractic practice. Chiropractors see a client base that consists mainly of people with back or neck pain [71] and are sought by the public for the treatment these problems [44,55]. In one population based survey, chiropractors and physical therapists were the second and third most utilized practitioners respectively for the treatment of chronic neck pain [55].

The effort to provide clear consistent messaging to relevant health professionals and the public regarding treatments with demonstrated effect as well as those without or even impeding recovery must continue and occur in multiple formats and mediums. This will help with the expenditure and appropriate allocation of healthcare dollars to minimize over-treatment with ineffective therapies or under-treatment of patients presenting with more complex conditions.

Limitations

This survey has limitations that should be considered when interpreting the results. Our survey was cross-sectional and therefore provides a one-time perspective of general treatment trends. The benefit of this is that it can be revisited over time and results compared to detect change. We are also aware that our sample was not proportional and over-represented Canadian clinicians compared to other countries. It also was largely representative of the chiropractic and physical therapy professions. Our snowball sampling technique was limited by the associations known within our network and likely resulted in the exclusion of several relevant associations, that had we been able to sample, their input could have altered our results. Also we cannot be certain of our response rate due to the limitations of the information that we were able to receive from the organizations that distributed the survey link. We are aware of the potential for significant variation in the numbers of people that actually received the link and therefore the response rate provided is likely a very conservative one, yet still quite low. Those who choose to participate in survey research may represent a systematically different type of practitioner than those who don't choose to participate. This survey was descriptive and to our knowledge the first of its kind. We did not conduct a Bonferroni correction to our results therefore allowing for the possibility that some reported differences in professions are due to chance. The results should not be considered generalizable but rather hypothesis generating to be further explored in future studies. Therefore, transferring the conclusions of this study to disciplines may not be appropriate.

Conclusions

Our survey respondents indicated that they widely use interventions with a strong evidence base for effectiveness and that they also use a variety of other interventions with limited support or conflicting evidence. This suggests there is a need for research to fill gaps in evidence that are associated with variable practice patterns and knowledge translation to reduce the usage of some interventions that have been shown to be ineffective. Examining the consistency or lack of it between available evidence and current treatment patterns can influence guideline dissemination as well as other interventions,

such as payment reform, to improve the effectiveness of current care for neck pain.

Endnote

[a]LimeSurvey software, Survey Service & Consulting, Hamburg, Germany.

Competing interests
The authors declare that they have no competing interests.

Authors' contributions
LC provided input at all stages of survey development, conducted the analysis, drafted the manuscript and incorporated feedback from all co-authors. JCM, ARG, DM and PLS provided input at all stages of survey development and provided feedback on the analysis and on the draft of the manuscript. All have given final approval for publication.

Acknowledgements
ICON is a multi-disciplinary collaborative group that includes scientist-authors (listed below) and support staff (Margaret Lomotan) that conduct knowledge synthesis and translation aimed at reducing the burden of neck pain. The ICON authors provided direction of the project; input into the survey questions and review of the findings/manuscript and includes (in alphabetical order): Gert Bronfort, Norm Buckley, Lisa Carlesso, Linda Carroll, Pierre Côté, Jeanette Ezzo, Paulo Ferreira, Tim Flynn, Charlie Goldsmith, Anita Gross, Ted Haines, Jan Hartvigsen, Wayne Hing, Gwendolen Jull, Faith Kaplan, Ron Kaplan, Helge Kasch, Justin Kenardy, Per Kjær, Janet Lowcock, Joy MacDermid, Jordan Miller, Margareta Nordin, Paul Peloso, Jan Pool, Duncan Reid, Sidney Rubinstein, P. Lina Santaguida, Anne Söderlund, Natalie Spearing, Michele Sterling, Grace Szeto, Robert Teasell, Arianne Verhagen, David M. Walton, Marc White.
Lisa Carlesso is supported by a Canadian Health Research Institute Fellowship.

ICON (International Collaboration on Neck)

- This work was supported by Canadian Institutes of Health Research (CIHR) grant(s) FRN: KRS-102084 and FRN: 114380.

Author details
[1]Toronto Western Research Institute, University Health Network, 399 Bathurst Street - MP11-328, Toronto, Ontario M5T 2S8, Canada. [2]School of Rehabilitation Sciences McMaster University, Hamilton, Ontario, Canada. [3]Clinical Research Lab, Hand and Upper Limb Centre, St. Joseph's Health Centre, London, Ontario, Canada. [4]School of Physical Therapy, Western University, London, Ontario, Canada. [5]Department of Clinical Epidemiology and Biostatistics, Hamilton, Ontario, Canada.

References
1. About systematic evidence reviews and clinical practice guidelines. In http://www.nhlbi.nih.gov/guidelines/about.htm.
2. Anderson-Peacock E, Blouin JS, Bryans R, Danis N, Furlan A, Marcoux H, Potter B, Ruegg R, Gross Stein J, White E: Chiropractic clinical practice guideline: evidence-based treatment of adult neck pain not due to whiplash. JCCA J Can Chiropr Assoc 2005, 49:158–209.
3. Bono CM, Ghiselli G, Gilbert TJ, Kreiner DS, Reitman C, Summers JT, Baisden JL, Easa J, Fernand R, Lamer T, Matz PG, Mazanec DJ, Resnick DK, Shaffer WO, Sharma AK, Timmons RB, Toton JF, North American Spine S: An evidence-based clinical guideline for the diagnosis and treatment of cervical radiculopathy from degenerative disorders. Spine J 2011, 11:64–72.
4. Childs JD, Cleland JA, Elliott JM, Teyhen DS, Wainner RS, Whitman JM, Sopky BJ, Godges JJ, Flynn TW, American Physical Therapy A: Neck pain: clinical practice guidelines linked to the International Classification of Functioning, Disability, and Health from the Orthopedic Section of the American Physical Therapy Association. J Orthop Sports Phys Ther 2008, 38:A1–A34.
5. Chou R, Huffman LH, American Pain S, American College of P: Nonpharmacologic therapies for acute and chronic low back pain: a review of the evidence for

an American Pain Society/American College of Physicians clinical practice guideline. *Ann Intern Med* 2007, **147**:492–504.

6. Hoy DG, Protani M, De R, Buchbinder R: **The epidemiology of neck pain.** *Best Pract Res Clin Rheumatol* 2010, **24**:783–792.

7. Martin BI, Deyo RA, Mirza SK, Turner JA, Comstock BA, Hollingworth W, Sullivan SD: **Expenditures and health status among adults with back and neck problems.** *JAMA* 2008, **299**:656–664.

8. Croft PR, Lewis M, Papageorgiou AC, Thomas E, Jayson MI, Macfarlane GJ, Silman AJ: **Risk factors for neck pain: a longitudinal study in the general population.** *Pain* 2001, **93**:317–325.

9. Harkness EF, Macfarlane GJ, Silman AJ, McBeth J: **Is musculoskeletal pain more common now than 40 years ago?: two population-based cross-sectional studies.** *Rheumatology (Oxford)* 2005, **44**:890–895.

10. Haldeman S, Carroll L, Cassidy JD: **Findings from the bone and joint decade 2000 to 2010 task force on neck pain and its associated disorders.** *J Occup Environ Med* 2010, **52**:424–427.

11. Borghouts JA, Koes BW, Vondeling H, Bouter LM: **Cost-of-illness of neck pain in The Netherlands in 1996.** *Pain* 1999, **80**:629–636.

12. Sterling M, Kenardy J: **Physical and psychological aspects of whiplash: important considerations for primary care assessment.** *Man Ther* 2008, **13**:93–102.

13. Thompson DP, Urmston M, Oldham JA, Woby SR: **The association between cognitive factors, pain and disability in patients with idiopathic chronic neck pain.** *Disabil Rehabil* 2010, **32**:1758–1767.

14. Webb R, Brammah T, Lunt M, Urwin M, Allison T, Symmons D: **Prevalence and predictors of intense, chronic, and disabling neck and back pain in the UK general population.** *Spine (Phila Pa 1976)* 2003, **28**:1195–1202.

15. Lee KC, Chiu TT, Lam TH: **The role of fear-avoidance beliefs in patients with neck pain: relationships with current and future disability and work capacity.** *Clin Rehabil* 2007, **21**:812–821.

16. Gross A, Goldsmith C, Hoving J, Haines T, Peloso P, Aker P, Santaguida P, Myers C: **Conservative management of mechanical neck disorders: a systematic review.** *J Rheumatol* 2007, **34**:1083–1102.

17. Miller J, Gross A, D'Sylva J, Burnie SJ, Goldsmith CH, Graham N, Haines T, Bronfort G, Hoving JL: **Manual therapy and exercise for neck pain: a systematic review.** *Man Ther* 2010, **15**:334–354.

18. Gross AR, Hoving JL, Haines TA, Goldsmith CH, Kay T, Aker P, Bronfort G: **Manipulation and mobilisation for mechanical neck disorders.** *Cochrane Database Syst Rev* 2004, **1**:CD004249.

19. Gross AR, Hoving JL, Haines TA, Goldsmith CH, Kay T, Aker P, Bronfort G: **A Cochrane review of manipulation and mobilization for mechanical neck disorders.** *Spine* 2004, **29**:1541–1548.

20. Vernon HT, Humphreys BK, Hagino CA: **A systematic review of conservative treatments for acute neck pain not due to whiplash.** *J Manipulative Physiol Ther* 2005, **28**:443–448.

21. Vernon H, Humphreys BK: **Manual therapy for neck pain: an overview of randomized clinical trials and systematic reviews.** *Eura Medicophys* 2007, **43**:91–118.

22. Bronfort G, Haas M, Evans RL, Bouter LM: **Efficacy of spinal manipulation and mobilization for low back pain and neck pain: a systematic review and best evidence synthesis.** *Spine J* 2004, **4**:335–356.

23. Kroeling P, Gross A, Goldsmith CH, Burnie SJ, Haines T, Graham N, Brant A: **Electrotherapy for neck pain.** *Cochrane Database Syst Rev* 2009, **4**:CD004251.

24. Graham N, Gross A, Goldsmith CH, Klaber Moffett J, Haines T, Burnie SJ, Peloso PM: **Mechanical traction for neck pain with or without radiculopathy.** *Cochrane Database Syst Rev* 2008, **3**:CD006408.

25. Gross AR, Haines T, Goldsmith CH, Santaguida L, McLaughlin LM, Peloso P, Burnie S, Hoving J, Cervical Overview G: **Knowledge to action: a challenge for neck pain treatment.** *J Orthop Sports Phys Ther* 2009, **39**:351–363.

26. Gross AR, Kaplan F, Huang S, Khan M, Santaguida PL, Carlesso LC, Macdermid JC, Walton DM, Kenardy J, Soderlund A, Verhagen A, Hartvigsen J: **Psychological care, patient education, orthotics, ergonomics and prevention strategies for neck pain: an systematic overview update as part of the ICON project.** *Open Orthop J* 2013, **7**:530–561.

27. Graham N, Gross AR, Carlesso LC, Santaguida PL, Macdermid JC, Walton D, Ho E: **An ICON overview on physical modalities for neck pain and associated disorders.** *Open Orthop J* 2013, **7**:440–460.

28. Charles C, Gafni A, Whelan T: **Shared decision-making in the medical encounter: what does it mean? (or it takes at least two to tango).** *Soc Sci Med* 1997, **44**:681–692.

29. May SJ: **Patient satisfaction with management of back pain. Part 2 an explorative, qualitative study into patients' satisfaction with physiotherapy.** *Physiotherapy* 2001, **87**:10–20.

30. Oostendorp RA, Rutten GM, Dommerholt J, der Sanden MW N-v, Harting J: **Guideline-based development and practice test of quality indicators for physiotherapy care in patients with neck pain.** *J Eval Clin Pract* 2013, **19**(6):1044–1053.

31. Streiner DL, Norman GR: *Health measurement scales: a practical guide to their development and use.* 4th edition. New York: Oxford University Press; 2008.

32. CCA membership demographics survey. In http://www.chiropracticcanada.ca/en-us/members/practice-building/survey-highlights/demographics.aspx.

33. Canadian Physiotherapy Association: *Member Services.* 2013.

34. The MacKenzie Institute International: *The MacKenzie Method.* http://www.mckenziemdt.org/approach.cfm?section=int.

35. Kay TM, Gross A, Goldsmith CH, Rutherford S, Voth S, Hoving JL, Bronfort G, Santaguida PL: **Exercises for mechanical neck disorders.** *Cochrane Database Syst Rev* 2012, **8**, CD004250.

36. Gross A, Miller J, D'Sylva J, Burnie SJ, Goldsmith CH, Graham N, Haines T, Bronfort G, Hoving JL, COG: **Manipulation or mobilisation for neck pain: a cochrane review.** *Man Ther* 2010, **15**:315–333.

37. D'Sylva J, Miller J, Gross A, Burnie SJ, Goldsmith CH, Graham N, Haines T, Bronfort G, Hoving JL, for the Cervical Overview G: **Manual therapy with or without physical medicine modalities for neck pain: a systematic review.** *Man Ther* 2010, **15**:415–433.

38. Furlan AD, Yazdi F, Tsertsvadze A, Gross A, Van Tulder M, Santaguida L, Gagnier J, Ammendolia C, Dryden T, Doucette S, Skidmore B, Daniel R, Ostermann T, Tsouros S: **A systematic review and meta-analysis of efficacy, cost-effectiveness, and safety of selected complementary and alternative medicine for neck and low-back pain.** *Evid Based Complement Alternat Med* 2012, **2012**:953139.

39. Driessen MT, Proper KI, van Tulder MW, Anema JR, Bongers PM, van der Beek AJ: **The effectiveness of physical and organisational ergonomic interventions on low back pain and neck pain: a systematic review.** *Occup Environ Med* 2010, **67**:277–285.

40. Verhagen AP, Karels C, Bierma-Zeinstra SM, Feleus A, Dahaghin S, Burdorf A, De Vet HC, Koes BW: **Ergonomic and physiotherapeutic interventions for treating work-related complaints of the arm, neck or shoulder in adults. A Cochrane systematic review.** *Eura Medicophys* 2007, **43**:391–405.

41. Brosseau L, Wells GA, Tugwell P, Casimiro L, Novikov M, Loew L, Sredic D, Clement S, Gravelle A, Hua K, Kresic D, Lakic A, Menard G, Cote P, Leblanc G, Sonier M, Cloutier A, McEwan J, Poitras S, Furlan A, Gross A, Dryden T, Muckenheim R, Cote R, Pare V, Rouhani A, Leonard G, Finestone HM, Laferriere L, Dagenais S, *et al*: **Ottawa Panel evidence-based clinical practice guidelines on therapeutic massage for neck pain.** *J Bodyw Mov Ther* 2012, **16**:300–325.

42. Patel KC, Gross A, Graham N, Goldsmith CH, Ezzo J, Morien A, Peloso PM: **Massage for mechanical neck disorders.** *Cochrane Database Syst Rev* 2012, **9**, CD004871.

43. Bronfort G, Haas M, Evans R, Leininger B, Triano J: **Effectiveness of manual therapies: the UK evidence report.** *Chiropr Osteopathy* 2010, **18**:3.

44. Wolsko PM, Eisenberg DM, Davis RB, Kessler R, Phillips RS: **Patterns and perceptions of care for treatment of back and neck pain: results of a national survey.** *Spine (Phila Pa 1976)* 2003, **28**:292–297. discussion 298.

45. Sherman KJ, Cherkin DC, Connelly MT, Erro J, Savetsky JB, Davis RB, Eisenberg DM: **Complementary and alternative medical therapies for chronic low back pain: what treatments are patients willing to try?** *BMC Complement Altern Med* 2004, **4**:9.

46. Cote P, van der Velde G, Cassidy JD, Carroll LJ, Hogg-Johnson S, Holm LW, Carragee EJ, Haldeman S, Nordin M, Hurwitz EL, Guzman J, Peloso PM, Bone, Joint Decade -2010 Task Force on Neck P, Its Associated D: **The burden and determinants of neck pain in workers: results of the bone and joint decade 2000-2010 task force on neck pain and its associated disorders.** *Spine (Phila Pa 1976)* 2008, **33**:S60–S74.

47. Hoe VC, Urquhart DM, Kelsall HL, Sim MR: **Ergonomic design and training for preventing work-related musculoskeletal disorders of the upper limb and neck in adults.** *Cochrane Database Syst Rev* 2012, **8**, CD008570.

48. Walton DM, Macdermid JC, Giorgianni AA, Mascarenhas JC, West SC, Zammit CA: **Risk factors for persistent problems following acute whiplash injury: update of a systematic review and meta-analysis.** *J Orthop Sports Phys Ther* 2013, **43**:31–43.

49. Sterling M, Pedler A: **A neuropathic pain component is common in acute whiplash and associated with a more complex clinical presentation.** *Man Ther* 2009, **14:**173–179.

50. Graham N, Gross AR, Goldsmith C, Cervical Overview G: **Mechanical traction for mechanical neck disorders: a systematic review.** *J Rehabil Med* 2006, **38:**145–152.

51. Hurwitz EL, Carragee EJ, van der Velde G, Carroll LJ, Nordin M, Guzman J, Peloso PM, Holm LW, Cote P, Hogg-Johnson S, Cassidy JD, Haldeman S, Bone, Joint Decade - Task Force on Neck P, Its Associated D: **Treatment of neck pain: noninvasive interventions: results of the bone and joint decade 2000-2010 task force on neck pain and its associated disorders.** *Spine (Phila Pa 1976)* 2008, **33:**S123–S152.

52. Shields N, Capper J, Polak T, Taylor N: **Are cervical pillows effective in reducing neck pain?** *N Z J Physiother* 2006, **34:**3–9.

53. Teasell RW, McClure JA, Walton D, Pretty J, Salter K, Meyer M, Sequeira K, Death B: **A research synthesis of therapeutic interventions for whiplash-associated disorder (WAD): part 2 - interventions for acute WAD.** *Pain Res Manag* 2010, **15:**295–304.

54. Gross AR, Dziengo S, Boers O, Goldsmith CH, Graham N, Lilge L, Burnie S, White R: **Low Level Laser Therapy (LLLT) for Neck Pain: a systematic review and meta-regression.** *Open Orthop J* 2013, **7:**396–419.

55. Goode AP, Freburger J, Carey T: **Prevalence, practice patterns, and evidence for chronic neck pain.** *Arthritis Care Res (Hoboken)* 2010, **62:**1594–1601.

56. Mootz RD, Cherkin DC, Odegard CE, Eisenberg DM, Barassi JP, Deyo RA: **Characteristics of chiropractic practitioners, patients, and encounters in Massachusetts and Arizona.** *J Manipulative Physiol Ther* 2005, **28:**645–653.

57. Elliott JM, Noteboom JT, Flynn TW, Sterling M: **Characterization of acute and chronic whiplash-associated disorders.** *J Orthop Sports Phys Ther* 2009, **39:**312–323.

58. Boyles R, Toy P, Mellon J Jr, Hayes M, Hammer B: **Effectiveness of manual physical therapy in the treatment of cervical radiculopathy: a systematic review.** *J Manipulative Physiol Ther* 2011, **19:**135–142.

59. Falla D, Jull G, Russell T, Vicenzino B, Hodges P: **Effect of neck exercise on sitting posture in patients with chronic neck pain.** *Phys Ther* 2007, **87:**408–417.

60. Jull G, Falla D, Treleaven J, Hodges P, Vicenzino B: **Retraining cervical joint position sense: the effect of two exercise regimes.** *J Orthop Res* 2007, **25:**404–412.

61. Jull GA, Falla D, Vicenzino B, Hodges PW: **The effect of therapeutic exercise on activation of the deep cervical flexor muscles in people with chronic neck pain.** *Man Ther* 2009, **14:**696–701.

62. Louw A, Diener I, Butler DS, Puentedura EJ: **The effect of neuroscience education on pain, disability, anxiety, and stress in chronic musculoskeletal pain.** *Arch Phys Med Rehabil* 2011, **92:**2041–2056.

63. Moseley GL: **Widespread brain activity during an abdominal task markedly reduced after pain physiology education: fMRI evaluation of a single patient with chronic low back pain.** *Aust J Physiother* 2005, **51:**49–52.

64. Carlesso L, Bartlett D, Padfield B, Chesworth B: **Cervical manipulation and informed consent: Canadian manipulative physiotherapists opinions on communicating risk.** *Physiother Can* 2007, **59:**86–96.

65. Carlesso L, Rivett D: **Manipulative practice in the cervical spine: a survey of IFOMPT member countries.** *J Manipulative Physiol Ther* 2011, **19:**66–70.

66. Adams G, Sim J: **A survey of UK manual therapists' practice of and attitudes towards manipulation and its complications.** *Physiother Res Int* 1998, **3:**206–227.

67. Sweeney A, Doody C: **Manual therapy for the cervical spine and reported adverse effects: a survey of Irish manipulative physiotherapists.** *Man Ther* 2010, **15:**32–36.

68. Jull G: **Use of high and low velocity cervical manipulative therapy procedures by Australian manipulative physiotherapists.** *Aust J Physiother* 2002, **48:**189–193.

69. Gleberzon B, Stuber K: **Frequency of use of diagnostic and manual therapeutic procedures of the spine taught at the Canadian Memorial Chiropractic College: a preliminary survey of Ontario chiropractors. Part 1 - practice characteristics and demographic profiles.** *J Can Chiropr Assoc* 2013, **57:**32–41.

70. Rupert RL: **A survey of practice patterns and the health promotion and prevention attitudes of US chiropractors. Maintenance care: part I.** *J Manipulative Physiol Ther* 2000, **23:**1–9.

71. Cherkin DC, Deyo RA, Sherman KJ, Hart LG, Street JH, Hrbek A, Davis RB, Cramer E, Milliman B, Booker J, Mootz R, Barassi J, Kahn JR, Kaptchuk TJ, Eisenberg DM: **Characteristics of visits to licensed acupuncturists, chiropractors, massage therapists, and naturopathic physicians.** *J Am Board Fam Pract* 2002, **15:**463–472.

7

The effect of spinal manipulation on deep experimental muscle pain in healthy volunteers

Søren O'Neill[2,1]*, Øystein Ødegaard-Olsen[1] and Beate Søvde[3]

Abstract

Background: High-velocity low-amplitude (HVLA) spinal manipulation is commonly used in the treatment of spinal pain syndromes. The mechanisms by which HVLA-manipulation might reduce spinal pain are not well understood, but often assumed to relate to the reduction of biomechanical dysfunction. It is also possible however, that HVLA-manipulation involves a segmental or generalized inhibitory effect on nociception, irrespective of biomechanical function. In the current study it was investigated whether a local analgesic effect of HVLA-manipulation on deep muscle pain could be detected, in healthy individuals.

Methods and materials: Local, para-spinal muscle pain was induced by injection of 0.5 ml sterile, hyper-tonic saline on two separate occasions 1 week apart. Immediately following the injection, treatment was administered as either a) HVLA-manipulation or b) placebo treatment, in a randomized cross-over design. Both interventions were conducted by an experienced chiropractor with minimum 6 years of clinical experience. Participants and the researcher collecting data were blinded to the treatment allocation. Pain scores following saline injection were measured by computerized visual analogue pain scale (VAS) (0-100 VAS, 1 Hz) and summarized as a) Pain duration, b) Maximum VAS, c) Time to maximum VAS and d) Summarized VAS (area under the curve). Data analysis was performed as two-way analysis of variance with treatment allocation and session number as explanatory variables.

Results: Twenty-nine healthy adults (mean age 24.5 years) participated, 13 women and 16 men. Complete data was available for 28 participants. Analysis of variance revealed no statistically significant difference between active and placebo manipulation on any of the four pain measures.

Conclusion: The current findings do not support the theory that HVLA-manipulation has a non-specific, reflex-mediated local or generalized analgesic effect on experimentally induced deep muscle pain. This in turn suggests, that any clinical analgesic effect of HVLA-manipulation is likely related to the amelioration of a pre-existing painful problem, such as reduction of biomechanical dysfunction.

Background

Spinal manipulation is commonly used in an effort to alleviate musculoskeletal pain, but the exact mechanisms by which such treatments can reduce pain are not well understood. It is commonly assumed however, that when pain arises from biomechanical dysfunction, spinal manipulation may affect pain relief through the reduction of such dysfunction. Pain relief following spinal manipulation is thus assumed to indicate curative treatment of painful biomechanical dysfunction.

A number of clinical studies now indicate, that spinal manipulation may be a prudent choice for patients with musculoskeletal pain, not least spinal pain syndromes [1]. It is difficult however, to reliably identify those patients who are most likely to benefit from spinal manipulation and it is also a challenge to demonstrate the presence of biomechanical dysfunction in a valid and reliable manner [2, 3].

*Correspondence: soren@oneill.dk
[2] Institute of Regional Health Research, University of Southern Denmark, Campusvej 55, 5230 Odense, DK, Denmark
[1] Spine Centre of Southern Denmark, Lillebælt Hospital, Østre Hougvej 55, 5500 Middelfart, DK, Denmark
Full list of author information is available at the end of the article

A pragmatic solution which has been suggested, is a trial of a few treatments to assess the potential benefit of further spinal manipulation for a given patient [4, 5]. This is perfectly sensible, assuming that pain relief with 2–4 such treatments indicates reduction of some underlying painful mechanical lesion or dysfunction. However, if spinal manipulation has non-specific, reflex-mediated pain-inhibitory effects irrespective of the underlying cause of nociception, such pain relief may in fact simply mask the symptoms of other painful disorders, which are not appropriately treated with *high-velocity, low-amplitude* (HVLA) manipulation. In other words: If spinal manipulation has substantial local or regional, non-specific analgesic effects irrespective of the cause of pain, such treatment could potentially obfuscate serious pathology.

Any such non-specific, reflex-mediated pain-inhibitory effect is likely to be neurophysiological in nature and neural mechanisms have played a central role in many of the theoretical models of spinal manipulation. By the same token, the first detailed theoretical model of a central reflex-mediated nociceptive modulatory mechanism focused specifically on the impact of mechano-sensory input on nociceptive processing (the pain-gate theory proposed by Melzack and Wall [6]). In more recent years several studies have demonstrated that mechanical stimulation such as joint manipulation/mobilization can inhibit pain: In laboratory animal models of inflammatory joint pain Sluka and Wright [7] and Skyba et al. [8] demonstrated a hypoalgesic effect with joint mobilization, and showed that this effect is mediated by serotonin and noradrenaline sensitive pathways. Extra-cellular thalamic recordings of nociceptive specific and wide-dynamic-range neurons (which are known to be involved in pain processing in states of central pain hypersensitivity) in rats has demonstrated that HVLA manipulation raises the mechanical response threshold, and furthermore that variations in the manipulation amplitude, but not duration affects the resulting hypoalgesia [9, 10]. Song et al. [11] demonstrated an effect of daily manipulations over a week (by Activator*) on pain from nerve-root inflammation, assessed by both behavioral pain measures and intracellular recordings in rats. These findings and other like them provide objective evidence of a central nociceptive inhibitory effect of mechanical stimuli in laboratory animals, which appear to be reliant on serotonin and noradrenaline sensitive pathways, thus hinting at a descending pain control mechanism from the periaquaductal gray matter and rostro-ventral medial medulla of the brain stem (see Lewis et al. [12] for a recent review of conditioned pain modulation in chronic pain).

Obviously, the translational value of animal models in pain research can be questioned [13, 14] but human research supports the presence of hypoalgesic effects of manipulation which are not mediated by (segmental) opioid sensitive pathways [15] and the findings of hypoalgesia, sympathetic facilitation and changes in motor-control by Vicenzino et al. [16, 17] and Sterling et al. [18] support a mechanism of descending inhibitory control from the brain stem. The later study by Bishop et al. [19] which demonstrated changes in thermal summation pain both segmentally and caudal to the manipulation also support descending inhibition as a likely mechanism of HVLA induced hypoalgesia.

It seems plausible then, that HVLA manipulation could exert a diffuse hypoalgesic effect on the basis of descending inhibitory control from the brain stem. A number of factors may have influenced previous findings, including (but not limited to) the study population, the time scale within which the effect of HVLA-manipulation is sought and the method with which pain sensitivity has been examined.

Whereas the specific cause and nature of pain in clinical spinal pain states is often undetermined, experimental pain can be induced in a manner which is controlled and well understood – researchers inducing experimental pain know the precise nature and tissue site of the pain they have induced and research indicates that spinal manipulation has a significant analgesic effect on such experimental pain whether induced by pressure, mechanical stretching, capsaicin or electrical stimulation [20, 21]. Most studies however, have examined and demonstrated that the effect is evident at the same spinal level or in the neighboring region of the experimental pain stimulus and HVLA manipulation.

The literature summarized by the reviews by Millan et al. [20] and Coronado et al. [21] examines the effects of spinal manipulation on *experimental* pain. Some of the reviewed literature is on healthy volunteers [19, 22–29], but most [16–18, 30–44] of the studies actually examine populations of patients with *clinical* pain conditions ranging from mechanical neck pain and low back pain to tender-points and latent trigger points. It is therefor possible, that any observed local hypoalgesic effect of spinal manipulation in those studies, is due to an effect on the underlying painful clinical condition itself or changes in central pain modulation specifically related to those clinical conditions.

In order to gain a better understanding of the mechanisms by which spinal manipulation may afford such hypoalgesic effects, it is necessary to distinguish between effects inherent to the manipulation itself, and effects mediated by the potential influence on an underlying clinical pain condition – is any observed difference in pain sensitivity caused by a diffuse anti-nociceptive effect of manipulation, or by reduction of some underlying (mechanical) painful condition, such as latent trigger points?

Furthermore, the manner in which experimental pain sensitivity is tested may prove important. Research suggests that different aspects of the pain experience are not simple correlates [45–50]; deep and superficial pain sensitivity may vary, as may sensitivity to different pain modalities (thermal, chemical, mechanical, etc) and the choice of pain indicators (thresholds, distribution, duration, modulation, quality, etc) may also be important.

The purpose of this study was examine the immediate, local, deep-tissue hypoalgesic effect of spinal manipulation in healthy volunteers with no assumption of underlying painful clinical or sub-clinical conditions.

Method and materials
Design
A randomized, controlled, crossover study.

Recruitment
Participants were recruited from the student population of the chiropractic degree program at the University of Southern Denmark. Only healthy volunteers without known contraindications to spinal manipulation were invited to participate.

As part of the university degree program, all chiropractic students are evaluated by a certified chiropractor during their 3rd semester, in order to detect possible contradictions for HVLA manipulations. Four study participants were recruited from the 2nd semester and prior to study participation these were interviewed and examined for contraindications for HVLA manipulation by a senior chiropractor at The Spinecentre of Southern Denmark, Lillebaelt Hospital, Denmark.

Participants with chronic pain, previous back surgery, current back problems, somatic or psychological conditions were excluded.

Study participants were recruited through verbal information in the classroom and written information was sent electronically to those who expressed an interest in participating.

The Regional Scientific Ethical Committee for Southern Denmark approved the study (S-0080137) and written consent was obtained from all participants.

Experimental procedure
The experiment was carried out at the Spinecentre of Southern Denmark, Lillebaelt Hospital. Two assistants (graduate students) and two senior chiropractors from the department conducted the study.

Participants were informed that they would receive two effective, but different treatments and that the aim of the study was to compare any difference in effectiveness between them. All participants were treated on two separate occasions at least 1 week apart and treatment sessions were identical apart from the actual manual treatment performed: a) active HVLA-manipulation treatment, and b) placebo treatment with an Activator instrument. Participants were not informed that one of the treatments was a placebo.

Treatments at both the first and second session were directed at the 6th thoracic level. Allocation of treatment was done randomly according to a pre-hoc computer generated list in which treatment and session was randomized, but balanced.

On each occasion, in preparation of the test procedure, assistant 1 (BS) identified the spinous process of the 6th thoracic segment through palpation (counting down from the bony landmark of the C7 spinous process). The T6 segment was marked with a pen and anesthetic cream (EMLA cream, Astra Zeneca – an eutectic mixture of the local anesthetics Lidocain and Prilocain) was applied para-spinally on the right side of the T6 spinous process and covered by a patch with self-adhesive borders (Tegaderm, 5×7 cm) to keep the cream in place. The anesthetic cream was applied to ensure that experimental pain was induced primarily from deep tissues and not from needle-puncture of superficial structures.

After 20 min, assistant 2 (ØØO) removed the patch, wiped off the anesthetic cream and instructed the participant in the use of the computerized visual analogue pain scale, before asking the participant to lie prone on a chiropractic treatment table.

The injection point was the same for all participants; para-spinally at T6 (center of the anesthetized area) which was wiped down twice with alcohol swaps, as per standard aseptic injection technique. Assistant 2 proceeded to aspirate and gradually (over approx 2 s) inject 0.5 ml sterile hyper-tonic saline solution (Sodium SAD 1 mmol/ml) at room temperature, into the right T6 paraspinal musculature at approximately 2 cm depth. Immediately thereafter, assistant 2 left the room and one of the two senior chiropractors delivered the allocated treatment.

Placebo treatment was performed immediately next to the injection site. The chiropractor stabilized the chosen segment with the left hand, while holding the activator in the right hand, placing it on the anesthetized skin on the right side of the transverse process. The participant was asked to take a deep breath. Upon exhalation the Activator was pressed twice, releasing two 'click' sounds, while giving no mechanical impulse (amplitude $= 0$ mm).

HVLA-manipulation was performed with bilateral thenar contact (Carver bridge) on both transverse processes on the T6 segment. The participant was asked to take a deep breath and upon exhalation the HVLA manipulation was administered over the segment resulting in a mechanical impulse, in most instances with an accompanying articular cavitation.

Immediately after administering the treatment, the chiropractor left the room and (the blinded) assistant 2 returned. Assistant 2 ensured, that the participant indicated the intensity of pain from the saline injection as it developed over time (computerized VAS). The computerized VAS consisted of a scale marked 'No pain' at one end and 'Worst possible pain' at the other, corresponding to a value between 0 and 100 respectively. The VAS was sampled with a frequency of 1 Hz and data was stored electronically, allowing for a time-series of VAS measurements (see Fig. 1 for an illustration). During the recording, there was complete silence and no activity in the treatment room.

Data recording was considered complete when the patient indicated that the pain declined to near 0 – typically within 3–5 min.

The participants were all chiropractic students with personal knowledge of spinal manipulative procedures, which challenges the validity of the chosen placebo treatment. For that reason, upon completion of the experimental part of the study, 14 participants were randomly selected for a phone interview and questioned if they had, at any point been aware that one of the treatments was a placebo treatment.

Data

The VAS data was summarized as four outcome variables: a) duration of pain, b) max VAS value, c) time from pain onset to max VAS value and d) accumulated area under the curve (VAS over time). See Fig. 1 for an illustration.

Statistical analysis

Data are presented as median values with minimum, maximum and 1st and 3rd quartiles. The results are analyzed with two-way Anova with treatment allocation and session number as explanatory variables. Homogeneity of variance was analyzed with Fligner-Killeen test. An alpha level of 5 % was considered statistically significant. Analysis was performed using R version 3.0.2 (2013-09-25) for Linux [51].

Results

A total of 29 participants took part in the study; 13 women and 16 men (mean age 24.5 years).

No complications or side effects were reported by any of the participants and there were no dropouts. Due to technical computer problems however, raw data for 1 participant (male) was lost, leaving complete data for both sessions for 28 subjects.

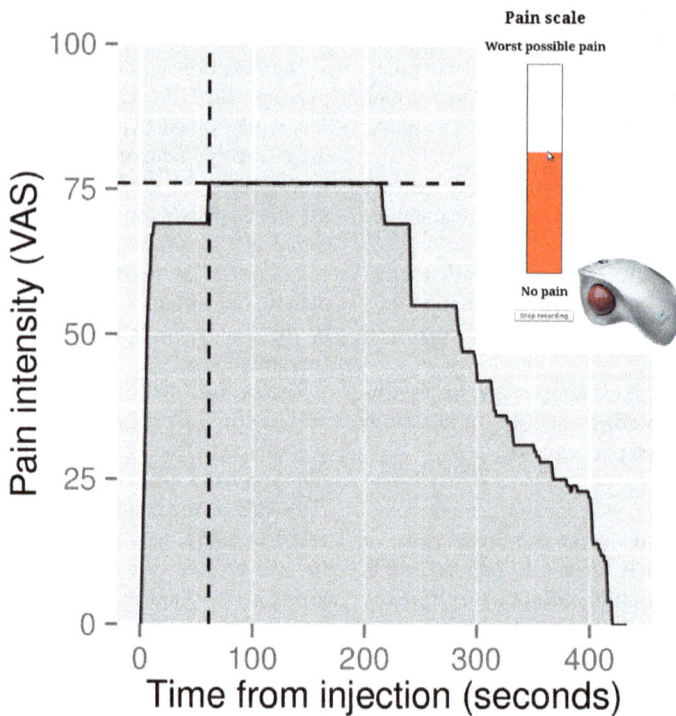

Fig. 1 Illustration of computerized VAS data. Pain intensity was measured using an on-screen visual analogue pain scale (insert in figure) controlled by the participant with a common computer trackball. The pain intensity was sampled with a frequency of 1 Hz and the resulting time-series data is illustred in the graph

Fourteen (14) participants received the active treatment on the first session (and placebo on the second), and vice versa.

The median duration of saline induced pain was 219 s (min = 101, 1. quartile = 178, 3. quartile = 274, max = 433), the median maximum VAS was 48 VAS (min = 7, 1.quartile = 35, 3.quartile = 66, max = 98), the median time from pain onset to max VAS was 44.5 s (min = 1, 1.quartile = 27, 3.quartile = 90.25, max = 143) and the median area-under-the-curve was 6117 VAS×seconds (min = 1019, 1.quartile = 3572, 3.quartile = 9182, max = 25010).

Fligner-Killeen test of homogeneity of variance for each of the four outcome variables, by each of the two explanatory variables yielded P values between 0.26 and 0.92, i.e. no heteroscedasticity of variance was observed.

Two-way analysis of variance revealed no significant differences in the 4 outcome variables by either explanatory variable, with one exception: A significant effect (p = 0.005) of session number on duration of pain was found, with longer duration of pain on the first session (mean = 256 s, 95 % QI [227;285]) compared to the second session (mean = 202 s, 95 % QI [178;226]).

A post-hoc power-calculation (based on paired t-test) revealed, that with n = 28, alpha = 0.05 and beta = 0.8, a moderate effect size (0.55) would have been detected if present.

None of the 14 randomly selected participants interviewed following the experiment indicated that they had any suspicion that the Activator treatment had been a placebo treatment.

Discussion

If the effects of HVLA-manipulation was due primarily to an immediate, non-specific and reflex-mediated inhibition of nociception, we would have expected to observe a difference in saline induced pain in the current study between active and placebo treatment, but no such difference was observed.

Current findings in relation to previous publications

At first, the present findings appear to be in contrast to most of the published literature on HVLA-manipulation and experimentally induced pain, as summarized in the two recent reviews by Millan et al. and Coronado et al. [20, 21]. The authors reported significant pain inhibitory effects of HVLA-manipulation on experimentally induced pain.

However, the published literature was mostly based on populations with clinical or sub-clinical conditions [16–18, 30–44], i.e. patients with clinical pain states such as neck and low back pain, or non-clinical populations in which HVLA-manipulation was directed at tissues identified as pain hypersensitive (tender-points,

trigger points). In those instances, it is unclear whether any effect of HVLA-manipulation should be ascribed to a non-specific reflex-mediated pain-inhibitory effect of the manual procedure itself, or a specific effect on the (sub-)clinical condition. In the present study, manipulation was not directed at any such clinical or sub-clinical condition and all participants were tested (arbitrarily) at the T6 segment. Any effect of HVLA-manipulation, had it been observed in the present study could thus have been ascribed to such non-specific, reflex-mediated pain inhibition.

Of the previous studies investigating healthy, pain free participants [19, 22–29] reviewed by Millan et al. and Coronado et al., the majority relied on pressure-pain thresholds and reported contradictory findings: Fernández-de-las-Peñas et al. [22, 23] used placebo-controlled designs and demonstrated an increase in pressure pain thresholds following cervical manipulation. This is in contrast to the controlled studies by Hamilton [25] and Soon [27], who reported no effect of manipulation on pressure pain thresholds. The study by Bishop et al. [19] which also involved a control group found a difference in thermal sensory summation between groups, but no difference in pressure pain or thermal pain thresholds.

The studies by Krouwel et al. [26] and Willet et al. [29] are harder to interpret as they did not involve clear-cut control groups: There is a tendency for experimental pain sensitivity to be higher on the first test, compared to subsequent tests which was also the finding in several of the papers discussed here – this underlines the importance of a control group in paired *before/after* pain sensitivity studies. In any case, the studies by Krouwel et al. [26] and Willet et al. [29] are similar in several respects, and while they both include a treatment group receiving simple sustained (*quasi-static*) pressure which could be interpreted as a minimalist intervention control group, this is not clearly stated. In any case, no group differences in pain thresholds are reported in either study.

Finally, the studies by George et al. [24] and Terrett and Vernon [28] both employed superficial pain stimuli (thermal and electrical, respectively). Whereas Terrett and Vernon reported a 140 % increase in superficial pain tolerance thresholds following manipulation, George et al. reported only few differences between those receiving manipulation, performing extension exercises or simply riding a stationary bicycle. Clearly, the literature on manipulation induced hypoalgesia in *healthy, pain-free subjects* is not concordant.

Care should be exercised when comparing animal and human pain research, but as described in the *Background* section, animal research indicates the presence of a non-specific anti-nociceptive effect of manipulation, possibly based on descending inhibitory control. The current findings did not demonstrate such an effect.

Differences between the present methodology and previous publications

The present study differs from the previously published literature on HVLA manipulation in the choice of pain stimulus: intra-muscular injection of hyper-tonic saline. Most of the previously published studies have used either pressure pain thresholds or superficial (skin) stimuli [20, 21]. Injection of hyper-tonic saline is a common experimental model of muscle pain [52], albeit less common than the ubiquitous pressure algometer. Slater et al. [53] also induced experimental pain by injection of hyper-tonic saline, albeit in adjunct to *delayed onset muscle soreness (DOMS)* of the extensor carpi radialis muscle and reported no difference in saline pain intensity, nor in pressure pain sensitivity following *mobilization-with-movement* manual therapy compared to placebo. In this respect, the present study is in alignment with the methodology and findings of Slater et al.

Although the specific seat and nature of most clinical spinal pain states for which spinal manipulation is used is unknown, it is rarely thought to originate in superficial structures, such as skin, subcutaneous connective tissues, etc. Furthermore, spinal manipulation is typically administered in an attempt to affect deep tissues such as facet joints, intervertebral disks and segmental musculature, but obviously also affects superficial tissues. The use of intra-muscular injection of hyper-tonic saline and a superficial anesthetic cream in the present study was chosen to ensure that the pain stimulus was indeed primarily delivered to deep spinal tissues.

The anesthetic cream was applied to reduced the superficial pain of the needle puncture and thus ensure that the induced experimental pain stemmed primarily from the deep intra-muscular saline. Whereas the cream will not have affected the deep experimental pain to any appreciable degree, it could arguably have affected the *profile* of sensory input in relation to the manipulation. The current study was not designed to cast light on any (potential) effect of superficial sensation or anesthesia on the effects of spinal manipulation, but this might be worth investigating in future research.

Conversely, the clinical pain for which HVLA spinal manual therapy is delivered, is of longer duration than the experimental pain induced in the current study – typically 2–4 min. This is a potential limitation of the current design and if, as some animal research indicates HVLA manipulation exerts anti-nociceptive effects through descending inhibitory control, a much longer time-frame is likely necessary to demonstrate such effects.

As there is no consensus on which experimental pain stimulus best simulate clinical pain or which tests most reliably reveals changes in pain sensitivity, a selection of diverse pain stimuli and measures are often recommended. In the present study only a single pain stimuli was used, however it could be argued that deep muscle pain more closely resembles clinical back pain than mechanical pressure or superficial thermal or electrical stimuli. The outcome measures used in the present study were related to several aspects of the pain experience: pain onset, intensity and duration. Other aspects such as pain detection- and tolerance threshold, spatial distribution, qualitative pain description, conditioned pain modulation and others could equally have been relevant, but as always a balance had to be struck between feasibility and methodological rigor.

Several studies in the pain literature conclude that pain sensitivity is complex and multi-modal, and that adequate assessment requires a battery of different quantitative sensory tests of pain sensitivity [45–50, 54]. The only study published on the *generalizability* of quantitative sensory testing of experimental pain [54], suggests that composite pain scores, such as those affected by e.g. both pain intensity and duration, offer greater generalizability than single scores such as e.g. pain threshold. We can not exclude however, that group differences could have been revealed by other quantitative sensory pain tests.

As an incidental finding, significantly longer pain duration on the first session, compared to the second session, was observed. This is not unusual in experimental pain research and is likely due to a degree of anxiety and unfamiliarity with the pain stimulus in the first session. For this reason some researchers employ an 'introductory'-session to familiarize study participants with the stimulus, some time well in advance of the actual study. This was not the case in the present study; instead the effect was countered by random allocation of treatments to session 1 and 2.

Study population

A potential limitation of the current study was the study population: students recruited from the chiropractic program at the University of Southern Denmark. This represents a potential bias, as the study population has prior knowledge of manipulative techniques and therefor might be in a position to recognize the placebo treatment as such. The study population was chosen for practicality, availability and economy, despite the potential sources of bias. According to Vernon et al. [55] it is difficult, but possible to construct a valid placebo treatment for manual procedures if it meets the following criteria; 1) the intervention should have no significant treatment effect and 2) the subject should be unable to determine whether they have received a sham treatment. All participants in the current study were unaware of the order of treatment and the existence of a placebo intervention, and none of the 14 participants, randomly chosen for interview after the study were aware of the use of a placebo treatment. We would thus argue that the inactivated Activator treatment represents a true placebo treatment in the current study.

Interpretation of findings

The current findings should not be over-interpreted. They indicate however, that HVLA-manipulation does not affect an immediate non-specific, reflex-mediated inhibition of deep-tissue segmental pain. Indirectly the findings thus lend support to the assumption that pain relief from HVLA-manipulation is likely to represent reduction of pain from some underlying painful condition, e.g. biomechanical dysfunction. This, in turn, suggests that the approach recommended by Leboeuf-Yde et al. and Axén et al. [4, 5], with a trial of 2–4 treatments to assess the effect of HVLA-manipulation is indeed a pragmatic and safe one. As stated above however, necessary choices regarding pain stimulus, pain measures, time frame etc should temper the conclusions based on a single study.

Future studies should take into consideration both the study population, the test- and treatment-sites and the chosen outcome measures. When quantifying experimentally induced pain in participants with painful clinical conditions, it becomes difficult to separate the intrinsic effects of HVLA manipulation from those of a clinical effect on the underlying cause of pain. Furthermore, if the intent is to disentangle the underlying neurological mechanisms of HVLA-manipulation induced hypoalgesia, test sites should be chosen which are appropriate for the hypothesis; local, segmental or generalized effects. And finally, the choice of pain measures is important and a battery of tests covering both different pain modalities and response domains is to be preferred.

Conclusion

The current study indicates, that HVLA-manipulation does not have an immediate non-specific, reflex-mediated local hypoalgesic effect on experimentally induced deep para-spinal muscle pain in healthy volunteers after skin anesthesia.

Competing interests
The authors declare that they have no competing interests.

Author's contributions
All authors contributed to the study design. ØØO and BS contributed to data collection and analysis. ØØO and SON contributed to manuscript preparation. All authors read and approved the final manuscript.

Author details
[1]Spine Centre of Southern Denmark, Lillebælt Hospital, Østre Hougvej 55, 5500 Middelfart, DK, Denmark. [2]Institute of Regional Health Research, University of Southern Denmark, Campusvej 55, 5230 Odense, DK, Denmark. [3]Stathelle Healthcentre, Brugata 10, 3960 Stathelle, Norway.

References
1. Clar C, Tsertsvadze A, Court R, Hundt GL, Clarke A, Sutcliffe P. Clinical effectiveness of manual therapy for the management of musculoskeletal and non-musculoskeletal conditions: systematic review and update of UK evidence report. Chiropr man ther. 2014;22(1):12. Accessed 2014-10-09.
2. Hestœk L, Leboeuf-Yde C. Are chiropractic tests for the lumbo-pelvic spine reliable and valid? a systematic critical literature review. J Manipulative Physiol Ther. 2000;23(4):258–75. Accessed 2014-10-17.
3. Huijbregts PA. Spinal motion palpation: A review of reliability studies. J Man Manip Ther. 2002;10(1):24–39. Accessed 2014-10-17.
4. Leboeuf-Yde C, Grønstvedt A, Borge JA, Lothe J, Magnesen E, Nilsson Ø, et al. The nordic back pain subpopulation program: demographic and clinical predictors for outcome in patients receiving chiropractic treatment for persistent low back pain. J Manipulative Physiol Ther. 2004;27(8):493–502.
5. Axén I, Jones JJ, Rosenbaum A, Lövgren PW, Halasz L, Larsen K, et al. The nordic back pain subpopulation program: validation and improvement of a predictive model for treatment outcome in patients with low back pain receiving chiropractic treatment. J Manipulative Physiol Ther. 2005;28(6):381–5.
6. Melzack R, Wall PD. Pain mechanisms: a new theory. Science (New York, N Y). 1965;150(3699):971–9.
7. Sluka KA, Wright A. Knee joint mobilization reduces secondary mechanical hyperalgesia induced by capsaicin injection into the ankle joint. Eur J Pain. 2001;5(1):81–7. doi:10.1053/eujp.2000.0223. Accessed 2015-05-19.
8. Skyba DA, Radhakrishnan R, Rohlwing JJ, Wright A, Sluka KA. Joint manipulation reduces hyperalgesia by activation of monoamine receptors but not opioid or GABA receptors in the spinal cord. Pain. 2003;106(1–2):159–68.
9. Reed WR, Pickar JG, Sozio RS, Long CR. Effect of spinal manipulation thrust magnitude on trunk mechanical activation thresholds of lateral thalamic neurons. J Manip Physiol Ther. 2014;37(5):277–86. doi:10.1016/j.jmpt.2014.04.001.
10. Reed WR, Sozio R, Pickar JG, Onifer SM. Effect of spinal manipulation thrust duration on trunk mechanical activation thresholds of nociceptive-specific lateral thalamic neurons. J Manipulative Physiol Ther. 2014;37(8):552–60. doi:10.1016/j.jmpt.2014.08.006.
11. Song XJ, Gan Q, Cao JL, Wang ZB, Rupert RL. Spinal manipulation reduces pain and hyperalgesia after lumbar intervertebral foramen inflammation in the rat. J Manip Physiol Ther. 2006;29(1):5–13. doi:10.1016/j.jmpt.2005.10.001.
12. Lewis GN, Rice DA, McNair PJ. Conditioned pain modulation in populations with chronic pain: a systematic review and meta-analysis. J Pain. 2012;13(10):936–44.
13. Mogil JS. Animal models of pain: progress and challenges. Nat Rev Neurosci. 2009;10(4):283–94. doi:10.1038/nrn2606. Accessed 2015-05-26.
14. Olesen AE, Andresen T, Staahl C, Drewes AM. Human experimental pain models for assessing the therapeutic efficacy of analgesic drugs. Pharmacol Rev. 2012;64(3):722–79. doi:10.1124/pr.111.005447. Accessed 2015-05-26.
15. Paungmali A, O'Leary S, Souvlis T, Vicenzino B. Naloxone fails to antagonize initial hypoalgesic effect of a manual therapy treatment for lateral epicondylalgia. J Manip Physiol Ther. 2004;27(3):180–5. doi:10.1016/j.jmpt.2003.12.022.
16. Vicenzino B, Collins D, Wright A. The initial effects of a cervical spine manipulative physiotherapy treatment on the pain and dysfunction of lateral epicondylalgia. Pain. 1996;68(1):69–74.
17. Vicenzino B, Collins D, Benson H, Wright A. An investigation of the interrelationship between manipulative therapy-induced hypoalgesia and sympathoexcitation. J Manipulative Physiol Ther. 1998;21(7):448–53.
18. Sterling M, Jull G, Wright A. Cervical mobilisation: concurrent effects on pain, sympathetic nervous system activity and motor activity. Man Ther. 2001;6(2). doi:10.1054/math.2000.0378.
19. Bishop MD, Beneciuk JM, George SZ. Immediate reduction in temporal sensory summation after thoracic spinal manipulation. Spine J. 2011;11(5):440–6. doi:10.1016/j.spinee.2011.03.001.

20. Millan M, Leboeuf-Yde C, Budgell B, Amorim M-A. The effect of spinal manipulative therapy on experimentally induced pain: a systematic literature review. Chiropr Man Therap. 2012;20(1):26.

21. Coronado RA, Gay CW, Bialosky JE, Carnaby GD, Bishop MD, George SZ. Changes in pain sensitivity following spinal manipulation: A systematic review and meta-analysis. J Electromyogr Kinesiol. 2012;22(5):752–67. Accessed 2014-10-09.

22. Fernandez-de-Las-Penas C, Alonso-Blanco C, Cleland JA, Rodriguez-Blanco C, Alburquerque-Sendin F. Changes in pressure pain thresholds over C5-C6 zygapophyseal joint after a cervicothoracic junction manipulation in healthy subjects. J Manipulative Physiol Ther. 2008;31(5):332–7. doi:10.1016/j.jmpt.2008.04.006.

23. Fernandez-de-las-Penas C, Perez-de-Heredia M, Brea-Rivero M, Miangolarra-Page JC. Immediate effects on pressure pain threshold following a single cervical spine manipulation in healthy subjects. J Orthop Sports Phys Ther. 2007;37(6):325–9. doi:10.2519/jospt.2007.2542.

24. George SZ, Bishop MD, Bialosky JE, Zeppieri GJ, Robinson ME. Immediate effects of spinal manipulation on thermal pain sensitivity: an experimental study. BMC Musculoskelet Disord. 2006;7:68. doi:10.1186/1471-2474-7-68.

25. Hamilton L, Boswell C, Fryer G. The effects of high-velocity, low-amplitude manipulation and muscle energy technique on suboccipital tenderness. Int J Osteopathic Med. 2007;10(2–3):42–9. doi:10.1016/j.ijosm.2007.08.002. Accessed 2015-04-29.

26. Krouwel O, Hebron C, Willett E. An investigation into the potential hypoalgesic effects of different amplitudes of PA mobilisations on the lumbar spine as measured by pressure pain thresholds (PPT). Man Ther. 2010;15(1):7–12. doi:10.1016/j.math.2009.05.013.

27. Soon BTC, Schmid AB, Fridriksson EJ, Gresslos E, Cheong P, Wright A. A crossover study on the effect of cervical mobilization on motor function and pressure pain threshold in pain-free individuals. J Manipulative Physiol Ther. 2010;33(9):652–8. doi:10.1016/j.jmpt.2010.08.014.

28. Terrett AC, Vernon H. Manipulation and pain tolerance. A controlled study of the effect of spinal manipulation on paraspinal cutaneous pain tolerance levels. Am J Phys Med. 1984;63(5):217–25.

29. Willett E, Hebron C, Krouwel O. The initial effects of different rates of lumbar mobilisations on pressure pain thresholds in asymptomatic subjects. Man Ther. 2010;15(2):173–8. doi:10.1016/j.math.2009.10.005.

30. Bialosky JE, Bishop MD, Robinson ME, Zeppieri GJ, George SZ. Spinal manipulative therapy has an immediate effect on thermal pain sensitivity in people with low back pain: a randomized controlled trial. Phys Ther. 2009;89(12):1292–1303. doi:10.2522/ptj.20090058.

31. Côté P, Mior SA, Vernon H. The short-term effect of a spinal manipulation on pain/pressure threshold in patients with chronic mechanical low back pain. J Manipulative Physiol Ther. 1994;17(6):364–8.

32. de Camargo VM, Alburquerque-Sendin F, Berzin F, Stefanelli VC, de Souza DPR, Fernandez-de-las-Penas C. Immediate effects on electromyographic activity and pressure pain thresholds after a cervical manipulation in mechanical neck pain: a randomized controlled trial. J Manipulative Physiol Ther. 2011;34(4):211–20. doi:10.1016/j.jmpt.2011.02.002.

33. Fernandez-Carnero J, Cleland JA, Arbizu RLT. Examination of motor and hypoalgesic effects of cervical vs thoracic spine manipulation in patients with lateral epicondylalgia: a clinical trial. J Manipulative Physiol Ther. 2011;34(7):432–40. doi:10.1016/j.jmpt.2011.05.019.

34. Fernandez-Carnero J, Fernandez-de-las-Penas C, Cleland JA. Immediate hypoalgesic and motor effects after a single cervical spine manipulation in subjects with lateral epicondylalgia. J Manipulative Physiol Ther. 2008;31(9):675–81. doi:10.1016/j.jmpt.2008.10.005.

35. Fryer G, Carub J, McIver S. The effect of manipulation and mobilisation on pressure pain thresholds in the thoracic spine. J Osteopathic Med. 2004;7(1):8–14. doi:10.1016/S1443-8461(04)80003-0.

36. Mansilla-Ferragut P, Fernandez-de-Las Penas C, Alburquerque-Sendin F, Cleland JA, Bosca-Gandia JJ. Immediate effects of atlanto-occipital joint manipulation on active mouth opening and pressure pain sensitivity in women with mechanical neck pain. J Manipulative Physiol Ther. 2009;32(2):101–6. doi:10.1016/j.jmpt.2008.12.003.

37. Mohammadian P, Gonsalves A, Tsai C, Hummel T, Carpenter T. Areas of capsaicin-induced secondary hyperalgesia and allodynia are reduced by a single chiropractic adjustment: a preliminary study. J Manipulative Physiol Ther. 2004;27(6):381–7. doi:10.1016/j.jmpt.2004.05.002.

38. Oliveira-Campelo NM, Rubens-Rebelatto J, Marti N-Vallejo FJ, Alburquerque-Sendi N F, Fernandez-de-Las-Penas C. The immediate effects of atlanto-occipital joint manipulation and suboccipital muscle inhibition technique on active mouth opening and pressure pain sensitivity over latent myofascial trigger points in the masticatory muscles. J Orthop Sports Phys Ther. 2010;40(5):310–7. doi:10.2519/jospt.2010.3257.

39. Parkin-Smith GF, Penter CS. A clinical trial investigating the effect of two manipulative approaches in the treatment of mechanical neck pain: a pilot study. J Neuromusculoskeletal Syst. 1998;1998(6):6–16.

40. Ruiz-Saez M, Fernandez-de-las-Penas C, Blanco CR, Martinez-Segura R, Garcia-Leon R. Changes in pressure pain sensitivity in latent myofascial trigger points in the upper trapezius muscle after a cervical spine manipulation in pain-free subjects. J Manipulative Physiol Ther. 2007;30(8):578–83. doi:10.1016/j.jmpt.2007.07.014.

41. Shearar KA, Colloca CJ, White HL. A randomized clinical trial of manual versus mechanical force manipulation in the treatment of sacroiliac joint syndrome. J Manipulative Physiol Ther. 2005;28(7):493–501. doi:10.1016/j.jmpt.2005.07.006.

42. Thomson O, Haig L, Mansfield H. The effects of high-velocity low-amplitude thrust manipulation and mobilisation techniques on pressure pain threshold in the lumbar spine. Int J of Osteopath Med. 2009;12(2):56–62. doi:10.1016/j.ijosm.2008.07.003. Accessed 2015-04-29.

43. van Schalkwyk R, Parkin-Smith GF. A clinical trial investigating the possible effect of the supine cervical rotatory manipulation and the supine lateral break manipulation in the treatment of mechanical neck pain: a pilot study. J Manipulative Physiol Ther. 2000;23(5):324–31.

44. Vernon HT, Aker P, Burns S, Viljakaanen S, Short L. Pressure pain threshold evaluation of the effect of spinal manipulation in the treatment of chronic neck pain: a pilot study. J Manipulative Physiol Ther. 1990;13(1):13–16.

45. Janal MN, Glusman M, Kuhl JP, Clark WC. On the absence of correlation between responses to noxious heat, cold, electrical and ischemic stimulation. Pain. 1994;58(3):403–11.

46. Lautenbacher S, Rollman GB, McCain GA. Multi-method assessment of experimental and clinical pain in patients with fibromyalgia. Pain. 1994;59(1):45–53.

47. Hastie BA, Riley JL, Robinson ME, Glover T, Campbell CM, Staud R, et al. Cluster analysis of multiple experimental pain modalities. Pain. 2005;116(3):227–37.

48. Greenspan JD, Slade GD, Bair E, Dubner R, Fillingim RB, Ohrbach R, et al. Pain sensitivity risk factors for chronic TMD: Descriptive data and empirically identified domains from the OPPERA case control study. J Pain. 2011;12(11):61–74.

49. Neziri AY, Curatolo M, Nääjesch E, Scaramozzino P, Andersen OK, Arendt-Nielsen L, et al. Factor analysis of responses to thermal, electrical, and mechanical painful stimuli supports the importance of multi-modal pain assessment. Pain. 2011;152(5):1146–55.

50. O'Neill S, Manniche C, Graven-Nielsen T, Arendt-Nielsen L. Association between a composite score of pain sensitivity and clinical parameters in low-back pain. Clin J Pain. 2014;30(10):831–8.

51. R Core Team. R: a language and environment for statistical computing. Vienna, Austria: R Foundation for Statistical Computing; 2013. http://www.R-project.org/.

52. Graven-Nielsen T, Arendt-Nielsen L. Assessment of mechanisms in localized and widespread musculoskeletal pain. Nat Rev Rheumatol. 2010;6(10):599–606. doi:10.1038/nrrheum.2010.107. Accessed 2015-05-16.

53. Slater H, Arendt-Nielsen L, Wright A, Graven-Nielsen T. Effects of a manual therapy technique in experimental lateral epicondylalgia. Man Ther. 2006;11(2):107–17. doi:10.1016/j.math.2005.04.005. Accessed 2015-07-09.

54. O'Neill S, O'Neill L. Improving QST reliability – more raters, tests, or occasions? a multivariate generalizability study. J Pain. 2015;16(5):454–62. doi:10.1016/j.jpain.2015.01.476.

55. Vernon H, MacAdam K, Marshall V, Pion M, Sadowska M. Validation of a sham manipulative procedure for the cervical spine for use in clinical trials. J Manipulative Physiol Ther. 2005;28(9):662–6.

8

Foam pads properties and their effects on posturography in participants of different weight

Guy Gosselin[*] and Michael Fagan

Abstract

Background: Foam pads are increasingly used on force platforms during balance assessments in order to produce increased instability thereby permitting the measurement of enhanced posturographic parameters. A variety of foam pads providing different material properties have thus been used, although it is still unclear which characteristics produce the most effective and reliable tests. Furthermore, the effects of participant bodyweight on the performance of the foam pads and outcome of the test are unknown. This project investigated how different foam samples affected postural sway velocity in participants of different weights.

Method: Four foam types were tested according to a modified American Society for Testing and Materials standard method for testing flexible cellular materials. Thirty-six healthy male factory workers divided into three groups according to body mass were tested three times for each of the 13 randomly-selected experimental situations for changes in postural sway velocity in this cross-over study. Descriptive and inferential statistics were used to compare the results and evaluate the difference in sway velocity between mass groups.

Results: For the materials considered here, the modulus of elasticity of the foam pads when compressed by 25% of their original heights was inversely proportional to their density. The largest changes in postural sway velocity were measured when the pads of highest stiffness were used, with memory foam pads being the least likely to produce significant changes.

Conclusions: The type of foam pads used in posturography is indeed important. Our study shows that the samples with a higher modulus of elasticity produced the largest change in postural sway velocity during quiet stance. The results suggest that foam pads used for static computerised posturography should 1) possess a higher modulus of elasticity and 2) show linear deformation properties matched to the participants' weight.

Keywords: Balance, Foam pads, Posturography, Modulus of elasticity, Biomechanics

Background

Posturography has been shown to be useful in the workplace, for example to assess different-aged workers in physically demanding jobs [1], determine the effects of obesity on balance [2], to measure sleepiness and fatigue [3], and even to observe the effects of neurotoxicity due to workers exposure to organic solvent mixtures [4]. Furthermore, there is now a trend in western countries to increase the age of retirement [5]. This aging workforce may in some instances be placed at risk should their functional capacities such as balance become altered. Approximately one person in three over

the age of 65 has at least one fall a year and one person in five who falls after the age of 65 for reasons connected with balance dies in the year following the fall [6]. In addition obese adults fall nearly twice as often as their non-obese counterparts [7]. All this motivates researchers and clinicians to develop new ways to understand and quantify postural stability.

Postural stability is often assessed by measuring the centre of pressure (COP) which is a point where the vertical reaction forces of the ground act. It represents the weighted average of all pressures over the body in contact with the ground. As such, there are numerous COP measures such as average velocity of COP, COP excursion, average radial displacement of the COP, to name a few; however until recently it was not evident which measure

* Correspondence: g.gosselin@2010.hull.ac.uk
School of Engineering, University of Hull, Cottingham Road,
Kingston-upon-Hull HU6 7RX, UK

is optimal [8]. Mahdavi-Amiri et al. have shown that during static posturography the average velocity for a given stability condition, is more repeatable (less variable) between trials from a data collection session, and more discernible between the different stability conditions [9].

Many of the modern assessments systems use dynamic posturographic devices, which are sophisticated apparatus that introduce instability along with altered visual cues [10]. Unfortunately the high costs of such systems together with their large size prevent their general use in industry. Static computerised posturography represents a low-cost alternative, although the current high variability of results limits the accuracy of the conclusions that can be drawn from such assessments [11].

Recently, foam pads have been used on force platforms in order to induce increased instability thereby decreasing the coefficient of variation (CV) to a more acceptable level [12]. The use of foam pads in posturography is thought to exaggerate balance deficits by altering the reliability of somatosensory input from cutaneous mechanoreceptors on the plantar soles. Previous research looking at the effect of the surface on which posturography is performed has shown that the type of foam has different effects on balance [11,13]. Although it is still unclear which characteristics produce the optimal performance, De Berardino and colleagues suggested that using foam pads of higher stiffness was best for clinical use [11]. More specific information is therefore essential before a standardised protocol can be proposed. Foam pads used in posturography will behave as any other material when placed under load, i.e. the deflection will be proportional to both the force, by a property known as the stiffness of the structure, and proportional to the property of the material itself called the modulus of elasticity [14].

Few papers have reported the material characteristics of foam pads used in posturography. Blackburn (2003) [15] investigated the kinematic analysis of the hip and trunk during bilateral stance on firm foam and multiaxial support surfaces. In this instance the height of the foam blocks was not mentioned but the density was reported as 54.53 kg/m^3 [15]. Another study that looked into trunk sway measurements during stance and gait tasks in Parkinson's disease [16], used foam pads with a height of 10 cm and a density of 25 kg/m^3. Finally, Di Bernardino et al. [11] evaluated the postural effects of standing on two different types of rubber foam pads: a "monolayer" with a thickness of 10 cm and a density of 25 kg/m^3, and a "bilayer" pad with a thickness of 8 cm and a density of 100 kg/m^3. Their results show that the variability of static posturography parameters was significantly reduced by the use of both foam pads. However, the comparison of the two types was also statistically significant, with the bilayer type presenting the lowest CV in the results of 10%, compared with 14.4% for the monolayer.

Unfortunately, the bi-layer foam pad described by Di Berardino is a specialist product that it is not readily available outside of Italy.

To the best of our knowledge no one has investigated the postural effects of participants of different mass and the effects of plantar surface area on different types of foam. One would assume that the postural effects of standing on a specific foam pad sample would be different for lighter and heavier participants. Thus, this study's main purpose was to determine how a range of foam pads (including bi-layer foam pad combinations) influenced postural sway velocity during quiet stance for subjects of different body mass. The null hypothesis tested was: there is no difference in sway velocity when any of the foam pads are used.

Method

Foam pads material properties

The properties of the pads were measured using three tests based on ASTM test D-3574-11 [17]. Uniaxial compression was achieved using a screw driven test machine (LR 100 K, Lloyds Instrument, Bognor Regis, UK) with a 100 kN load cell (Figure 1). The press was remotely controlled via a desktop computer running Nexygen software (Lloyds Instrument, Bognor Regis, UK). Four foam pads were obtained from three sources: 1) rehabilitation material supplier, 2) online foam shop and 3) upholstery high street shop (Table 1). The pads had a size of 480 × 480 mm, with the exception of the rehabilitation balance pad which had a smaller size of 440 × 400 mm. The atmospheric pressure in the laboratory was 1015 hPa and the temperature was 22°C.

Test A: density test

The density of the uncored foam was calculated from the mass and volume of each specimen. The pad's dimensions

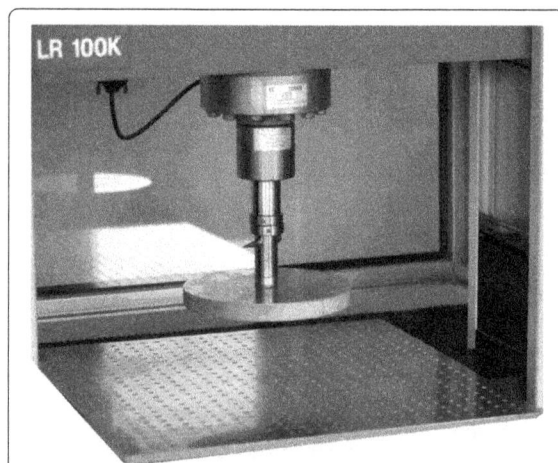

Figure 1 Screw driven test machine (LR 100 K, Lloyds Instrument, Bognor Regis, UK) with a 100 kN load cell showing the 203 mm indenter foot above the perforated horizontal support plate.

Table 1 Foam sample specification

Manufacturer	Model	Type	Size (mm)	Volume (m³)	Mass (kg)	Density kg/m³	E kPa
Vitafoam Ltd UK	Memory Foam Vasco 40 MF-75 mm	Urethane Open-Cell	480 x 480 x 75	0.01728	1.07	63.5	16.1
Vitafoam Ltd UK	Memory Foam Vasco 40 MF-100 mm	Urethane Open-Cell	480 x 480 x 100	0.02304	1.46	63.5	16.1
Vitafoam Ltd UK	Reflex 35 M Ups-100 mm	Urethane Open-Cell	480 x 480 x 100	0.02304	0.86	37.3	44.9
Airex AG Speciality Foams Industrie, Switzerland	Balance Pads BP-50 mm	Polyurethane Closed-cell	440 x 400 x 50	0.0088	0.34	38.6	217.9

The density was calculated by dividing the mass by the volume. E was measured using the data provided by the indentation force deflection test when the specimen was compressed by 25% of its original height.

(m³) were measured with the use of a millimetric measuring tape. The mean mass (kg) was recorded as the average of five measurements with an electronic scale (± 1 g) (Model 1089 BKWHDR, Salter, Hamburg). The density was calculated by the formula:

$$\text{Density} = \text{M/V}$$

where: M = mass of specimen, kg, and V = volume of specimen, m³.

Test B: indentation force deflection test (IFD)

Based on ASTM standard D-3574-11, this test consisted of measuring the force necessary to produce a predefined indentation in the foam. A flat circular indenter with a 203 mm diameter foot was used to apply a load on the specimen which was supported on a level horizontal plate that was perforated with approximately 6.5 mm holes on approximately 20 mm centres to allow for rapid escape of air during the tests. From the data obtained, the modulus of elasticity was calculated for each specimen with the following formula:

$$E = \frac{\sigma}{\varepsilon} = \frac{\frac{F}{A_0}}{\frac{\Delta L}{L_0}} \cdots \text{N/m}^2$$

where:

E is the Young's modulus (modulus of elasticity);
σ is the stress applied on the pad;
ε is the strain measured from the application of σ;
F is the force exerted on the foam pad
A_0 is the original cross-sectional area of the indenter through which the force is applied;
ΔL is the amount by which the height of the pad changes;
L_0 is the original height of the pad.

Procedure

The specimen was placed such that the indenter was in the centre of the apparatus' supporting plate. The area to be tested was preflexed twice by lowering the indenter's foot to a total deflection of 75% of the full part thickness at a rate of 250 ± 25 mm/min. The specimen was allowed to rest 6 ± 1 min after the preflex. The indenter was then brought into contact with the specimen by applying a 4.5 N load to the indenter's foot. The specimen was further indented at a rate of 50 ± 5 mm/min to a displacement equal to 25% of the original thickness. The force was then adjusted to retain this displacement for 60 ± 3 s at which point the force measurement was taken. Without unloading the specimen, the deflection was increased to 65% deflection and once more the force was adjusted to retain this displacement for 60 ± 3 s when the force was recorded.

Test C: modified indentation residual gage length test – specified force (MIRGL)

The traditional "indentation residual gage length" test force (IRGL) used to measure the thickness of the pad under a fixed force of 110 N and 220 N on a 203 mm diameter circular indenter foot [17]. However, these loads were not sufficient to represent the force of an adult standing on the foam pads. For this reason, the ASTM method was modified to use fixed loads of 110 N, 220 N 330 N, 440 N, 550 N, 660 N, 770 N, 880 N, 990 N, 1100 N, 1210 N and 1320 N. Furthermore, we tested the materials with two indenter sizes: 203 mm diameter and 406 mm diameter.

Procedure

The specimen was preflexed twice with a 330 N force applied at 200 ± 20 mm/min and then allowed to rest after load removal 180 ± 5 sec. Foam pads were tested either as single layer pads (MF: memory foam; Uph: upholstery foam; BP: balance pad) or a combination of two different size bi-layer pads. The first one being a large bi-layer of 0.25 m² surface board (MFL: Memory foam large; UphL: Upholstery foam large; BPL: balance pad large) or with a small bi-layer of 0.09 m² surface board (MFS: Memory foam small; UphS: Upholstery foam small; BPS: balance pad small). The deflection was then recorded after the application of 110 N applied for 60 ± 3 sec. The load was then increased up to 1320 N in steps of 110 N, again holding for 60 ± 3 sec at each load increment. The procedures were repeated a second time with a 406 cm diameter indenter.

Posturography

Thirty-six healthy male factory workers (mean age = 39.7 years ± 9.3; mass = 88.4 kg ± 14.1; height = 1.78 m ± .034; BMI = 28 ± 3.1) volunteered to participate in this cross-over study. All participants were physically active and none had neurological, vestibular, visual or musculoskeletal complaints at the time of the experimentation. The participants were divided into three groups according to mass (Group 1: less than 60 kg, n = 5; Group 2: 60.1 kg to 89.9 kg, n = 23; Group 3: greater than 90 kg, n = 8). Ethical approval was obtained for the posturography assessment from the University's Ethics committee and the procedures followed were in accordance with the ethical standards of the Helsinki Declaration of 1975, as revised in 2013 [18]. All participants read the information sheet and signed the consent form.

Postural sway velocity was recorded with the use of a force platform (QPS-200, Midot Medical Technology) linked via a USB connector to a laptop computer and the signal processed with Posture Analyser software (Midot Medical Technology). Postural sway velocities provided by the Posture Analyser software were saved in separate files on a computer.

Procedure

Posturography was measured three times for each of the 13 randomly-selected experimental situations (no foam, four samples of mono-layered foam, and eight samples of bi-layered foam). The order of each test was determined by a random sequence generator (http://www.random.org/sequences/). The bi-layered form consisted of the foam pad covered by either a square 0.25 m² or 0.09 m² wooden 2 cm thick board. The values of the three posturographic records were averaged and used for analysis.

Participants were instructed to stand on the force platform with their feet together and eyes closed. Recording was started after 30 seconds of quiet stance. After recording was completed, participants were allowed to step off the platform and relax for one minute before the procedure

was repeated two additional times. Once the three posturographic recordings were completed, the participants were asked to stand off the force platform and the experimenter changed the foam sample according to the pre-determined sequence. Posturography was again recorded. Sampling was recorded for 30 seconds [19] at 30 Hz per channel.

Analysis

The overall posturographic data and the participants' posturographic data grouped by mass were both tested for normality using the Shapiro-Wilk test. Descriptive statistics presented the mean sway velocity ($\bar{x}$), Interquartile range, 95% Confidence Interval for $\bar{x}$ and sway velocity per mass category. Statistical tests were used to determine change in postural sway velocity. One-way repeated measures analyses of variance (ANOVA) with Greenhouse-Geisser corrections were used to compare postural sway velocity in the 13 experimental situations between 1) balance without foam surfaces and 2) with 12 other foam combinations. Wilcoxon-signed rank tests were used to evaluate the difference in sway velocity between mass groups. Levels of significance were set at 0.05 and the Bonferroni post-hoc test was used in the ANOVA and Wilcoxon-signed rank tests. Statistical analyses were performed using SPSS 17.0.

Results

The density of the tested samples varied from 63.5 kg/m³ for the Vitafoam memory foam down to 38.6 kg/m³ for the Airex balance pad. Conversely, the memory pads had a value of E of 16.1 kPa whilst the balance pad's E was 217.9 kPa (Table 1) when compressed by 25% of their original height.

The indentation force deflection test showed that memory foam pads necessitated much lower loads in order to produce a deflection of 25 and 65% of their original height. Conversely, pads with a larger E required a larger force in order to achieve the same deflection as seen in Table 2.

The deformations of the foam pads during the MIRGL test using the 203 mm indenter were non-linear with the exception of the balance pad which showed linearity

Table 2 Indentation force deflection test (IFD)

| | 203 mm diameter indenter | |
	Load (N) at 25% thickness reduction	Load (N) at 65% thickness reduction
MF-75 mm	65.2	169.5
MF-100 mm	74.7	200.6
Uph-100 mm	181.3	550.7
BP-50 mm	880.9	4861.2

Force necessary to produce 25% and 65% indentation on four different foam samples. MF-75 mm: memory foam 75 mm thickness; MF-100 mm: memory foam 100 mm; Uph: upholstery foam 100 mm thickness; BP: balance pad 50 mm thickness.

throughout the range of loads applied (Figure 2). Furthermore, both memory foam and upholstery pads were compressed to more than 75% of their original length when a load corresponding to an average male's weight of 770 N was used (Figure 2). The 406 cm indenter did not alter the memory foam's linearity during the MIRGL test, in contrast to the upholstery pad which showed a linear deformation from 660 N compression onwards with this larger indenter (Figure 3).

Posturography

The Shapiro-Wilk normality tests for changes in postural sway velocity in all participants suggested that normality was a reasonable assumption ($p > 0.05$). On the other hand, when participants' results were stratified by body mass, the velocity data was not normally distributed ($p < 0.05$). The average velocity, coefficient of variation, Interquartile range and average sway velocity according to body mass results according to each foam sample and indenter size are presented in Table 3.

A repeated measures ANOVA with a Greenhouse-Geisser correction determined that postural sway velocity differed significantly between surfaces measured ($F(1.984, 22.257) = 21926.764$, $P < 0.0001$). Post hoc tests using the Bonferroni correction revealed that postural sway velocity was significantly increased especially when standing on a monolayer upholstery foam and on a monolayer balance pad ($75.6 \pm .18.7$ mm/s and 78.7 ± 13.5 mm/s respectively) (Table 4).

Wilcoxon signed-rank tests with Bonferroni corrections showed that in three experimental situations, the postural sway velocities were significantly different in participants of different masses (<60 kg vs 60-89 kg, upholstery foam, $Z = -6.156$, $p = .009$; 60 kg vs >90 kg, upholstery foam,

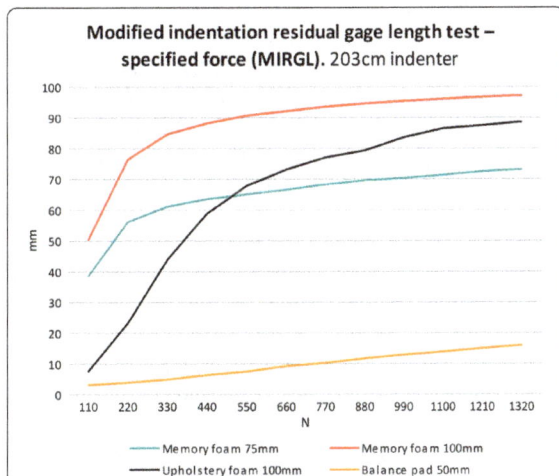

Figure 2 Results from the modified indentation residual length test using the 203 mm indenter foot.

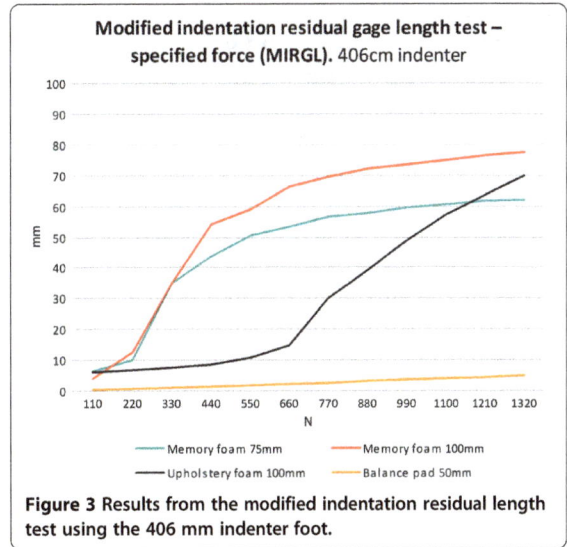

Figure 3 Results from the modified indentation residual length test using the 406 mm indenter foot.

$Z = -1.950$, $p = .012$; <60 kg vs 60-89 kg, upholstery foam and large board, $Z = -2.646$, $p = .010$; 60-89 kg vs >90 kg, upholstery foam and large board, $Z = -2.521$, $p = .012$).

Discussion

The objective of this project was to determine which type of foam pads were the most effective to enhance postural disturbances according to participant's weight.

Foam pads

Balance during quiet stance has been shown to be a good representation of overall system health, but not a good measure of underlying pathophysiology due to numerous contributing factors potentially affecting balance. Static posturography can be altered in different ways in order to challenge the participants to maintain a stable posture for example, narrowing the base of support by having the feet close to each other, decreasing visual feedback (closing eyes), altering the standing surface to decrease proprioceptive feedback, or introducing an accessory task or action during balance recording [20]. An increased average centre of pressure change has been associated with aging, obesity, neuropathy, Parkinson's disease, vestibular loss, stroke etc. [7,21-23]. The usefulness in using foam pads to decrease cutaneous plantar proprioception during posturographic measurement is fairly well established [11,24-26]. However, the types of foam pads used in previous experimentation has differed and it is difficult to compare results between studies. Through compression testing of different types of open cell foams using ASTM standard D-3574-95, our study has shown that stiffness varies as the material specimen cross-section changes in size relative to the indenter. We have demonstrated that foams pads, with the exception of the balance pad and the

Table 3 Mean, coefficient of variation, interquartile range and confidence intervals for overall posturographic results and participants' results stratified by body mass

	x̄ (SD) mm/s	CV	IQR	95% CI for x̄		<60 kg		60-89 kg		>90 kg	
						x̄	Mdn	x̄	Mdn	x̄	Mdn
No foam	25.1 (5.2)	0.21	18.7	21.1	27.7	29.1	21	24.0	28.5	24	28.5
MF-75 mm	23.4 (6.1)	0.26	15.5	19.7	22.6	27.1	18	22.3	27.1	21	25.5
MF-100 mm	22.3 (4.9)	0.22	14.7	18.4	21.4	26.1	17	21.2	25.8	20	24.5
Uph-100 mm	75.6 (7.4)	0.10	23.2	69.2	85.7	81.9	82	82.1	49.5	45	49.5
BP-50 mm	78.7 (7.1)	0.09	23.7	74.1	82.7	83.2	79	82.0	66.5	62	66.5
MFL-75 mm	27.0 (4.6)	0.17	18.3	23.1	27.7	30.9	24	26.1	28.8	24.3	28.8
MFL-100 mm	32.8 (6.9)	0.21	18.7	28.8	29.7	36.8	36	31.4	30.5	26	30.5
UphL-100 mm	64.5 (6.3)	0.10	24.5	59.3	67.7	69.7	64	57.0	81.4	76	81.4
BPL-50 mm	33.0 (2.5)	0.08	19.75	29.2	33.7	36.9	30	33.0	32.5	28	32.5
MFS-75 mm	25.5 (6.6)	0,25	19.1	21.4	26.8	29.6	21.4	24.4	28.7	24.1	28.6
MFS-100 mm	29.0 (5.3)	0.18	18.5	24.5	42.7	33.4	39	24.6	28.6	23.5	28.0
UphS-100 mm	48.4 (3.7)	0.07	20.5	43.6	44.7	53.3	41	44.0	63.5	59	63.5
BPS-50 mm	34.0 (3.1)	0.09	19.8	30.0	34.7	38.1	31	34.0	33.5	29	33.5

x̄ (SD) = average velocity and its standard deviation. IQR = Interquartile range. CI – 95% confidence interval for the average velocity of sway.
MF: memory foam; Uph: upholstery foam; BP: balance pad; Large bi-layer with a surface of 0. 25 m² board: MFL: Memory foam large; UphL: Upholstery foam large; BPL: balance pad large; Small bi-layer with a surface of 0.09 m²: MFS: Memory foam small; UphS: Upholstery foam small; BPS: balance pad small.

upholstery foam with the 406 mm indenter, did not show linear deformation throughout the range of loads used in the MIRGL with both the 203 mm and 406 mm indenters. Both memory foam pads failed to resist the compression at relatively low loads which suggested they would not provide sufficient resistance to compression during posturography for healthy adult participants. Their compression slopes during the MIRGL clearly show a trend towards asymptotic displacement beyond 220 N for the memory foam and beyond 660 N compression for the mono-layer upholstery foam. Non-linear stress–strain relationships were observed

Table 4 ANOVA Pairwise comparison between velocity of sway without foam and with different foam surfaces

		p	95% CI for difference with no foam	
Mono-layer	MF-75 mm	ns	−0.3	3.7
	MF-100 mm	.002	0.6	5.0
	Uph-100 mm	.000	−61.0	−39.9
	BP-50 mm	.000	−58.8	−48.2
Bi-layer 0.09 m²	MFL-75 mm	.030	−3.6	−0.08
	MFL-100 mm	ns	−15.1	−0.2
	UphL-100 mm	.000	−44.5	−34.1
	BPL-50Lmm	.000	−9.2	−6.5
Bi-layer 0.25 m²	MFS-75 mm	ns	−2.2	0.8
	MFS-100 mm	ns	−8.4	0.6
	UphS-100 mm	.000	−27.2	−19.3
	BPS-50 mm	.000	−10.2	−7.5

ns = not significant.

due to the changes in the foam geometry at high strains. When the foam is highly compressed the foam volume tends to zero and the stiffness tends to infinity. Patel suggested that such large compression (as observed with the memory foam here) would result in the participants coming in to close contract with the rigid surface beneath the foam [13]. The balance pad showed a largely linear response throughout the loads applied during the MIRGL test. Conversely, the upholstery foam exhibited a bi-linear type of behaviour when compressed with the 406 mm diameter indenter. It supported the load with minimum deformation up to 660 N, at which point it gave way and deformed with a lower stiffness up to the maximum load.

Our results show that foam pads can indeed increase the postural sway velocity of healthy participants, in some cases significantly. Participants standing on foam pads did elevate their centre of mass by nearly 50 mm corresponding to less than 3% of the participants' average height. The force platform used in this project consisted of 4 weighing plates, and the CoP is calculated from the resultant force, with the velocity calculated by the change in the CoP position. It is therefore unlikely that elevating the centre of mass would have affected appreciably the postural sway velocity results. When participant data were stratified according to mass, results showed that the balance pad did still produce the largest increase in sway velocity in Groups 1 and 2, in the heavier Group 3 (mass > 90 kg), the large bi-layer upholstery foam pad had the largest effect. The pairwise comparison between sway velocities without foam and with foam surfaces showed a large confidence interval, which can be attributed to the separation of participants into smaller groups according to mass. The null hypothesis stating "there is no difference in sway velocity when any of the foam pads are used" can thus be rejected. Furthermore, our participants were male factory workers with a mean BMI of 28 which is slightly higher than the UK male average [27]. Athletes presenting the same mass but with a more mesomorphic body type might have provided different results.

It is interesting to note that not only was there no significant difference between posturographic results between "no foam" and samples of 75 mm and 100 mm thick memory foam samples, but the sway velocity was somewhat improved when memory foam pad were used. A learning effect explanation can be excluded in view of the random order of the test conducted. We concluded that because the participants' feet had a smaller cross-sectional area than the pads onto which they were standing on and the fact that our participants nearly flattened the pads meant a shear force was created between the material and the sides of the feet as the specimen deformed. This would have increased the surface area of contact between the foam pads and the side of the feet which in turn would most likely have increased proprioception thereby providing additional cues and improving balance. With participants of larger mass, as the deflection increased, the memory foam could actually have provided an advantage in the posturographic task. Thus, when selecting a type of foam pad to be used in posturography, it is recommended that investigators select samples appropriate to their participants' weight. For instance, in the selection of foam pads for individuals weighting more than 900 N, a bi-layer upholstery foam pad of around 37.3 kPa and 44.9 kPa such as used in our experiment would be the appropriate choice. Additionally, it may be of importance to select a foam pad presenting limited deflection under loading in order to avoid contact of the feet with the sides of the material.

Conclusion

The Balance pad produced the largest postural sway velocity in participants with less than 90 kg mass whilst the bi-layer upholstery sample (406 mm indenter) produced the largest changes in participants above 90 kg of mass. The results suggest that foam pads selected for static computerised posturography: 1) could possess a modulus of elasticity of around 40 kg/m^3, and 2) show linear deformation properties matched to the participants' weight.

Competing interests
The authors declare that they have no competing interests.

Authors' contributions
GG designed, executed and analysed the entire experiment and prepared the manuscript. MF assisted in design and testing materials. Both authors read and approved the final manuscript.

References
1. Punakallio A. Balance abilities of different-aged workers in physically demanding jobs. J Occup Rehabil. 2003;13(1):33–43.
2. Wu X, Madigan ML. Impaired plantar sensitivity among the obese is associated with increased postural sway. Neurosci Lett. 2014;583:49–54.
3. Forsman P, Wallin A, Haeggstrom E. Validation of a posturographic approach to monitor sleepiness. J Biomech. 2010;43(16):3214–6.
4. Zarnyslowska-Szmytke E, Sliwinska-Kowalska M. The influence of organic solvents on hearing and balance: a literature review. Med Pr. 2013;64(1):83–102.
5. Munnell A. What is the Average Retirement Age? Chestnut Hill, MA: Centre for Retirement Research, Boston College; 2011.
6. St-Pierre F. Analysis of Static and/or Dynamic Posture on a Force Platform (Posturography). St-Denis la Plaine, France: Department of Medical and Surgical Procedures Assessment, Haute Authorite de Sante; 2007.
7. Mitchell RJ, Lord SR, Harvey LA, Close JCT. Obesity and falls in older people: mediating effects of disease, sedentary behaviour, mood, pain and medication use. Arch Gerontol Geriatr 2014 Sep 22. doi:10.1016/j.archger.2014.09.006. [Epub ahead of print].
8. Chaudhry H, Bukiet B, Ji Z, Findley T. Measurement of balance in computer posturography: comparison of methods–a brief review. J Bodyw Mov Ther. 2011;15(1):82–91.
9. Mahdavi-Amiri N, Bidabadi N. Constrained nonlinear least squares: a superlinearly convergent projected structured secant method. Int J Electrical Comput Syst. 2012;1(1):1–8.
10. Wade C, Davis J, Weimar WH. Balance and exposure to an elevated sloped surface. Gait Posture. 2014;39(1):599–605.
11. Di Berardino F, Filipponi E, Barozzi S, Giordano G, Alpini D, Cesarani A. The use of rubber foam pads and "sensory ratios" to reduce variability in static posturography assessment. Gait Posture. 2009;29(1):158–60.
12. Gosselin G, Fagan MJ. The effects of cervical muscle fatigue on balance - a study with elite amateur rugby league players. J Sports Sci Med. 2014;13(2):329–37.
13. Patel M, Fransson PA, Lush D, Gomez S. The effect of foam surface properties on postural stability assessment while standing. Gait Posture. 2008;28(4):649–56.
14. Todd BA, Smith SL, Vongpaseuth T. Polyurethane foams: effects of specimen size when determining cushioning stiffness. J Rehabil Res Dev. 1998;35(2):219–24.
15. Blackburn JT, Riemann BL, Myers JB, Lephart SM. Kinematic analysis of the hip and trunk during bilateral stance on firm, foam, and multiaxial support surfaces. Clin Biomech (Bristol, Avon). 2003;18(7):655–61.
16. Adkin AL, Bloem BR, Allum JH. Trunk sway measurements during stance and gait tasks in Parkinson's disease. Gait Posture. 2005;22(3):240–9.
17. D-3574-11 AS. Standard Methods of Testing Flexible Cellular Materials—Slab, Bonded and Molded Urethane Foams. Philadelphia: American Society for Testing and Materials; 2012. p. 18.
18. World Medical A. World medical association Declaration of Helsinki: ethical principles for medical research involving human subjects. JAMA. 2013;310(20):2191–4.
19. Prosperini L, Fortuna D, Gianni C, Leonardi L, Pozzilli C. The diagnostic accuracy of static posturography in predicting accidental falls in people with multiple sclerosis. Neurorehabil Neural Repair. 2013;27(1):45–52.
20. Mancini M, Horak FB. The relevance of clinical balance assessment tools to differentiate balance deficits. Eur J Phys Rehabil Med. 2010;46(2):239–48.
21. Prieto T. Measures of postural steadiness: differences between healthy young and elderly adults. IEEE Trans Biomed Eng. 1996;43(9):956–66.
22. Hung J-W, Chou C-X, Hsieh Y-W, Wu W-C, Yu M-Y, Chen P-C, et al. Randomized comparison trial of balance training by using exergaming and conventional weight-shift therapy in patients with chronic stroke. Arch Phys Med Rehabil. 2014;95(9):1629–37.
23. Nardone A, Godi M, Artuso A, Schieppati M. Balance rehabilitation by moving platform and exercises in patients with neuropathy or vestibular deficit. Arch Phys Med Rehabil. 2010;91(12):1869–77.

24. Chiang JH, Wu G. The influence of foam surfaces on biomechanical variables contributing to postural control. Gait Posture. 1997;5(3):239–45.
25. Allum JH, Honegger F. Interactions between vestibular and proprioceptive inputs triggering and modulating human balance-correcting responses differ across muscles. Exp Brain Res. 1998;121(4):478–94.
26. Liu B, Kong W. Reliability of foam posturography in assessment of postural balance in the patients with vertigo. Front Med China. 2008;2(4):361–5.
27. Finucane MM, Stevens GA, Cowan MJ, Danaei G, Lin JK, Paciorek CJ, et al. National, regional, and global trends in body-mass index since 1980: systematic analysis of health examination surveys and epidemiological studies with 960 country-years and 9.1 million participants. Lancet. 2011;377 (9765):557–67.

9

Attainment rate as a surrogate indicator of the intervertebral neutral zone length in lateral bending: an in vitro proof of concept study

Alexander C Breen[1*], Mihai Dupac[1] and Neil Osborne[2]

Abstract

Background: Lumbar segmental instability is often considered to be a cause of chronic low back pain. However, defining its measurement has been largely limited to laboratory studies. These have characterised segmental stability as the intrinsic resistance of spine specimens to initial bending moments by quantifying the dynamic neutral zone. However these measurements have been impossible to obtain in vivo without invasive procedures, preventing the assessment of intervertebral stability in patients. Quantitative fluoroscopy (QF), measures the initial velocity of the attainment of intervertebral rotational motion in patients, which may to some extent be representative of the dynamic neutral zone. This study sought to explore the possible relationship between the dynamic neutral zone and intervertebral rotational attainment rate as measured with (QF) in an in vitro preparation. The purpose was to find out if further work into this concept is worth pursuing.

Method: This study used passive recumbent QF in a multi-segmental porcine model. This assessed the intrinsic intervertebral responses to a minimal coronal plane bending moment as measured with a digital force guage. Bending moments about each intervertebral joint were calculated and correlated with the rate at which global motion was attained at each intervertebral segment in the first 10° of global motion where the intervertebral joint was rotating.

Results: Unlike previous studies of single segment specimens, a neutral zone was found to exist during lateral bending. The initial attainment rates for left and right lateral flexion were comparable to previously published in vivo values for healthy controls. Substantial and highly significant levels of correlation between initial attainment rate and neutral zone were found for left (Rho = 0.75, $P = 0.0002$) and combined left-right bending (Rho = 0.72, $P = 0.0001$) and moderate ones for right alone (Rho = 0.55, $P = 0.0012$).

Conclusions: This study found good correlation between the initial intervertebral attainment rate and the dynamic neutral zone, thereby opening the possibility to detect segmental instability from clinical studies. However the results must be treated with caution. Further studies with multiple specimens and adding sagittal plane motion are warranted.

Background

Low back pain (LBP) is a growing problem which is responsible for major population disability [1]. In the absence of a specific pathological or neurological cause, most LBP is classified as 'non-specific' and is often assumed to be mechanical if the pain is made better or worse by movement or position [2–4]. Lumbar

segmental instability is thought to be an important factor in this, but for which there is no single definition or clinically available method for detection in patients [5, 6]. However, a generally accepted definition of clinical instability is "loss of the normal pattern of spinal motion causing pain and/or neurologic dysfunction" [7]. Many laboratory studies have explored this in terms of the neutral zone (NZ), which is the size of the zone of displacement when the bending moment is minimal [8, 9]. This measure has been found to be a more sensitive motion parameter in defining the onset and progression

* Correspondence: alexbreen@aecc.ac.uk
[1]School of Design Engineering and Computing, Bournemouth University, Bournemouth, BH1 5BB, UK
Full list of author information is available at the end of the article

of spinal injury than the elastic zone or range of motion [10]. However, the measurement of the NZ has traditionally been impossible to obtain in vivo without invasive procedures, preventing its use in patient assessment.

A number of studies have used quantitative fluoroscopy (QF) for the measurement of inter-vertebral motion *in vivo* [11–15]. QF provides continuous intervertebral motion information in both flexion-extension and lateral flexion. Patients lie passively on a robotic passive motion platform (Fig. 1a, b) which bends them at a standardised range and velocity while fluoroscopic sequences of inter-vertebral motion are obtained for measurement using image processing codes. This patient orientation minimises muscle activity and allows the intrinsic passive holding element (disc and ligament) restraints to be characterised.

QF has been used *in vivo* to study lumbar intervertebral motion patients and healthy controls [15]. An early version of this technology used weight bearing cineradiography and manual image registration to measure sagittal intervertebral angular motion as trunk motion progressed and claimed to be a surrogate for the NZ [16]. Later studies using fluoroscopy described this parameter as "the slope of the IVFE curve" and "the intervertebral attainment rate" [11, 13, 17].

Although most studies have concentrated on flexion-extension motion, lateral flexion has also been linked to segmental instability [18, 19]. Furthermore, lateral flexion stability has been shown both to be affected by discectomy and altered in lower limb amputees [20, 21].

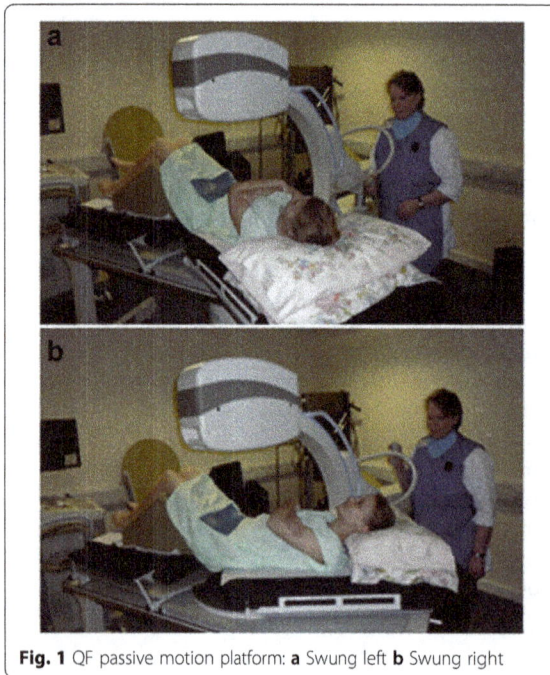

Fig. 1 QF passive motion platform: **a** Swung left **b** Swung right

Studies by our group used the ratios of the intersegmental bending gradients in the initial 10° of standardised trunk lateral flexion to express the initial attainment rate in an attempt to obtain a more standardised NZ surrogate [15] (Fig. 2).

Both the initial attainment rate and the NZ are expressions of intervertebral laxity. If a relationship is found to exist between them, it would provide evidence of the criterion validity of the former and demonstrate that this *in vivo* assessment of intrinsic lumbar segmental robustness might be used as a relatively non-invasive diagnostic tool in patients with persistent back disability where stability is in question. This study therefore sought to explore a methodology for determining this using a multi-segmented porcine lumbar spine with segments L1 to L5. The bending moments, intervertebral motion and global motion were recorded together using QF, using the same procedures as in lateral flexion QF studies of patients.

Methods
Apparatus
A fresh 5-segment porcine lumbar spine (L1 to L5) was prepared as recommended for the biomechanical testing of vertebral specimens [22] The porcine spine is said to have an anatomy that geometrically and biomechanically resembles that of the human spine [23, 24]. The paraspinal muscles were completely excised and all ligamentous components, including the interspinous ligament were preserved [24]. The specimen was preserved wrapped in saline-soaked gauze, covered in cling film and frozen for storage. It was thawed over 12 h before testing, mounted in a horizontal testing frame with the L1 and L5 vertebrae secured by metal halos and circumferential bolts. The same robotic horizontal motion platform used to provide controlled passive motion in patients receiving quantitative fluoroscopy examinations was used for testing (Atlas Clinical Ltd.) (Fig. 2). L1 was attached to the movable segment of the platform and L5 to the fixed segment.

A digital force guage (Omega Engineering Ltd DFG35-10, range 50 N, resolution 0.05 N, sampled at 125Hz) was rigidly connected to the movable part of the motion platform holding the superior vertebral segment. The motion of a connecting rod forced the specimen through a 40° arc, as applied in patient protocols [25], simultaneously transmitting continuous force data from the rod to a laptop computer. The force data were co-ordinated with the digital time stamp output of the motion platform's motor, which moved the specimen at a uniform velocity of 6° per second at a standardised ramp-up speed over the first second of the motion. This velocity derived from the need to replicate the image recording protocol used in patients, where trade-offs on tolerance, safety and X-ray exposure led to a consensus on these settings [25].

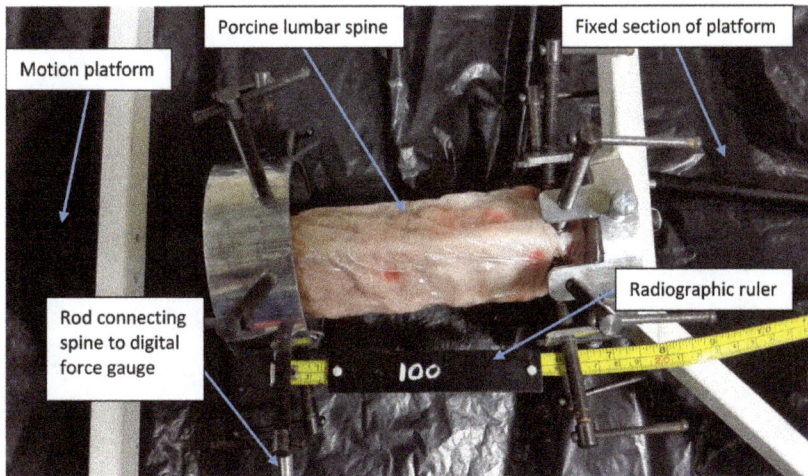

Fig. 2 Porcine lumbar spine testing apparatus and motion platform seen from above

Data collection

Fluoroscopic sequences of left and right lateral flexion were recorded at 15 frames per second over 15 s using a Siemens Arcadis Avantic fluoroscope VC10A portable C-arm fluoroscope (CE012), whose primary beam was centred on the disc space between the L3 and L4 vertebrae of the specimen. The image field included all 5 segments in all frames so that each vertebra could be tracked and the fluoroscope incorporated automatic distortion correction. Before recording the motion, a calibration image was acquired using a radiographic ruler comprising of two metallic beads of known diameter (4.4 mm) set 100 mm apart into a plastic bar and placed adjacent to the porcine spine and perpendicular to the primary-ray beam in the image field. A single fluoroscopic image was acquired so that this could be used as a scaling factor to calculate the distances between objects in the image sequences.

As in the protocol for patient recordings, the spine was preconditioned by performing four consecutive out and return lateral flexion sequences increasing from 10° up to 40° to replicate this. Ten consecutive recordings were then made of 40° left lateral flexion sequences. The spine was then replaced in a 'neutral' position where the force applied by the motion platform was as close to zero as possible. The same procedure was followed for right lateral flexion, however, due to the configuration of the apparatus only a maximum of 30° was achievable for right lateral flexion.

Image analysis

Outlines of the vertebral body borders of the first image were marked using the computer's cursor in the first of each sequence of images in a manner identical to

the patient mark-up protocol. The positions each of the vertebrae in each of the fluoroscopic images were calculated using automated frame to frame registration codes written in Matlab (The Mathworks Ltd. Cambridge) producing continuous tracking of each vertebral body image throughout the sequences [12]. Trackings were verified visually by a trained operator and the means of the positions of each vertebral section were generated as an output. Average angular motion was smoothed by Tikhonov regularization to reduce inter image variation as with the analysis in living subjects [26, 27].

The changing intervertebral angles of the specimen were co-ordinated with the timing and position of the motion platform. The intervertebral angles of the specimen when the motion platform reached 10°, the moments applied at each intervertebral joint and the motion platform rotation were recorded dynamically. The positions of the point of load application/measurement and the individual joint centres were derived from the trackings of each vertebra in each image frame. Since the centres of rotation between vertebrae are not generally to be found in the joint centre and due to the elasticity of the intervertebral joint, these distances varied slightly during motion and were incorporated into the continuous calculation of moments as detailed below. Forces and moments could not be measured directly at each joint, therefore estimation of forces and moments of forces were derived from the kinematics and inertial properties of the spine by applying the process of inverse dynamics. Modelling the spine as a series of free bending rods of negligible thickness and with uniform mass distribution, an estimation of forces and moments was derived based on

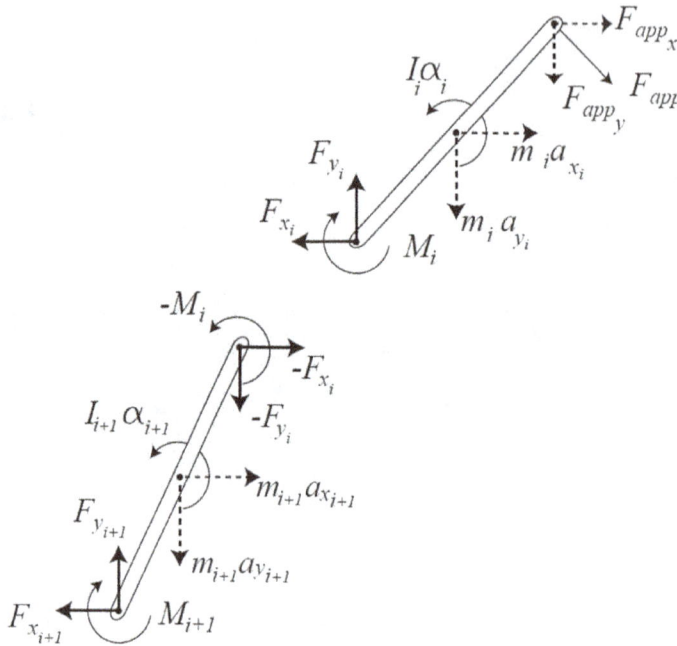

Fig. 3 Mechanical model of two successive vertebrae, modelled as having negligible thickness and uniform mass distribution. The figure shows action and reaction forces, net moments of force, and all linear and angular accelerations. Gravitational forces are ignored as they are not applicable in the plane of motion

D'Alembert's principle (Fig. 3). One can write the Newton-Euler equations as:

$$\sum \mathbf{F} = m_i \mathbf{a}_i \Leftrightarrow (-\mathbf{F}_{i-1}) + \mathbf{F}_i + m_i \mathbf{g} = m_i \mathbf{a}_i \qquad (1)$$

$$\sum \mathbf{M} = I_i \boldsymbol{\alpha}_i \Leftrightarrow (-\mathbf{M}_{i-1}) + \mathbf{r}_{i-1} \times (-\mathbf{F}_{i-1}) + \mathbf{M}_i + \mathbf{r}_i \times \mathbf{F}_i$$
$$= I_i \boldsymbol{\alpha}_i$$
$$(2)$$

where $\mathbf{F}_{app}$ is the applied force, $\mathbf{F}_i$ is the reaction force, $\mathbf{r}_i$ is the distance from the segment centre of mass to $\mathbf{F}_i$, since the geometrical centre is considered to be the

centre of mass – $\mathbf{r}_i$ is the distance from the segment centre of mass to $\mathbf{F}_{app}$, m_i is the mass of segment i, g is gravity vector, $\boldsymbol{\alpha}_i$ is the angular acceleration, Ii is the moment of inertia and × represents the vector (cross) product. Since gravity is acting perpendicular to the plane of measurement it can be ignored as in Fig. 3.

From Equations 1 and 2 one can calculate each reaction force ($\mathbf{F}_i$) and joint moment ($\mathbf{M}_i$) acting on each vertebra of the spine.

Initial attainment rate was calculated as the ratio of the slopes of the first 10° of platform rotation and intervertebral rotation over the contemporaneous outward

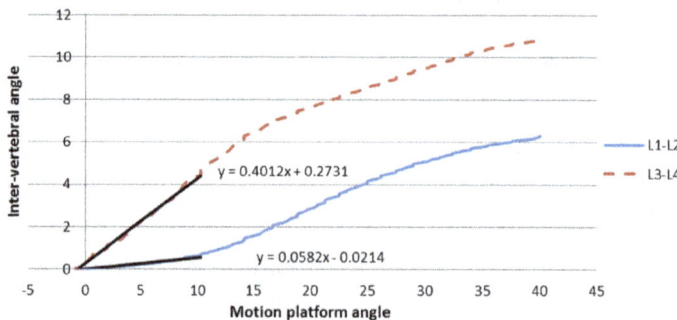

Fig. 4 Examples of initial attainment rate calculation: Gradients of inter-vertebral and platform motion in first 10 degrees of platform motion (two intervertebral levels)

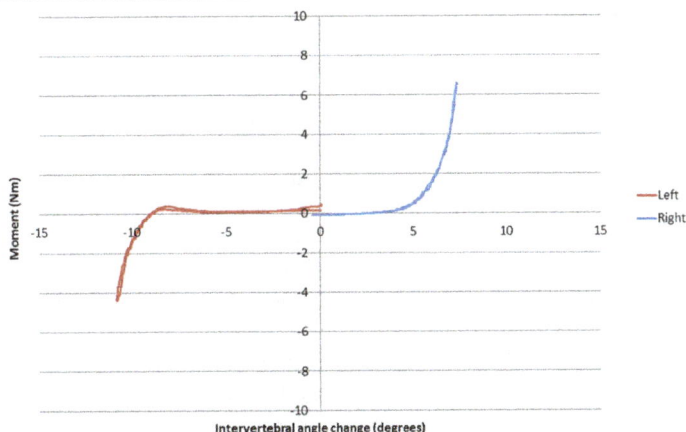

Fig. 5 Example of a force deformation curve from an L3-4 motion segment undergoing left and right lateral flexion

displacement of the latter (Fig. 3). If the motion segment did not rotate by at least 2.5° over this part of the motion (being twice the inter-observer error of the measurement of rotational deformation with this method) the segment was considered stiff and the initial attainment rate was not calculated [25] (Fig. 4).

The dynamic NZ was taken to be the inter-vertebral angle at the end of the region confined by a slope of +0.05 Nm/degree [28]. Samples of the force-deformation curves for all levels and directions in the specimen were examined to confirm that this was a reasonable assumption for this experiment (Fig. 5).

Statistical analysis

All data were tested for normality using the Shapiro-Wilk test. The inter-vertebral angle at 10° of platform motion, the dynamic NZs and the initial attainment rates were calculated for each intervertebral level and direction. Correlations between the dynamic NZs and the initial attainment rates in each segment were determined for the pooled data ($n = 52$) and for left and right separately using the Spearman rank correlation coefficient for non-normally distributed data. The cut-off for statistical significance was set at a P value of 0.05.

Results

The mean (SD) (L1-5) ranges of motion for each direction, as measured on the fluoroscopic images were: left 33.5°(1.2) and right 28.3°(0.9), which represented 83 % and 94 % of platform motion respectively. The initial attainment rates for left and right lateral flexion and the pooled data are shown in Table 1.

The levels of nonparametric correlation between initial attainment rate and dynamic NZ (Fig. 5) were substantial and highly significant for left and combined left-right and moderate for right alone [29] (Table 2).

Discussion
Main result

These results are similar to previously published in vivo values for healthy human controls [15] and suggest that there is a relationship between the initial attainment rate and the dynamic NZ. The range of upper quartiles for initial attainment rate (0.204–0.413) were comparable to the upper reference ranges found *in vivo* (0.290–0.429) [15]. However, initial attainment rate and the dynamic NZ are not usually perfectly coincident because they do not measure the same thing; NZ reflects resistance to a pure moment and attainment rate the inter-vertebral motion velocity compared to trunk motion. Furthermore,

Table 1 Median segmental initial attainment rates for left and right lateral flexion

Left					Right				
	Median	Upper quartile	Lower Quartile	N		Median	Upper quartile	Lower quartile	N
L1-2	-	-	-	0	L1-2	0.204	0.351	0.271	7
L2-3	0.310	0.319	0.302	10	L2-3	0.331	0.342	0.300	10
L3-4	0.406	0.413	0.383	10	L3-4	0.339	0.344	0.333	10
L4-5	-	-	-	0	L4-5	0.239	0.248	0.236	6

Table 2 Correlations between initial attainment rate and dynamic NZ for pooled levels (L1-2 to L4-5)

	Rho[a]	2-sided p	Number
Left and Right	0.72	0.0001	52
Right	0.55	0.0012	32
Left	0.75	0.0002	20

[a]Spearman's rank correlation

it is not suggested that the NZ can be calculated from the initial attainment rate, but merely that they are linked in a way that would allow the order of NZ length to be determined from a set of specimens or patients based on initial attainment rate results. In this experiment, they both appear to reflect the intrinsic restraining properties of the inter-vertebral linkages, although the differences need further explanation. In addition, the 10° cut-off used historically to define initial attainment was arbitrary. A better justified calculation may be provided by considering the subsequent work of Smit et al. [30].

Learning points as an exploratory study

Some of the motion of the frame (40°) was not transferred to the vertebral segments, as 6.5° (left) and 1.5° (right) respectively were lost. This may be due to the use of retaining bolt heads into the bone, calling for a better fixation method. This may have affected the correlations. In addition, two of the segments (L1-2 and L4-5 left) did not reach the required 2.5° required for initial attainment rate to be reported (Table 1). This is likely to be a prevailing feature of multi-segmental examinations, especially if segmental levels are not challenged. Future experimental setups should ensure that equal ranges of the motion platform are obtained.

In calculating the point of inter-vertebral motion from which initial attainment rate measurement begins,

fluctuations can occur. If these are prominent, the initial attainment rate value may alter and the method chosen for smoothing to obtain an average value, as well as the ramp-up speed, could affect initial attainment rate values. An international forum on the use of QF suggested this preferred smoothing function but that these values should be kept under review [25–27].

Another question might be why there was not symmetry in the measurement results. The dynamic NZs were generally of a greater order for left lateral flexion, (median left = 7.17°, median right = 4.70°) but over a higher range (range left = 5.90°, range right = 6.49°). This might be the result of lower ranges of right global bending during pre-conditioning and repeated motion and/or alternatively, greater laxity at L3-4 in left lateral flexion (representing the upper cluster in Fig. 6) as a physiological variant. Further studies using multiple specimens and symmetrical testing should clarify this.

Relevance to clinical studies

In patient and volunteer research studies, the presence of a greater volume of soft tissue between the motion frame and the segment will add noise to the calculation of the initial attainment rate. It might be expected that laxity would be associated with a greater overall range of the segment, but may also be affected by the soft tissue mass. The extent of this might be explored *in vivo* by comparing the initial attainment rates to the overall segmental ranges obtained using QF and to body-mass index.

An additional major challenge in passive system spine kinematics research lies in the complexity of upright motion. This adds the influence of unaccounted variations arising from muscle motor control and body segment mass. However, it also extends the scope of the kind of stability parameters that can be considered.

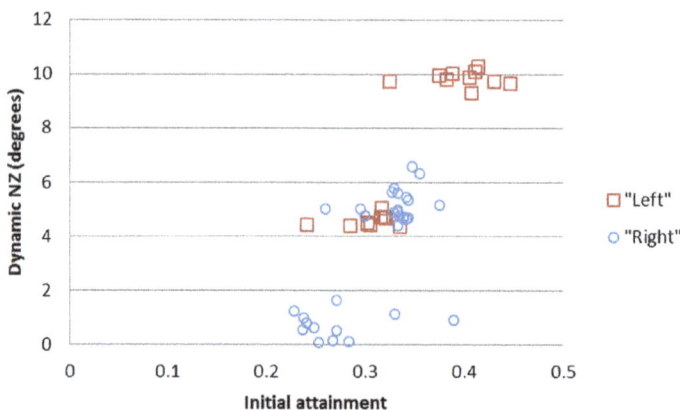

Fig. 6 Scatter plot of dynamic NZ (degrees) against initial attainment for left and right lateral flexion

Suggestions for further work

The present studies were limited to lateral flexion, where in some circumstances stability may be important. However, the greatest interest in stability, especially for purposes of surgical decisions, focuses on the sagittal plane, where translation is the main kinematic measure used in estimating stability [5]. Studies of the correlation between this and initial attainment rate in the sagittal plane would further inform the use of initial attainment rate in the assessment of patients for segmental laxity.

Conclusion

The ability to measure inter-vertebral laxity in patients with QF is a step forward in the assessment of chronic back pain where mechanics is thought to be important. This study used the passive recumbent QF protocol in a multi-segmental porcine model for assessing the intrinsic intervertebral responses to a minimal bending moment. It found there to be good correlation between the initial attainment rate and the dynamic NZ, thereby opening the possibility to measure passive system intervertebral laxity in clinical studies. However, this was an exploratory study based on repeated measurements in a single specimen, albeit a multilevel one. Therefore, the results, although likely to be important, should be treated with caution. Further, multi-specimen *in vitro* studies are now warranted.

Competing interests
The authors declare that they have no competing interests.

Authors' contribution
AB carried out the specimen experiments, analysed the results and drafted themanuscript. All authors read and approved the final manuscript.

Author details
[1]School of Design Engineering and Computing, Bournemouth University, Bournemouth, BH1 5BB, UK. [2]Anglo-European College of Chiropractic, Bournemouth, BH5 2DF, UK.

References

1. Hoy D, March L, Brooks P, Blyth F, Woolf A, Bain C, et al. The global burden of low back pain: estimates from the Global Burden of Disease 2010 study. Ann Rheum Dis. 2014;73(6):968–74.
2. NICE Back pain - low (without radiculopathy) - Management. Clinic Knowledge Summaries, 2015. http://cks.nice.org.uk/back-pain-low-without-radiculopathy.
3. Deyo RA, Dworkin SF, Amtmann D, Andersson G, Borenstein D, Carragee E, et al. Report of the National Institutes of Health Task Force on Research Standards for Chronic Low Back Pain. J Manipulative Physiol Ther. 2014;37(7):449–67.
4. Campbell J, Colvin LA. Management of Back Pain. Br Med J. 2013;347(Dec 5):f3148.
5. Kanemura A, Doita M, Kasahara K, Sumi M, Kurosaka M, Iguchi T. The influence of sagittal instability factors on clinical lumbar spinal symptoms. J Spinal Disord Tech. 2009;22(7):479–85.
6. Steiger F, Becker H-J, Standaert CJ, Nalague F, Vader J-P, Porchet F, et al. Surgery in lumbar degenerative spondylolisthesis: indications, outcomes and complications. A systematic review. Eur Spine J. 2014;23:945–73.
7. Panjabi MM. Clinical spinal instability and low back pain. J Electromyogr Kinesiol. 2003;13(4):371–9.
8. Panjabi MM. The stabilising system of the spine - Part 2: Neutral zone and instability hypothesis. J Spinal Disord. 1992;5(4):390–7.
9. Crawford NR, Peles JD, Dickman CA. The spinal lax zone and neutral zone: measurement techniques and parameter comparisons. J Spinal Disord. 1998;11:416–29.
10. Oxland TR, Panjabi MM. The onset and progression of spinal injury: A demonstration of neutral zone sensitivity. J Biomech. 1992;25(10):1165–72.
11. Wong KWN, Leong JCY, Chan M-K, Lu WW. The flexion-extension profile of lumbar spine in 100 healthy volunteers. Spine. 2004;29(15):1636–41.
12. Breen A, Muggleton J, Mellor F. An objective spinal motion imaging assessment (OSMIA): reliability, accuracy and exposure data. BMC Musculoskelet Disord. 2006;7(1):1–10.
13. Teyhen DS, Flynn TW, Childs JD, Kuklo TR, Rosner MK, Polly DW, et al. Fluoroscopic Video to Identify Aberrant Lumbar Motion. Spine. 2007;32(7):E220–E9.
14. Ahmadi A, Maroufi N, Behtash H, Zekavat H, Parnianpour M. Kinematic analysis of dynamic lumbar motion in patients with lumbar segmental instability using digital videofluoroscopy. Eur Spine J. 2009;18:1677–85.
15. Mellor F, Muggleton JM, Bagust J, Mason W, Thomas PW, Breen AC. Mid-lumbar lateral flexion stability measured in healthy volunteers by in-vivo fluoroscopy. Spine. 2009;34(22):E811–E7.
16. Kanayama M, Abumi K, Kaneda K, Tadano S, Ukai T. Phase Lag of the Intersegmental Motion in Flexion-Extension of the Lumbar and Lumbosacral Spine: An In Vivo Study. Spine. 1996;21(12):1416–22.
17. Wong K, Luk K, Leong J, Wong S, Wong K. Continuous dynamic spinal motion analysis. Spine. 2006;31(4):414–9.
18. Miles M, Sullivan WE. Lateral bending at the lumbar and lumbosacral joints. Anat Rec. 1961;139(3):387–98.
19. Kirkaldy-Willis WH, Farfan HF. Instability of the lumbar spine. Clin Orthop Relat Res. 1982;165:110–23.
20. Goel VK, Nishiyama K, Weinstein J, Liu YK. Mechanical properties of lumbar spinal motion segments as affected by partial disc removal. Spine. 1986;11:1008–12.
21. Hendershot BD. Alterations and Asymmetries in Trunk Mechanics and Neuromuscular Control among Persons with Lower-Limb Amputation: Exploring Potential Pathways of Low Back Pain. Blacksburg: Virginia Polytechnic Institute and State University; 2012.
22. Wilke HJ, Wenger K, Claes L. Testing criteria for spinal implants: recommendatons for the standardization of in vitro stability testing of spinal implants. Eur Spine J. 1998;7:148–54.
23. Busscher I, van der Veen AJ, van Dieen JH, Kingma I, Verkerke GJ, Veldhuizen AG. In Vitro Biomechanical Characteristics of the Spine: A comparison between Human and Porcine Spinal Segments. Spine. 2010;35(2):E35–42.
24. Tai C, Hsieh P, Chen W, Chen L, Chen W, Lai P. Biomechanical comparison of lumbar spine instability between laminectomy and bilateral laminotomy for spinal stenosis syndrome-an experimental study in porcine model. BMC Musculoskelet Disord. 2008;9:84.
25. Breen AC, Teyhan DS, Mellor FE, Breen AC, Wong KWN, Deitz A. Measurement of InterVertebral Motion Using Quantitative Fluoroscopy: Report of an International Forum and Proposal for Use in the Assessment of Degenerative Disc Disease in the Lumbar Spine. Adv Orthop. 2012;2012:802350.
26. Eilers PH. A perfect smoother. Anal Chem. 2003;75(14):3631–6. Epub 2003/10/23.
27. Lubansky AS, Yeow YL, Leong Y-K, Wickramasinghe SR, Han B. A general method of computing the derivative of experimental data. AIChE J. 2006;52(1):323–32.
28. Thompson RE, Barker TM, Pearcy MJ. Defining the Neutral Zone of sheep intervertebral joints during dynamic motions: an in vitro study. Clin Biomech. 2003;18:89–98.
29. Landis JR, Koch GG. The Measurement of Observer Agreement for Categorical Data. Biometrics. 1977;33(1):159–74.
30. Smit TH, van Tunen MSLM, van der Veen AJ, Kingma I, van Dieen JH. Quantifying Intervertebral disc mechanics: a new definition of the neutral zone. BMC Musculoskelet Disord. 2011;12:38.

10

Wearing American Football helmets increases cervicocephalic kinaesthetic awareness in "elite" American Football players but not controls

Peter W. McCarthy[1*], Phillip J. Hume[2], Andrew I. Heusch[1] and Sally D. Lark[3]

Abstract

Background: While there have been investigations into the reduced neck injury rate of wearing protective helmets, there is little information on its effects on normal kinaesthetic neck function. This study aims to quantify the kinaesthetic and movement effects of the American football helmet.

Methods: Fifteen British Collegiate American football players (mean age 22.2, SD 1.9; BMI kg.m^2 26.3, SD 3.7) were age and size matched to 11 non-American football playing university students (mean age 22.5, SD 3.6; BMI 24.3, SD 3.3 kg.m^2). Both groups had their active cervical range of motion and head repositioning accuracy measured during neck flexion/extension using a modified cervical range of motion device and a similarly modified football helmet.

Results: Wearing helmets significantly reduced active cervical range of motion in extension in both groups ($P = 0.007$ and $P = 0.001$ Controls and American Footballers respectively). While both groups had similar repositioning when not wearing a helmet (flexion $P = 0.99$; extension $P = 0.52$), when wearing helmets, American football players appeared to be more accurate in relation to cervical kinaesthetic repositioning (ANOVA: $P = 0.077$: flexion effect size =0.84; extension effect size =0.38).

Conclusions: Wearing American football helmets significantly reduces the active cervical range of motion in extension, along with a change in the neutral head position. American footballers have a greater accuracy in repositioning their head from flexion (potentially enhanced proprioception) when wearing a helmet. This finding might allow development of a simple objective test to help discern presence of minor concussive or cervical musculoskeletal injury on or off the field.

Keywords: Neck function, Proprioception, Sports, Protective equipment

Background

Afferent proprioceptive information is important for sensorimotor control of posture and movement [1]. Joint disease and other musculoskeletal conditions can associate with altered proprioceptive functioning [2–4] which, in extreme cases such as following joint injection in the neck can result in ataxia; ipsilateral hypotonia of the arm and leg and a strong sensation of falling or tilting [1]. Although extreme, this highlights the potential for lesser changes in neural feedback to affect the fine motor control crucial for elite performance.

American Football (AF) is the third highest source of sports injuries being responsible for over one million reported injuries a year within the United States alone [5]. Concussion appears the most common injury type, with 17.78–26.95 concussive and neck neurologic injuries per 10,000 athlete exposures [6]. Injuries to the cervical spine are the most common catastrophic injuries in AF [7], and the second highest cause of death within the sport over the period 1977–2001 [8]. Consequently strict rules and considerable protective clothing have reduced the severity of impacts to the head and body [7, 9, 10]. Cumulative

* Correspondence: peter.mccarthy@southwales.ac.uk
[1]Faculty of Life Sciences and Education, University of South Wales, Pontypridd, Mid-Glamorgan, Wales CF37 1DL, UK
Full list of author information is available at the end of the article

effects of more frequent lesser neuro-musculoskeletal trauma (e.g., minor head injury) tend to be ignored in contact sports that require repetitive short bursts of maximal effort (American Football and Rugby football).

Embedding use of protective equipment into training and gameplay helps familiarization and adaptation. However, equipment may have predictable additional effects (visual and auditory impairment) and less immediately apparent postural adaptations, decreased cervical spine function (range of motion [ROM] and cervicocephalic kinaesthetic repositioning: [CKR]). In elite professional Rugby football players cervical spine range of motion appears related to both game play and time in the sport [11, 12]. In apparent contrast, AF players [13] have a greater active cervical range of motion (ACROM). However, to the author's knowledge, there is no information available concerning the possible consequences of wearing a protective helmet in terms of its' added mass, displaced centre of gravity and neutral head position and CKR.

There is evidence of deficits in CKR (interchangeable with the term proprioceptive deficits) resulting from trauma, such as in whiplash [14]; however, Rugby players also had a significantly decreased ability to reposition the head to a neutral position following neck extension [11] or rotation [15]. If the helmet is truly protective, AF players, who are subject to similar forces (impact and shear forces) to Rugby, should not have the same degree of deficit in CKR seen in the Rugby player [11, 12, 16].

The aim of this study was to determine whether the wearing of protective headgear by AF players influences active range of motion in the neck and CKR as assessed by head repositioning.

Method

The population size for this study was determined from previous studies of active cervical range of motion (ACROM and CKR effect sizes 0.3 to 1.2) [11]. Fifteen AF player volunteers (22.2 SD 1.9 years) were recruited from the British Collegiate American Football League. All players came from one of the national semi-finalist teams (Cardiff University Cobras, Southampton University Stags England), with nine volunteers having represented Great Britain at the collegiate level (equates to playing in the National Collegiate Athletic Association [NCAA] Division III within the USA). For inclusion in this study each player had to have had a minimum of 3 years playing experience of full contact, kitted AF. Further criteria included participants being currently asymptomatic for neck pain or discomfort. A screening questionnaire was completed by all recruited participants to determine presence of current or previous neck trauma, surgery or disorders that may exclude them from participating in the study or influence the results: e.g., dizziness, tinnitus, diabetes mellitus, asthma, hypertension, headaches/migraines.

Initially 15 age and size matched control volunteers were recruited, however only 11 of these fulfilled the inclusion criteria ($n = 11$; 22.5 SD 3.6 years). Controls were trained athletes who participated in non-contact amateur competitive sports such as triathlon, swimming, water polo and basketball. All participants volunteered and gave written informed consent after receiving verbal and written information about the study, which was approved by the ethics committee of the School of Applied Sciences, University of Glamorgan, and follows the Helsinki Declaration ethical guidelines.

The method employed here is based on that described previously [11]. The protocol will be described in 3 sections: anthropometrics, assessment with a cervical range of motion (CROM) device, and helmeted assessment. The study presentation order regarding CROM or helmet measurements was randomised between participants to remove potential order effects.

Anthropometric measures: neck girth (Hoechstmass HM-82203 Rollfix Tape Measure; Cranlea, Bourneville UK), body mass (floor scales model 761, Seca GmBH, Germany) and height (stadiometer model 202, Seca GmBH, Germany) were recorded. Participants sat in a chair which was height adjustable, so that their hips, knees and ankle angles were all set to ~90° SD 5°, as assessed by a professional quality JAMAR E-Z Read goniometer (Physiomed, Manchester, UK). The chair was positioned so that the vertex of the participants' head was 1 m (SD 5 %) from a custom made wall mounted chart (Fig. 1a) that was to receive light from a laser either mounted onto the CROM device (Performance Attainment Associates, Lindstrom MN, USA) or AF helmet with face guard (see below and Fig. 1b & c for details). The participants were instructed not to arch their thoracolumbar spine during extension, to ensure only neck muscles were engaged in the flexion-extension movements. A biofeedback cuff (Stabilizer™ pressure bio-feedback, Chattanooga group, Encore Medical Texas, USA) was placed between the posterior upper thoracic spine region and the back of the chair and inflated to 40 mm Hg. Measurements were repeated if the pressure deviated by >2 mm Hg during head movements. Each participant was guided through a warm-up and familiarization session (the equivalent of three repeated trials) before assessment began.

To measure ACROM, a cotton bandana was tied around the head (above the brow anteriorly and tied posteriorly above the occiput), to cushion the body of a CROM device and ensure stability regardless of idiosyncrasy associated with head/skull morphology. The CROM was placed onto the head as described by the manufacturers: the magnetic yolk was not used in these experiments, as rotation was not measured in this study. CROM devices have been used extensively in this type of research and have been shown to have sufficient accuracy [17], validity [18, 19], and reliability [20] for studies of ACROM such as this.

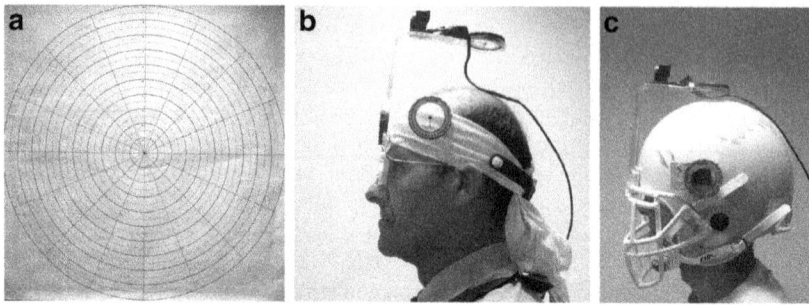

Fig. 1 This figure shows the measurement chart target for quantifying repositioning error (**a**) and the cervical range of motion (CROM) devices used for assessing unhelmeted (**b**) and helmeted (**c**) range of motion. Figure 1a shows the wall chart *in situ* illustrating the concentric evenly placed circles about the (0, 0) centre point with a laser light visible between rings labelled 1 and 2 above the centre spot. In Fig. 1b, the modified CROM can be seen showing the side mounted gravity goniometer and the rotational arm suspended above vertex of the subject's head which holds the mounted pencil laser. The final element (1c) shows the modified American football helmet with the rotational arm of the CROM mounted on the front of the helmet and gravity goniometer on the side in line with the vertex of the helmet. In all cases, the rotational arm of the goniometer was only used as a stable point to mount the pencil laser

This CROM device had a custom made laser block (Perspex block containing a pencil laser (class 3a: 650 nm: miraclebeam™ Pacoima, CA) mounted (screwed) on the rotational arm slightly forward of the position which would overly the vertex (Fig. 1b). This was used for assessment of CKR using the CROM or adapted helmet.

The participants' ACROM in full flexion and full extension was assessed as follows: the participant was asked to maximally flex their head forwards by tucking in their chin to their chest, or extend their head back while maintaining their shoulders and mid-to lower back in a normal upright position (including their normal curvature). There was a 2 s hold at the end of each movement to establish the end point reading (angle). After each head movement, the participants were asked to return to their neutral starting position (looking directly ahead).

To assess ACROM wearing the football helmet a standard mid-sized AF helmet and grill was adapted as follows (Fig. 1c): an attachment for the rotational arm of the CROM was custom made of aluminium and bolted onto anterior midline of the helmet; between the two upper anterior grill anchor points. A further custom-made aluminium block was bolted on the left lateral aspect above the grill attachment point (in line with the vertex in the coronal plane). This was used to affix a gravity goniometer that had been extracted from a spare CROM device. Using the same type and manufacture of goniometer allowed the modified helmet assessment to have comparable reading accuracy to the CROM.

Laser repositioning was used in the assessment of CKR. Participants were asked to close their eyes and find a comfortable neutral head position, at which point the laser was switched on. Once the laser light was visible on the wall mounted chart (Fig. 1a), the chart was moved so that the laser light impacted the centre of the chart (position 0, 0). Following chart alignment, participants were instructed to repeat the flexion and extension movements (returning to their perceived neutral position between movements) keeping their eyes closed. Repositioning was assessed by returning to perceived neutral from both full flexion and full extension, with the order of head movement alternated to reduce any order effect. The CKR was recorded using an adaptation of the procedure reported by Revel [21]. Once the participant affirmed they had returned to neutral, the actual position of the laser on the wall chart was noted (distance from the centre, direction in relation to undershoot or overshoot as well as lateral deviation).

Data was tested for skewness and kurtosis and deemed to be normally distributed for statistical analysis. A repeated measures ANOVA was used to identify main effects, post-hoc analysis using the Paired Student's T-test for the helmet effect separately in each group (controls and AF). As direction of change was not immediately predictable, 2-tailed analysis was used. Probability values of 0.1 to 0.05 were considered as signifying strong trends and values <0.05 were deemed a significant change. Effect size (ES) was calculated using the method of Cohen's D [22]. Statistical analysis was performed using SPSS 18.0 for Windows.

Results

Age and anthropometric characteristics of the participants are shown in Table 1. Although the AF players appeared heavier than controls, this was not statistically significant instead showing a strong trend ($P = 0.085$). Both groups of participants had reportedly sustained similar numbers of concussive injuries overall and had similar ACROM in flexion and extension (t-test: $P = 0.62$ and $P = 0.63$ respectively). The main ACROM effects

Table 1 Anthropometric and Concussive Injury Measures

	Age (years)	Height (m)	Mass (kg)	BMI	Neck Girth (cm)	Concussive Head Injuries
Control (n = 11)	22.5 (3.6)	1.77 (9.6)	76.2 (11.9)	24.2 (3.3)	39.1 (2.3)	1.3 (0.5)
American Football players (n = 15)	22.2 (1.9)	1.81 (7.5)	87.1 (17.3)	26.3 (3.7)	39.0 (2.4)	1.5 (0.5)

Mean (±1 standard deviation) for the anthropometric measures and the number of concussion head injuries declared for Controls and American Football players

calculated from the repeated measures ANOVA reveal that wearing a helmet affects the ACROM ($P = 0.014$) with no difference between the controls and AF players ($P = 0.62$). Although wearing a helmet did not significantly alter the ACROM in flexion for both controls and AF players (paired t-tests: $P = 0.14$ and $P = 0.31$ respectively: Fig. 2a), it significantly decreased the ACROM in extension (paired t-tests: $P = 0.007$ [ES = 0.88] and $P = 0.001$ [ES = 1.02]; controls and AF players respectively: Fig. 2b). To determine whether the changes in ACROM were the result of a displacement in the neutral point, the ratio between flexion and extension (flexion/extension) was calculated (Table 2).

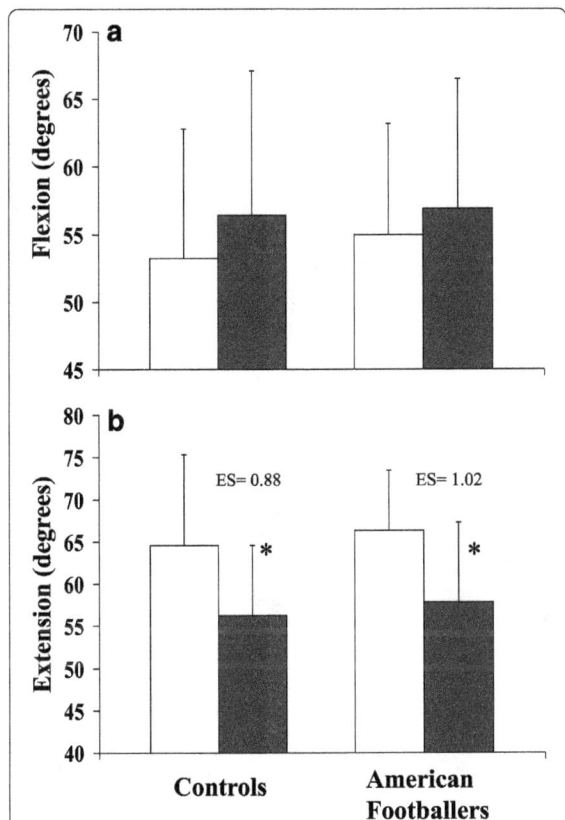

Fig. 2 Mean ± SD values for cervical range of motion in American football players and controls subjects in flexion (**a**) and extension (**b**) while either wearing a football helmet (*blocked bars*), or not (*unblocked bars*). * denotes a significant difference (*P* < 0.05) between wearing a helmet or not. Effect sizes (ES) are shown as helmet vs no helmet for each group

Generally, AF players had similar CK repositioning to the controls when not wearing a helmet (unpaired t-tests: returning from flexion $P = 0.99$, or extension $P = 0.52$). Wearing the helmet significantly enhanced the CK repositioning ability (ANOVA: $P = 0.04$: Fig. 3a and b). However, AF players appeared to be more accurate than the controls in relation to CK when wearing the helmet (ANOVA: $P = 0.077$). The CK of the control participants appeared unaffected either returning from flexion (paired t-test: $P = 0.93$) or extension (paired t-test: $P = 0.6$). In contrast, wearing helmets enhanced the AF players CK: flexion with no helmet 3.1°, with helmet 1.9°, (paired t-test: $P = 0.054$: [ES = 0.84] Fig. 3a); extension with no helmet 3.2°, with helmet 2.6° (paired t-test: $P = 0.22$: [ES = 0.38] Fig. 3b). Direct comparison between controls and players showed that when returning from flexion, helmeted players had better CK than helmeted controls (ES = 0.71). All other comparisons had ES <0.20.

Discussion

Wearing an AF helmet appears to have affected the ACROM of the user regardless of group and the CK repositioning error to the benefit of the trained wearer. ACROM assessment revealed similar effects in both groups with the most noticeable being a significant decrease in extension. From a physical perspective, participants in this study were generally not significantly different between groups (Table 1). Additionally, neck girths were of similar circumference in both groups and were within the range reported [23] for young AF players; however, there was no neck circumference data available from older AF players for comparison.

A possible explanation for the decrease in extension and lack of significant change in flexion could be a re-alignment of the head so that the neutral point is further

Table 2 Flexion-Extension Ratios

		Helmet	No Helmet
Controls (n = 11)	range	0.75–1.39	0.61–1.15
	average	1.01 ± 0.21	0.85 ± 0.20
AF Players (n = 15)	range	0.57–1.62	0.59–1.30
	average	1.04 ± 0.21	0.87 ± 0.18

Ratios of the active cervical range of motion (ACROM) for amount of flexion compared to extension can be used as an indication of the subject's preferred neutral point under those conditions. Both groups were measured with and without an American footballers (AF) helmet. Both AF and control groups significantly changed their flexion-extension ratio whilst wearing the helmet (*p* < 0.01). Data is presented as mean ± 1 standard deviation; however the range is also presented to allow greater clarity regarding the changes seen

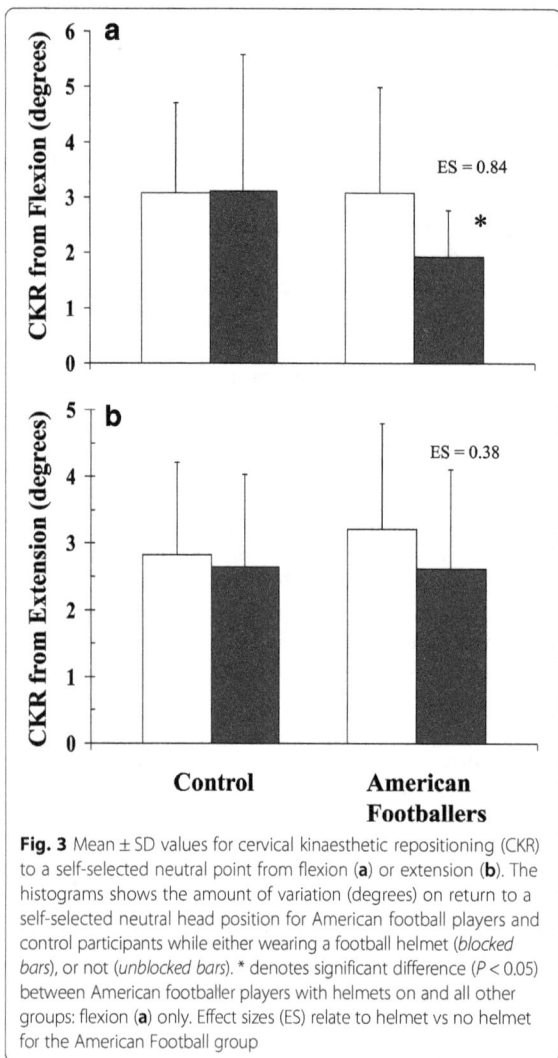

Fig. 3 Mean ± SD values for cervical kinaesthetic repositioning (CKR) to a self-selected neutral point from flexion (**a**) or extension (**b**). The histograms shows the amount of variation (degrees) on return to a self-selected neutral head position for American football players and control participants while either wearing a football helmet (*blocked bars*), or not (*unblocked bars*). * denotes significant difference (*P* < 0.05) between American footballer players with helmets on and all other groups: flexion (**a**) only. Effect sizes (ES) relate to helmet vs no helmet for the American Football group

increasing that for flexion, as can be seen in the significant change in flexion-extension ratio (Table 2). Interestingly, the reset neutral point became equidistant for flexion and extension, whereas without the helmet the ratio was in favour of flexion. Such a change in muscular balance over time might be expected to result in hypertonicity of the neck musculature which in turn might restrict return to the unhelmeted position; however, there was no apparent evidence for this in the data. Adaptations in either muscle length or tonicity related to the helmeted neutral position do not appear to have occurred in these younger AF players; as their unhelmeted and helmeted ACROM results are almost identical to the controls. It would be interesting to determine if older or elite professional AF players maintain this characteristic or show more permanent adaptation to helmet wear, in which case use of electromyography might help determine if increased muscle activity is involved in any change.

Although it was considered that the AF players might gain advantage from the prolonged use of the helmet in training and play, it was surprising to find that the controls did not suffer from a reduced repositioning accuracy when put into the unfamiliar situation of wearing the helmet (Fig. 3a and b). In addition to simply wearing the helmet, the adaptations made by the participant, such as a potential displacement of the neutral position (flexion:extension ratio; Table 2), would be expected to exacerbate potential for reduced repositioning accuracy. The *significantly* lower error in repositioning from flexion *(from 3.08° to 1.93°)* for the AF player population when wearing the helmet (*P* = 0.054: ES = 0.84) suggests that the regular wearing of the helmet can create an advantage in repositioning accuracy. The exact cause of this is unknown, but could include: mass of the helmet, displacement of the centre of gravity, and/or the specific training and repetitive use with some element of feedback or "reward" affecting neurological programming. While integration of all the afferent information is at a higher level of the vestibular nuclei, the vestibular system reflexes are closely coupled to cervicospinal reflexes and activation of the neck muscles increases vestibular responsiveness via the combined cervico-collic and vestibulo-collic reflexes. It has been proposed that sustained cervico-spinal reflex activation affords a prolonged after-effect to enhance the vestibulo-collic reflex (Pettorossi and Schieppati 2014) [24]. This would equate to the habituation of increased loading on the head and neck muscles by the helmet. Lack of equivalent change in the control group supports this hypothesis and suggests that incorporating useful feedback from wearing of the helmet might require a training period. The lack of difference between the AF players and the controls prior to putting on the helmet supports this conclusion. It might be worth considering whether there are general

into extension (Table 2) coupled with the physical restriction associated with wearing the helmet. If the change in flexion was equal and opposite to that in extension, one could surmise that this was due to neutral point deviation alone. However as the change was not equal and opposite, the additional difference could result from a physical restriction to movement caused by the helmet. The slight difference between Pearl and Mayer (1979) [23] and the results presented here regarding changes in flexion ACROM, tend to support this hypothesis: although, the presence of shoulder pads worn in the Pearl and Mayer [23] study could be considered to have contributed to an additional reduction in flexion range of motion. The effect of the helmet's mass appeared to have resulted in realignment of the head's neutral position on the cervical spine towards extension. Thereby decreasing available range for extension and benefits conferred by the enhanced CK repositioning to a self-selected neutral position when wearing the helmet. However, this was not apparent in the AF players available for this study when returning from extension (from 3.21° to 2.62°: $P = 0.22$: ES = 0.38). It is possible that a different result might be found with players of a higher standard (i.e. higher than National Collegiate Athletic Association Division III). Furthermore, there are a number of additional questions raised by these results: such as whether position of play has any specific relationship to changes in repositioning accuracy?

Although the effects of the helmet were tested without the participants being in full kit, a number of points can still be drawn from the results of the study. Primarily, wearing the helmet affects the flexion:extension ratio and reduces total available ACROM. Although this would be expected to cause adaptations in neck use for the player, these were not apparent in these younger players, but muscle length and strength changes along with associated cervical spine joint damage might accrue chronically so become apparent in older players. It has been well documented that such changes can result in symptoms such as headache [25]. However, although headache is very common in AF as a result of direct head contact [26], resolving the effects of adaptations in the neck muscles to the helmet alone will probably be too subtle or inconsequential to be determined by this method.

The enhanced CKR might have implications in the detection of neurological and musculoskeletal impairment in AF such as following minor concussion and or recovery from neck trauma [27]. Detection of minor concussion or determining full recovery are recognised problems in AF. Most methods employable during a game are limited and usually test for gross neurological compromise such as gross disturbance of proprioception, (standing and walking tests), which tend to miss the more subtle changes, making accurate determination of recovery difficult for the clinician. Furthermore, subjective tests such as those for pain tend to be hidden when elite players wish to remain on the field. There is evidence to support a relationship between presence of subclinical pain and changed cervicocephalic kinaesthetic sensibility [28] which strengthens the possible usefulness of a tool to objectify neurological damage on the field. Finding an objective tool to help determine level of neurological or musculoskeletal damage following a collision is important when taken into context with the additive effect of further head collisions which have more profound implications to outcome [29]. However, as fine neurological processing skills including CKR, can be easily lost following a concussive injury [30] or musculoskeletal damage akin to whiplash, the use of a simple testing system such as this, on a fully kitted player, might allow future development of a more reliable field based test for the presence of such damage following head collision in elite sport.

Conclusions

In conclusion wearing an AF helmet causes a significant reduction in extension ACROM in AF players and controls, as well as potentially disturbing the flexion:extension ratio. Constantly wearing a helmet results in AF players developing improved CK when returning from full flexion but not extension, short term wearing does not give any beneficial effects in terms of CK.

There is a need to determine the cause and extent of this improvement, also to determine whether player position/role and standard of play affects the size and direction of change.

Practical implications

- Applications of this research might help develop a sensitive proprioceptive test for AF players suffering from a concussive injury, which can be applied without removing the helmet.
- This research might be extrapolated to other helmet wearing sports and occupations.
- Future study of AF players might give an insight into enhancing proprioceptive skill acquisition in sport.

Abbreviations
ACROM: Active cervical range of motion; AF: American Football; CROM: Cervical range of motion; CKR: Cervicocephalic kinaesthetic repositioning; ROM: Range of motion; ES: Effect size.

Competing interests
The authors declare that they have no competing interests.

Authors' contributions
All authors were involved in the conception, design of the study, PH performed most of the data acquisition under supervision of PWM, analysis was performed by AIH, SL and PH and all authors played a part in data interpretation and construction of the manuscript. PWM devised the CKR testing methodology, all authors read and approved the final manuscript.

Acknowledgments
We would like to thank the support and participation of British Collegiate American Football League. We would also like to acknowledge the financial support of the Welsh Institute of Chiropractic and The University of South Wales. Study conducted at: University of Glamorgan (now University of South Wales), Welsh Institute of Chiropractic, Pontypridd, Wales, UK, CF37 1DL.

Author details
[1]Faculty of Life Sciences and Education, University of South Wales, Pontypridd, Mid-Glamorgan, Wales CF37 1DL, UK. [2]Anglo-European College of Chiropractic, Parkwood Road, Bournemouth, Dorset BH5 2DF, UK. [3]Massey University Wellington, College of Health, P O Box 756, Wellington 6140, New Zealand.

References
1. de Jong PTVM, de Jong JMBV, Cohen B, Jongkees LBW. Ataxia and nystagmus induced by injection of local anaesthetics in the neck. Ann Neurol. 1977;1:240–6. doi:10.1002/ana.410010307.

2. Baker V, Bennell K, Stillman B, Cowan S, Crossley K. Abnormal knee joint position sense in individuals with patellofemoral pain syndrome. J Orthop Res. 2002;20:208–14. doi:10.1016/S0736-0266(01)00106-1.

3. Newcomer KL, Laskowski ER, Yu B, Johnson JC, An K-N. Differences in repositioning error among patients with low back pain compared with control subjects. Spine. 2000;25:2488–93.

4. Treleaven J, Jull G, LowChoy N. The relationship of cervical joint position error to balance and eye movement disturbances in persistent whiplash. Man Ther. 2006;11:99–106. doi:10.1016/j.math.2005.04.003.

5. Watkins RG. Acute cervical spine injuries in the adult competitive athlete: football injuries (burners). Sports Med Arthrosc Rev. 1997;5:182–19.

6. Meeuwisse WH, Hagel BE, Mohtadi NGH, Butterwick DJ, Fick GH. The distribution of injuries in men's Canada west university football – a 5-year analysis. Am J Sport Med. 2000;28:516–23.

7. Booher JM, Thibodeau GA. Athletic Injury Assessment. 3rd ed. St Louis: Mosby; 1994.

8. Cantu RC, Mueller FO. Catastrophic spine injuries in American football, 1977–2001. Neurosurgery. 2003;53:358–63. doi:10.1227/01.NEU0000073422.01886.88.

9. Nightingale RW, McElhaney JH, Richardson WJ, Best TM, Myers BS. Experimental impact injury to the cervical spine: relating motion of the head and the mechanism of injury. J Bone Joint Surg Am. 1996;78:412–21.

10. Heck JF, Clarke KS, Peterson TR. National Athletic Trainers' Position Statement: Head-down contact and spearing in tackle football. J Athl Training. 2004;39:101–11.

11. Lark SD, McCarthy PW. Cervical range of motion and proprioception in rugby players versus non-rugby players. J Sport Sci. 2007;25:887–94. doi:10.1080/02640410600944543.

12. Lark SD, McCarthy PW. The effects of a single game of rugby on active cervical range of motion. J Sport Sci. 2009;27:491–7. doi:10.1080/02640410802632136.

13. Nyland J, Johnson D. Collegiate football players display more active cervical spine mobility than high school football players. J Athl Training. 2004;39:146–50.

14. Loudon JK, Ruhl M, Field E. Ability to reproduce head position after whiplash injury. Spine. 1997;22:865–8.

15. Pinsault N, Anxionnaz M, Vuillerme N. Cervical joint position sense in rugby players versus non-rugby players. Phys Ther Sport. 2010;11:66–70. doi:10.1016/j.ptsp.2010.02.004.

16. Lark SD, McCarthy PW. The effects of a rugby playing season on cervical range of motion. J Sport Sci. 2010;28:649–55. doi:10.1080/02640411003631968.

17. Ordway NR, Seymour R, Donelson RG, Hojnowski L, Lee E, Edwards TW. Cervical sagittal range-of-motion analysis using three methods: cervical range-of-motion device, 3space, and radiography. Spine. 1997;22:501–8.

18. Tousignant M, de Bellefeuille L, O'Donoughue S, Grahovac S. Criterion validity of the cervical range of motion (CROM) goniometer for cervical flexion and extension. Spine. 2000;25:324–30.

19. Youdas JW, Carey JR, Garrett TR. Reliability of measurements of cervical spine range of motion – comparison of three methods. Phys Ther. 1991;71:98–104. http://ptjournal.apta.org/content/71/2/98.

20. Dhimitri K, Brodeur S, Croteus M, Richard S, Seymour CJ. Reliability of the cervical range of motion device in measuring upper cervical motion. J Manual Manip Ther. 1998;6:31–6. doi:10.1179/jmt.1998.6.1.31.

21. Revel M, Andre-Deshays C, Minguet M. Cervicocephalic kinesthetic sensibility in patients with cervical pain. Arch Phys Med Rehab. 1991;72:288–91.

22. Cohen J. Statistical power analysis for the behavioural sciences. Secondth ed. New York: Lawrence Erlbaum Associates; 1988.

23. Pearl AJ, Mayer PW. Neck motion in the high school football player: Observations and suggestions for diminishing stresses on the neck. Am J Sport Med. 1979;7:231–3. doi:10.1177/036354657900700404.

24. Pettorossi VE, Schieppati M. Neck Proprioception Shapes Body Orientation and Perception of Motion. Frontiers in Human Neuroscience. 2014;8:895. doi:10.3389/fnhum.2014.00895.

25. Page P. Cervicogenic headaches: an evidence-led approach to clinical management. Int J Sports Physical Therapy. 2011;6:254–66.

26. Sallis RE, Jones K. Prevalence of headaches in football players. Med Sci Sport Exer. 2000;32:1820–4.

27. Guskiewicz KM. Postural stability assessment following concussion: one piece of the puzzle. Clin J Sport Med. 2001;11:182–9.

28. Lee H-Y, Wang J-D, Yao G, Wang S-F. Association between cervicocephalic kinesthetic sensibility and frequency of subclinical neck pain. Man Ther. 2008;13:419–25. doi:10.1016/j.math.2007.04.001.

29. Bey T, Ostick B. Second impact syndrome. West JEM. 2009;10:6–10. http://westjem.com/articles/second-impact-syndrome.html.

30. Iverson GL, Brooks BL, Collins MW, Lovell MR. Tracking neuropsychological recovery following concussion in sport. Brain Inj. 2006;20:245–52. doi:10.1080/02699050500487910.

11

Orthosis reduces breast pain and mechanical forces through natural and augmented breast tissue in women lying prone

Karin Ried[1*], Simon Armstrong[1], Avni Sali[1] and Patrick McLaughlin[2]

Abstract

Background: Breast implant displacement or rupture can cause aesthetic problems and serious medical complications. Activities with prone positioning and loading of the anterior chest wall, such as massage, chiropractic or osteopathic therapies may increase the risk of implant failure and can also cause discomfort in women with natural breast tissue. Here we test the effectiveness of a newly developed orthosis on pain, mechanical pressure and displacement of breast tissue in women with cosmetic augmentation, post-mastectomy reconstruction, lactating or natural breast tissue.

Methods: Thirty-two females volunteers, aged 25–56 years with augmented, reconstructed, natural or lactating breast tissue and cup sizes B-F, participated in this open-label clinical trial. We measured pain perception, peak pressure, maximum force, and breast tissue displacement using different sizes of the orthosis compared to no orthosis. Different densities of the orthosis were also tested in a subgroup of women (n = 7). Pain perception was rated using a validated 11-point visual-analogue scale. Peak pressure and maximum force were assessed using a bilateral set of capacitance-pliance® sensor strips whilst participants were load bearing in a prone position, and breast displacement was measured by magnetic-resonance-imaging.

Results: The orthosis significantly reduced pain, breast displacement and mechanical pressures in women with natural and augmented breast tissue in prone position. Greater relief of pain and greater reduction in mechanical forces were found with increased size and density of the orthosis. Use of the orthosis improved overall comfort by 64-100%, lowered peak pressure by up to 85% and maximum force by up to 96%. Medio-lateral displacement of breast tissue was reduced by 16%, resulting in a 51% desirable increase of breast tissue height.

Conclusion: Our study demonstrated that the newly developed orthosis significantly reduced pain, mechanical pressure and breast tissue displacement in women with augmented and natural breast tissue when lying prone. Our findings are of clinical significance, potentially reducing the risk of complication from prone activities in women with breast augmentation or reconstruction, as well as improving comfort whilst undergoing prone procedures.

Trial registration: Australia and New Zealand Clinical Trials Register, ACTRN12613000541707.

Keywords: Breast implant, Breast augmentation, Breast reconstruction, Implant rupture, Lactation, Orthosis, Pain, Mechanical forces, Pressure, Displacement

* Correspondence: karinried@niim.com.au
[1]National Institute of Integrative Medicine, Melbourne VIC 3122, Australia
Full list of author information is available at the end of the article

Background

Clinical and ongoing management following cancer mastectomy and reconstruction, cosmetic augmentation or normal variations in breast tissue structures can present a significant challenge. Some women experience discomfort and potential trauma in clinical settings, when participating in activities that load the anterior chest wall, such as massage, chiropractic or osteopathic therapies. Clinicians need to be aware of altered breast structures and considerations must be given to appropriately manage and accommodate these patients. A new orthosis has been developed to allow women with natural or augmented breast tissue to increase comfort and protection from mechanical forces in the clinical setting or in some recreational activities when lying prone [1].

Breast augmentation has been controversial, especially in light of the French Poly Implant Prothèse (PIP), leading to increased problems and causing anxiety in the perception of this medical field [2,3]. Recent improvements in implant technology and surgical approaches have assisted in improving the outcomes for many individuals. Implants are not for life and will require surgical revision and management [4,5]. Implant rupture rates vary and may be up to 57% at 11 years, with PIP implants rupturing 2–6 times more often than other implants [6]. The biodurability of the implant is of significant concern to patients [7]. In addition, recent court cases on breast implant damage due to manipulation by therapists were decided in favour of the patient [8].

Insertion of a foreign body produces a normal immune response of encapsulation of the object [9]. The body then requires time for the implant to 'settle', which can be an ongoing process when complicated by reconstructive, post mastectomy or radiation treatment [10].

Positioning or undertaking activities where loading through the tissues of the anterior chest wall occurs may alter the state of function of breast tissue and/or implant material. This can be highlighted by imaging techniques. Capsular contracture is the most common complication of breast augmentation and can result in collagen fibres of the implant pocket impacting the breast or implant material, which can lead to hardening and resultant asymmetry [11].

Our study investigated mechanical forces, displacement and subjective pain levels of women with natural and surgically altered breasts in the prone position, with and without an orthosis, of different sizes and densities.

Methods

Study design and participants

Our study comprised of a non-randomised open-label clinical trial of 32 female volunteers, aged 25–56 years, with breast cup sizes ranging from B-F. About two thirds had augmented breast tissues, most for aesthetic

purposes (n = 18), and a few had implants after mastectomy (n = 3). About one third of women in the trial had natural breast tissue, with normal (n = 7), lactating (n = 2), after lumpectomy (n = 1), or reconstruction by tram-flap (n = 1). All but one women in the augmented group had bilateral, complete, silicone implants, with no capsular contracture, which were performed by infra-mammary incision, either with submuscular positioning (n = 13) or subglandular positioning (n = 4). One women in the augmented group had a one-sided reconstruction after mastectomy (n = 1) (Table 1).

All measurements were taken with the participant lying prone for up to 1 hour during a single day of testing. Magnetic Resonance Imaging (MRI) was performed at Medical Imaging Australia (MIA Victoria) in East Melbourne (45 min), and mechanical forces (peak pressure and maximum pressure were tested at the Victoria University biomechanics lab (15 min). Transport was provided between the testing labs. Pain perception, tissue displacement measured by MRI (4 MRIs per participant) and mechanical forces during prone loading through the anterior chest and breast tissue without and with different sizes (sizes 1–3) of the orthosis were assessed in all participants. In addition, mechanical

Table 1 Baseline characteristics, N = 32

Characteristics	Mean	SD	Range
Age (yrs)	36.7	9.7	25-56
Height (cm)	166.7	7.3	150-179
Weight (kg)	64.2	7.1	51-80
BMI (kg/m²)	23.1	2.7	18-31.6
Cup-size	4	1.9	B-F
	N		
B	1		
C; CC	8;5		
D; DD	8;2		
E; EE	4;2		
F	2		
Type			
A) Augmentation[1]:			**Details**
Primary:	18		For aesthetic purposes (5.2 ± 3.0 yrs)
Reconstruction:	3		After mastectomy (4.3 ± 1.5 yrs)
B) Natural:			
Normal	7		
Lactating	2		2-3 months
Lumpectomy	1		3 months since operation
Tram flap	1		12 months since operation

[1]All silicone implants, bilateral, complete, no capsular contracture by infra-mammary incision, with submuscular positioning (n = 13), subglandular (n = 4), or reconstruction (n = 1).
Abbreviations: mth month, *n* number, *SD* standard deviation, *yrs* year.

forces were tested with different densities (soft, medium, firm) of the orthosis in a subgroup of women.

The study was approved by the Human Research Ethics Committee at the National Institute of Integrative Medicine, Melbourne, Australia.

The orthosis

Made from medical grade thermoplastic elastomer, the orthosis absorbs, deflects and displaces load, protecting the breast structure from trauma and reduces loading of adjacent tissues. The orthosis demonstrates unique elasticity, durability and elastic strain properties, whilst being capable of long term deformation under load. The orthosis is sterilisable in autoclaves and washable with isopropyl, making it suitable for clinical settings and multi-use environments.

The orthosis device loads the sternum, upper and lower rib cage and upper abdomen (Figure 1). Incremental increases in height, depth and width between the sizes of the orthosis provides allowances for different breast sizes and other structural variations and individual preferences. Size-3 of the orthosis is about 60% higher, 9% wider and 6% longer than the smallest size (size-1) (approximate dimensions of size-1 orthosis: W × L × H = 230 × 260 × 35 mm^3).

Pain

Comfort/pain levels were assessed without and with each of 3 sizes of the orthosis. Pain was assessed using a validated 11-point visual-analogue pain rating scale, ranging from 0='no pain' to 10='worst possible pain' [12,13].

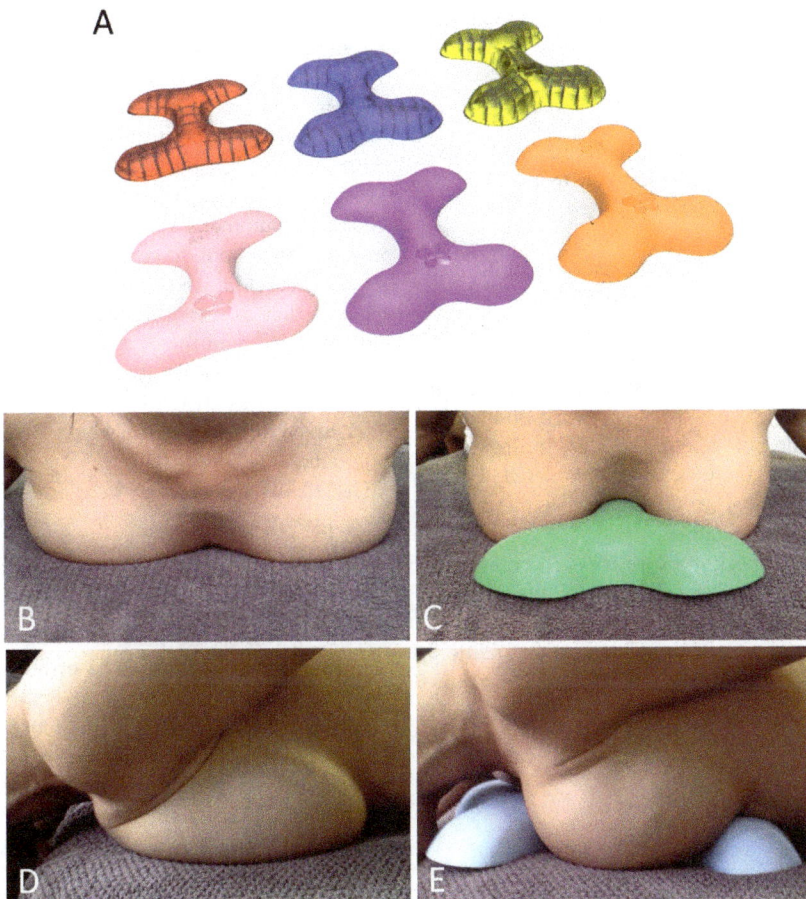

Figure 1 Orthosis in different sizes and densities, the transparent models illustrate the orthosis' ribbing for adjustment of firmness (A); Participant positioning on the orthosis in cephalic view (B), side view (C), lateral view without the orthosis (D) and with the orthosis (E).

Breast displacement and deformation, mechanical force and peak pressure

To measure breast tissue displacement and deformation we used Magnetic Resonance Imaging (MRI) in antero-posterior (AP) and medio-lateral (ML) planes. MRIs were performed to show segmental transverse and para-sagittal mid-breast views, providing linear measurements in millimetres (mm) of breast tissue displacement and compression (Siemens 1.5 T Magnetom Espree) [14].

Following MRI scans, mechanical force assessments were taken with subjects lying prone wearing a 15 kilogram load-vest, simulating therapeutic massage and manipulation loading. Bilateral capacitance pliance® sensor strips were used as a means of measuring force (Newton, N) and pressure (kilo pascal kPa) from the breast tissue. Two 8×25 cm sensor strips with sensor resolution of 1 sensor/cm^2 and a total measurement area of 400 cm^2, sensitive to 4 kPa at a sample rate of 50 Hz, were placed onto a standard treatment table under each of the participants' breasts. Sensors were aligned to a standardised scale assuring comparable positioning for all participants.

Sample size and analysis

A sample size of 30 was calculated to detect a difference of 5 ± 2.3 kPa of peak pressure or 25 ± 13 N of maximum force with the orthosis compared to no orthosis with a power of 80% and 95% confidence [1].

Statistical analyses were completed with SPSS Statistics program version 21.0 [15]. Statistical significance was set at $p < 0.05$. All data were analysed descriptively.

Perceived levels of pain using different sizes of the firm density orthosis compared to no orthosis were assessed by ANOVA repeated measures (General Linear Model univariate repeated measures) with Bonferroni adjustment. The ratio between any pain and no pain was tested by chi-square. Analyses were completed for all participants and by subgroups (primary augmentation, reconstruction, natural, lactating).

Maximum force and peak pressure for each breast side were compared between different sizes of the orthosis and no orthosis using the ANOVA Repeated Measures model for all participants and by subgroups. In addition, different densities of the orthosis as well as sizes compared to no orthosis were tested in a subset of patients (total n = 6; augmented n = 5; natural n = 1).

Results

Pain

All women reported a significant reduction of pain with the orthosis compared to no orthosis when lying prone ($p < 0.0001$; Table 2). The larger size orthosis provided generally greater relief than the smaller size, overall reducing pain sensation by 64-100%. In our patient group,

the size-3 orthosis provided complete relief and greatest comfort ($p < 0.0001$). Average pain perception with no orthosis was slightly higher in augmented patients compared with natural non-lactating patients. The patient with the tram-flap reconstruction did not have any sensation in the reconstructed breast tissue at all and therefore could not report any pain. Generally, smaller breast cup sizes achieved pain reductions with the smaller devices, compared to the larger breast cup sizes which required the larger devices to achieve adequate pain reduction. Comfort data was not captured with the different densities of the orthosis in the subgroup.

Mechanical forces

Peak pressure, maximum force and displacement of breast tissue were significantly reduced for all patients using the orthosis compared with no orthosis ($p < 0.001$; Table 3A; Figures 2 and 3). The larger size orthosis generally reduced mechanical forces more than the smaller size orthosis (Reduction of forces: Size-3 > Size-2 > Size-1 > no orthosis). The peak pressure reductions observed using the orthosis compared with no orthosis were between 58% and 85% for both breasts for all patients, and maximum force reduction ranged from 73-96%. Breast tissue displacement in the medio-lateral plane was reduced by 14-16%, resulting in a desired increase of 15-51% in the antero-posterior plane.

Table 3B summarises subgroup analysis results on peak pressure, maximum force and displacement by patients with or without implants, and by natural, lactating, primary augmentation or reconstruction. Reductions in peak pressure and maximum forces were similar in women with or without implants using the orthoses, while reduction of displacement was greater in women without implants. The effect of the orthosis on mechanical forces was comparable in all subgroups.

The effect of difference densities of the orthosis on peak pressure was tested in a subgroup of women (n = 7). Mean peak pressure dropped with increasing size and density of the orthosis, with firmer and larger orthosis providing greater decrease in mechanical forces (Figure 4). Almost no peak pressure was observed with the firmer variant of the size-3 orthosis in this group of women.

Table 4 provides a general guide for matching size and density of the orthosis to breast cup-size based on our findings and on clinical practice. Women with A-C cup-size breasts generally require a size-1 orthosis to provide protection. A size-3 orthosis can be used, although there is no functional gain in this group. Women with D-E cup-size require a size-2 orthosis as a minimum, and breast cup-sizes EE and above must only use a size-3 device or larger. Appropriate sizing of the orthosis is crucial as breast tissue and implant material must not load

Table 2 Effect of orthosis on pain scores

All participants (n = 31)[1]	Pain score		Orthosis vs no orthosis	Any pain vs no pain
	Mean (SD)	% change vs no orthosis	ANOVA; p-value	Chi-square; p-value
No orthosis	4.8 (1.9)			
Size-1	1.4 (1.0)	−71	<0.0001	0.02
Size-2	0.2 (0.4)	−96	<0.0001	<0.0001
Size-3	0	−100	<0.0001	<0.0001
Primary augmentation (n = 18)				
No orthosis	4.7 (1.8)			
Size-1	1.7 (1.0)	−64	<0.0001	
Size-2	0.2 (0.4)	−96	<0.0001	
Size-3	0	−100	<0.0001	
Reconstruction (n = 3)				
No orthosis	4.3 (0.6)		0.01	
Size-1	1.0 (0)	−77		
Size-1	0.3 (0.6)	−93	0.006	
Size-3	0	−100		
Natural (n = 7)				
No orthosis	4.0 (1.6)			
Size-1	1.3 (1.1)	−68	<0.0001	
Size-2	0.4 (0.5)	−90	<0.0001	
Size-3	0	−100	<0.0001	
Lactating (n = 2)				
No orthosis/Size-1/2/3	8/1.5/0/0	−81,-100		
Lumptectomy (n = 1)	9/0/0/0	−100		
TramFlap (n = 1)[1]	0/0/0/0	no pain sensation		

Participants experienced significantly less pain with the orthosis compared to no orthosis.
[1]The patient with the tram-flap reconstruction did not have any sensation in the breast, therefore did not experience any pain. This patient was excluded from the analysis of all patients.
Ns, not significant; vs, versus.

onto the device but be adjacent to it for correct uses allowing optimal protection (Figure 5).

Discussion

Our study demonstrated that the new orthosis significantly reduced pain, breast displacement and mechanical pressures in women with natural and augmented breast tissue when undergoing activities in prone position. Greatest comfort and complete pain relief was observed with the largest size-3 orthosis in our group of women with B-F cup-sizes. The orthosis allowed peak pressure to be lowered by up to 85%, maximum force by up to 96%, and medio-lateral displacement of breast tissue by up to 16%, which in turn resulted in up to 51% increase of breast tissue in the antero-posterior plane.

Natural breast tissue demonstrated a greater proportional protection from displacement and deformation with the orthosis compared to augmented individuals.

This can be attributed to the implant's fixed volume and inability to simulate natural human tissue movement.

The findings of this larger study are in line with our earlier pilot study [1]. Here we provide additional data on bilateral measurements and a variety of densities of the orthosis.

Our findings are clinically important to provide lactating women or women with natural painful breast tissue a safer and more comfortable option when undergoing prone activities, such as massage to relief back pain. Additionally, use of the orthosis in women with augmented breast tissue may reduce the risk of rupture or displacement of implant material during activities involving external pressure and mechanical loading of the breast tissues, often involved in massage, chiropractic, osteopathic, and physical therapy modalities [8].

Stiffness, fluidity, elasticity and density vary between tissue and implant material, causing shear strains parallel to the patient's plane of contact, and when reaching the

Table 3 Effect of orthosis on mechanical forces

Outcome	Participants	Side	No orthosis Mean (SD)	Size-1 Mean (SD)	Size-2 Mean (SD)	Size-3 Mean (SD)	Contrast	Change vs no orthosis %	ANOVA repeated measures p-value
A)									
Peak pressure (kPa)	All (n = 32)	left	14.9 (7.4)	6.0 (3.6)	4.5 (3.0)	2.3 (2.1)	S0 vs S1:	-60	<0.001
							S2:	-70	
							S3:	-85	
		right	15.8 (8.4)	6.6 (4.6)	4.8 (3.7)	2.3 (2.1)	S0 vs S1:	-58	<0.001
							S2:	-70	
							S3:	-85	
Max force (N)		left	55.0 (20.4)	14.7 (10.2)	6.9 (5.9)	2.3 (2.6)	S0 vs S1:	-73	<0.001
							S2	-87	
							:S3:	-96	
		right	58.8 (18.7)	15.1 (10.0)	7.3 (6.3)	2.7 (3.0)	S0 vs S1:	-74	<0.001
							S2:	-88	
							S3:	-95	
Displacement (cm)	All (n = 32)	ML	14.6 (1.9)	12.5 (1.8)	12.1 (1.7)	12.2 (1.4)	S0 vs S1:	-14	<0.001
		right					S2:	-17	
							S3:	-16	
		AP	4.1 (1.3)	4.7 (1.3)	5.4 (1.1)	6.2 (1.1)	S0 vs S1:	15	<0.001
		right					S2:	32	
							S3:	51	
B)	Subgroups								
Peak pressure (kPa)	Without implant (n = 11)	left	12.6 (4.6)	4.2 (3.7)	3.2 (3.2)	2.1 (2.5)	S0 vs S1:	-67	0.001
							S2:	-75	
							S3:	-83	
		right	13.2 (4.9)	4.8 (3.9)	3.3 (3.3)	2.0 (2.4)	S0 vs S1:	-64	0.006
							S2:	-75	0.001
							S3:	-85	0.001
	With implant (n = 20-21)[1]	left	16.1 (8.6)	6.6 (2.8)	5.1 (2.7)	2.5 (1.9)	S0 vs S1:	-59	0.002
							S2:	-68	<0.001
							S3:	-84	<0.001
		right	17.1 (9.5)	7.6 (4.8)	5.6 (3.7)	2.5 (2.0)	S0 vs S1:	-56	0.001
							S2:	-67	<0.001
							S3:	-85	<0.001

Table 3 Effect of orthosis on mechanical forces *(Continued)*

Max force (N)							
Without implant (n = 11)							
left	48.8 (14.4)	10.1 (11.9)	4.6 (6.5)	1.9 (3.3)	S0 vs S1:	−79	<0.001
					S2:	−91	
					S3:	−96	
right	61.4 (20.9)	18.1 (8.2)	8.9 (6.0)	3.0 (2.7)	S0 vs S1:	−71	<0.001
					S2:	−86	
					S3:	−95	
With implant (n = 20-21)[1]							
left	60.4 (20.7)	17.8 (8.0)	8.4 (5.1)	2.7 (2.2)	S0 vs S1:	−71	<0.001
					S2:	−86	
					S3:	−96	
right	53.6 (12.8)	9.4 (10.6)	4.3 (6.0)	2.0 (3.7)	S0 vs S1:	−82	<0.001
					S2:	−92	
					S3:	−96	
Displacement (cm)							
Without implant (n = 11)							
ML	14.5 (1.8)	12.3 (2.5)	11.4 (2.4)	13.2 (1.6)	S0 vs S1:	−15	0.023
right					S2:	−21	0.019
					S3:	−9	0.023
AP	3.1 (1.4)	4.1 (1.6)	5.0 (1.2)	6.4 (1.1)	S0 vs S1:	32	0.023
right					S2:	61	0.051
					S3:	106	0.002
With implant (n = 21)							
ML	14.6 (1.9)	12.7 (1.0)	12.4 (1.1)	11.9 (1.3)	S0 vs S1:	−13	0.001
right					S2:	−15	0.002
					S3:	−18	<0.001
AP	4.6 (0.9)	5.2 (0.9)	5.6 (1.1)	6.1 (1.1)	S0 vs S1:	13	0.002
right					S2:	22	<0.001
					S3:	33	<0.001
Peak pressure (kPa)							
Natural (n = 7)							
left	13.0 (2.8)	4.3 (4.1)	3.4 (3.4)	2.4 (2.4)	S0 vs S1:	−67	0.014
					S2:	−74	0.006
					S3:	−82	0.002
right	13.3 (3.6)	5.1 (4.4)	3.4 (3.4)	2.4 (2.4)	S0 vs S1:	−62	0.084
					S2:	−74	0.018
					S3:	−82	0.007
Lactating (n = 2)							
left	15.0 (11.3)	7.0 (0)	5.5 (2.1)	3.0 (4.2)	S0 vs S1:	−53	na
					S2:	−63	
					S3:	−80	

Table 3 Effect of orthosis on mechanical forces *(Continued)*

	right	16.0 (11.3)	7.0 (0)	6.0 (1.4)	2.5 (3.5)	S0 vs S1:	−56	na
						S2:	−63	
						S3:	−84	
Primary augmentation (n = 18)	left	16.6 (8.9)	6.7 (2.9)	5.1 (2.9)	2.4 (2.0)	S0 vs S1:	−60	0.003
						S2:	−69	0.001
						S3:	−86	<0.001
	right	16.6 (11.3)	7.0 (0)	6.0 (1.4)	2.5 (3.5)	S0 vs S1:	−58	0.003
						S2:	−64	0.001
						S3:	−85	<0.001
Reconstruction (n = 2-3)[1]	left (n = 2)	11.5 (0.7)	5.5 (0.7)	5.0 (0.7)	3.0 (0)	S0 vs S1:	−52	na
						S2:	−57	
						S3:	−74	
	right (n = 3)	20.3 (14.4)	12.7 (10.7)	9.0 (7.8)	2.0 (1.7)	S0 vs S1:	−37	na
						S2:	−56	
						S3:	−90	
Lumpectomy (n = 1)	left	8	0	0	0	S0 vs all:	−100	na
	right	10	0	0	0	S0 vs all:	−100	
Tram flap (n = 1)	left	10	2	0	0	S0 vs all:	−80,-100	na
	right	10	3	0	0	S0 vs all:	−70,-100	
Max force (N)								
Natural (n = 7)	left	52.3 (13.9)	11.6 (13.1)	5.0 (7.0)	2.1 (3.7)	S0 vs S1:	−78	0.005
						S2:	−90	0.001
						S3:	−96	0.001
	right	51.4 (12.0)	10.1 (11.4)	4.0 (5.6)	2.1 (4.1)	S0 vs S1:	−80	0.005
						S2:	−92	0.001
						S3:	−96	<0.001
Lactating (n = 2)	left	45.5 (17.7)	14.5 (12.0)	8.0 (8.5)	3.0 (4.2)	S0 vs S1:	−68	na
						S2:	−82	
						S3:	−93	
	right	47.0 (15.6)	15.0 (11.3)	9.5 (9.2)	3.5 (4.9)	S0 vs S1:	−68	na
						S2:	−80	
						S3:	−93	

Table 3 Effect of orthosis on mechanical forces *(Continued)*

	side							
Primary augmentation (n = 18)	left	59.0 (21.2)	17.5 (8.4)	8.2 (5.2)	2.6 (2.3)	S0 vs S1: / S2: / S3:	−70 / −86 / −96	<0.001
	right	60.8 (21.1)	18.1 (8.7)	9.2 (6.4)	2.9 (2.7)	S0 vs S1: / S2: / S3:	−70 / −85 / −95	<0.001
Reconstruction (n = 2-3)[1]	left	72.5 (13.4)	20.5 (5.0)	10.5 (5.0)	3.0 (1.4)	S0 vs S1: / S2: / S3:	−72 / −86 / −96	na
	right	65.0 (23.6)	18.3 (4.7)	7.3 (2.5)	4.0 (2.6)	S0 vs S1: / S2: / S3:	−72 / −89 / −94	na
Lumpecto	left	27	0	0	0	S0 vs all:	−100	na
my (n = 1)	right	70	0	0	0	S0 vs all:	−100	na
Tram flap	left	53	1	0	0	S0 vs all:	−98,−100	na
(n = 1)	right	66	2	0	0	S0 vs all:	−97,−100	na

A) All participants; B) Subgroups. All orthoses tested were of firm density.[1] One participant had a one sided (right side) implant after mastectomy. Subgroup analysis includes the participant's measures for the right side only.

AP, antero-posterior; kPa, kilopascal; ML, medio-lateral; N, Newton; n, number; na, not applicable; S0, no orthosis; S1, size-1 orthosis; S2, size-2 orthosis; S3, size-3 orthosis; vs, versus

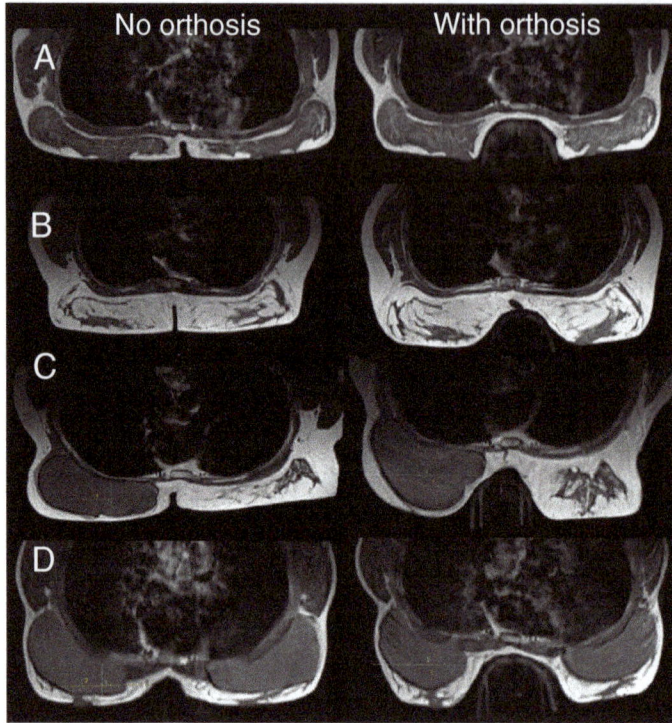

Figure 2 Assessment of breast displacement. MRI transverse view of natural breast C-cup **(A)**; lactating breast EE-cup **(B)**; unilateral reconstruction C-cup **(C)**; primary augmentation DD-cup **(D)**; all without (left panel) and with orthosis (right panel).

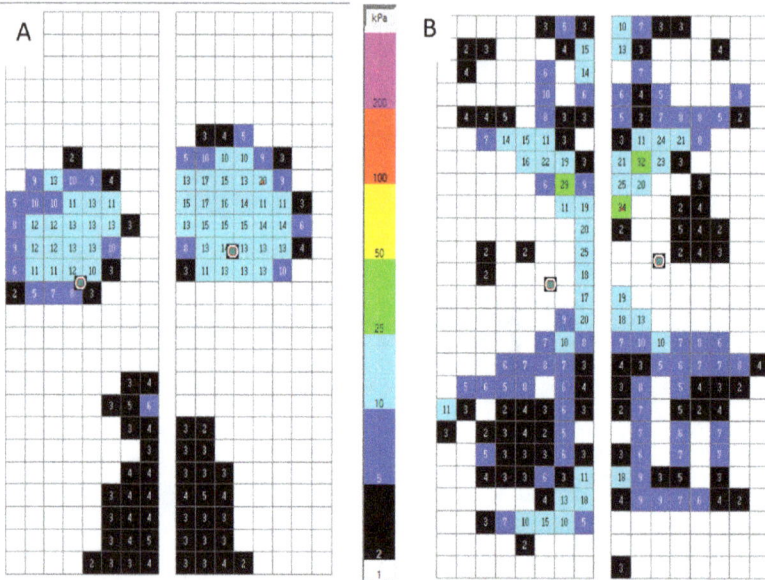

Figure 3 Assessment of mechanical forces. Plane view of loading through breast tissue without **(A)** and with the orthosis **(B)**, where pressure (kPa) is distributed along the orthosis.

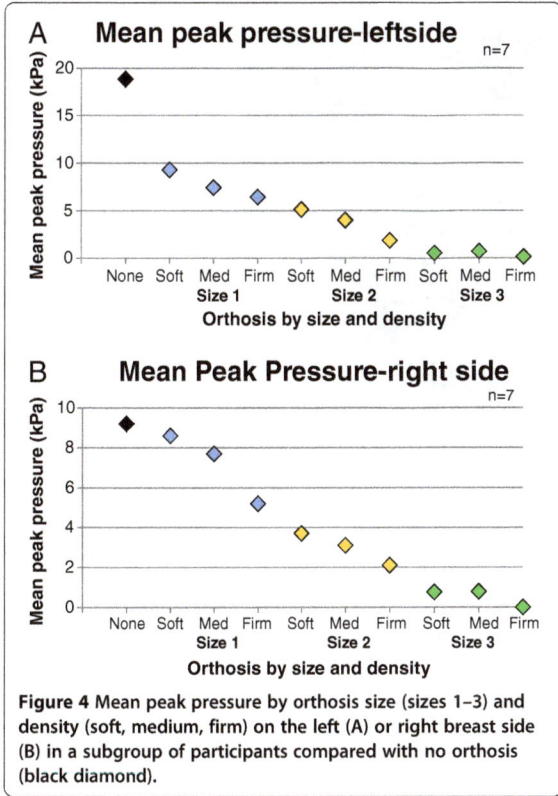

Figure 4 Mean peak pressure by orthosis size (sizes 1–3) and density (soft, medium, firm) on the left (A) or right breast side (B) in a subgroup of participants compared with no orthosis (black diamond).

Conversely, when human tissue fails and the implant moves, asymmetry such as a symmastia or 'uni-breast' is caused [17].

The newly developed orthosis' structure allows for specificity in load distribution, isolating pressure tolerant areas and relieving sensitive areas (Figure 1a). Further research is needed to capture the breast pain in relation to device density and duration of prone loading. In our study, patients were most comfortable lying prone on the size-3 firm orthosis during the 1 hour testing sessions. Our subgroup study suggests that the softer density device provides less loading protection, but additional studies are needed to ascertain whether softer varieties provide greater rib cage comfort when used for longer periods. In practice lighter subjects generally prefer the softer density device whilst heavier subjects prefer the firmer density device. Comfort and correct fit are key to the orthosis being superior to current methods of using towels, pillows and bolsters. The orthosis is reliable in its capacity, its use is repeatable and results are reproducible, which is important in litigious environments.

Professional fitting by an orthotist or primary healthcare practitioner is recommended to ensure appropriate use and maximum protection (Additional file 1). It is imperative that the altered and 'at risk' breast structures be exposed to minimal loading and therefore must be adjacent to the device. The orthosis should be part of ongoing management when breast tissue has been altered. It is advisable that patient have their own orthosis for use in day to day management.

Future research could test the orthosis in situations other than prone, for example in the upright positioning such as car seat travel to reduce the risk of breast implant rupture by the seat belt during an accident [18]. A light harness or fixation system could hold the orthosis in position against the torso. Further larger long-term

limits of elasticity the implant material or human tissue may rupture or tear. Patients who have undergone breast reconstruction using implants after breast cancer surgery are likely to have a higher failure rate than primary augmentation patients, as their residual natural tissues are generally more vulnerable [16]. Furthermore, as implant material has no neural innervation the individual may be unaware of the damage, known as silent rupture.

Table 4 Guidelines for size and density choice of orthosis by breast cup-size, as suggested (X), optional (O), and to avoid (white)

Breast cup size	Orthosis size-1				Orthosis size-2				Orthosis size-3			
	SSoft	Soft	Med	Firm	SSoft	Soft	Med	Firm	SSoft	Soft	Med	Firm
A+	X	X	X	X	O	O	O					
B+	X	X	X	X	X	O	O	O				
C+	O	O	X	X	X	X	X	X	O	O		
D+				X	X	X	X	X	X	O	O	O
E+					X	X	X	X	X	X	X	O
F+									X	X	X	X
G+									X	X	X	X
H+									X	X	X	X

Ssoft, supersoft; Med, medium.
The orthosis of supersoft density was not used in this trial.

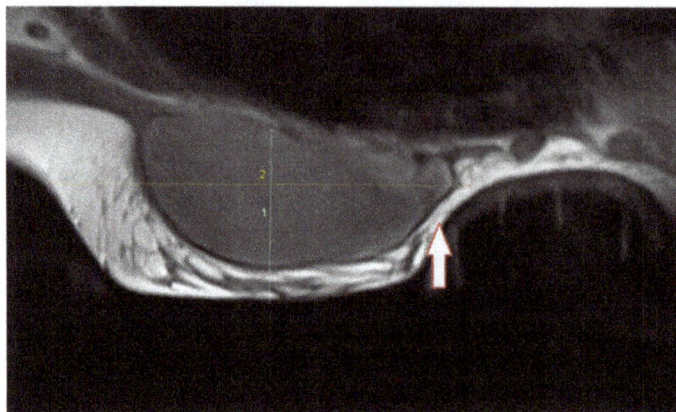

Figure 5 Sagittal MRI view mid-breast of an E-cup primary augmented individual in a size-1 device. The arrow points to the implant loading upon the orthosis, as it is too small. This must be avoided.

studies are needed to determine potential risk reduction in complication rates and breast implant longevity with regular use of the orthosis.

Conclusion

Our research demonstrates the new orthosis to significantly reduce pain, displacement and mechanical pressure in natural and augmented breast tissue in women undertaking prone activities with symmetrical loading across their back. This has significant implications in both clinical settings, and for general activities of the patient in prone position, e.g. massage, orthopaedic treatment. Our study has contributed to developing guidelines for fitting of optimal size and density of the orthosis to reduce loading and increase comfort, also in relation to breast size, and patient weight. In our study, larger and firmer options of the orthosis showed generally greater effectiveness in our group of women with breast cup-sizes B-F. Clinicians placing patients in prone positions are encouraged to use the orthosis. In patients with breast augmentation or reconstruction, to prevent litigation risks, as resultant breast structures are less deformable and may cause greater discomfort in the prone position. Post-operative fitting following breast surgery of any description is advisable to protect the altered tissues and allow for a more safe and comfortable return to activities of daily living.

Consent

Written informed consent was obtained from the participants for the publication of this report and any accompanying images.

Additional file

Additional file 1: Professional fitting guidelines of MammaGard orthosis. **Figure S1.** The manubrio-sternal joint is lying approximately adjacent to the MammaGard name logo (red circle). The logo is engraved on top of the orthosis (refer to Figure 1A in the main manuscript). **Figure S2.** The xiphoid process is adjacent to the butterfly logo (red circle). The logo is engraved on top of the orthosis (refer to Figure 1A in the main manuscript).

Competing interests
PM is consultant to novel.de, but none of the companies and centres accessed for this study were involved in the study design, data collection, analysis and preparation of the manuscript. No external or industry funding was received. The authors declare no conflict of interest.

Authors' contributions
All authors contributed to the design and planning of the study. SA and PM conceptualised the study, recruited participants, and collected data. KR analysed data and prepared the manuscript for publication with contributions from co-authors. All authors approved the final version.

Acknowledgements
We thank MammaGard Pty Ltd who supplied the orthosis, the Melbourne Specialist Imaging Centre for radiology expertise, College of Health and Biomedicine at Victoria University for biomechanics testing facilities, and the Defence Science and Technology Organisation (Novel.de) for loaning the pliance sensors. We are grateful to all the women who participated in the study. PM's role in this work was partly supported by the Australian Government funded Collaborative Research Networks Program at Victoria University.

Author details
[1]National Institute of Integrative Medicine, Melbourne VIC 3122, Australia. [2]College of Health and Biomedicine, Victoria University, Melbourne VIC 3001, Australia.

References
1. Armstrong S, Ried K, Sali A, McLaughlin P: A new orthosis reduces pain and mechanical forces in prone position in women with augmented or natural breast tissue: a pilot study. *J Plastic Reconstr Aesthet Surg* 2013, 66:e179–88.

2. Keogh B: *Poly Implant Prothese (PIP) breast implants: final report of the expert group.* UK: Department of Health, National Health Service (NHS); 2012.
3. Therapeutic Goods Administration: *PIP Breast Implants - TGA Update.* Canberra: Australian Government Department of Health and Ageing; 2012.
4. Therapeutic Goods Administration: *Breast Implant Information Booklet.* 4th edition. Canberra: Australian Government Department of Health and Ageing; 2001.
5. Food and Drug Administration: *FDA update on the safety of silicone gel-filled breast implants.* U.S: Center for Devices and Radiological Health; 2011.
6. Brown SL, Middleton MS, Berg WA, Soo MS, Pennello G: **Prevalence of rupture of silicone gel breast implants revealed on MR imaging in a population of women in Birmingham, Alabama.** *Am J Radiol* 2000, **175:**1057–1064.
7. Daniels A: **Silicone breast implant materials.** *Swiss Med Wkly* 2012, **142:**w13614.
8. Medical Observer: **Judge orders chiro to pay for twisted breast implant.** 2013. http://www.medicalobserver.com.au/news/judge-orders-chiro-to-pay-for-twisted-breast-implant.
9. Granchi D, Cavedagna D, Ciapetti G, Stea S, Schiavon P, Giuliani R, *et al:* **Silicone breast implants: the role of immune system on capsular contracture formation.** *J Biomed Mater Res* 1995, **29:**197–202.
10. Janowsky EC, Kupper LL, Hulka BS: **Meta-analyses of the relation between silicone breast implants and the risk of connective-tissue diseases.** *N Engl J Med* 2000, **342:**781–90.
11. Wong CH, Samuel M, Tan BK, Song C: **Capsular contracture in subglandular breast augmentation with textured versus smooth breast implants: a systematic review.** *Plast Reconstr Surg* 2006, **118:**1224–1236.
12. Farrar JT, Young JP Jr, LaMoreaux L, Werth JL, Poole RM: **Clinical importance of changes in chronic pain intensity measured on an 11-point numerical pain rating scale.** *Pain* 2001, **94:**149–158.
13. Breivik H, Borchgrevink PC, Allen SM, Rosseland LA, Romundstad L, Hals EK, *et al:* **Assessment of pain.** *Br J Anaesth* 2008, **101:**17–24.
14. *Magnetic Resonance Imaging Scanner Siemens 1.5T Magnetom Espree.* USA: Siemens; 2010.
15. IBM Corp: *IBM SPSS Statistics 21.0.* 2012.
16. Handel N, Cordray T, Gutierrez J, Jensen JA: **A long-term study of out-comes, complications, and patient satisfaction with breast implants.** *Plast Reconstr Surg* 2006, **117:**757–767.
17. Spear SL, Bogue DP, Thomassen JM: **Synmastia after breast augmentation.** *Plast Reconstr Surg* 2006, **118:**168S–171S.
18. Nordhoff LS Jr: **Frontal crashes: biomechanics and injuries. Chapter 16 in Motor Vehicle Collision Injuries.** In *Biomechanics Diagnosis and Management.* 2nd edition. MA, USA: Jones and Bartlett Publishers; 2005.

12

An anatomical study of arcuate foramen and its clinical implications: a case report

Salman Afsharpour[1*], Kathryn T. Hoiriis[2], R. Bruce Fox[3] and Samuel Demons[1]

Abstract

Background: The objective of this paper is to describe the relationship of the vertebral artery (VA) to the Atlas (C1) in the sub-occipital region in the presence of arcuate foramen; and discuss the clinical implications related to manual therapies and surgical implications related to screw placement. This study is an anatomical cadaveric case report of symmetrical bilateral lateral and dorsal arcuate foramina on the C1 dorsal arch.

Case Presentation: Out of 40 cadavers that were available for use in teaching anatomy in the university setting, three presented with anomalies of the C1 dorsal arch. The sub-occipital regions were skillfully prosected to preserve related structures, especially VAs, sub-occipital and greater occipital nerves. Visual observations, photographs, measurements, and radiographic examinations were performed between January 15, 2014 and August 25, 2014. One cadaver (Specimen A) presented with complete bilateral ossified arcuate foramina, and two presented with partial ossification of the atlanto-occipital membrane. Specimen A presented the bilateral anomaly which is almost symmetrical. The VAs were found passing through double foramina (lateral and dorsal) on each side.

Conclusions: Arcuate foramina have been shown to be commonly found anomalies with highly variable shapes and sizes, even in the same individual with a bilateral condition. This study found a rare type of the anomaly associated with the C1 dorsal arch, which protected the VA against manual pressure. However, VA, in this case, would be more susceptible to dissection. The presence of the arcuate foramen would also complicate screw placement during surgery. Clinical pre-screening for signs of vertebrobasilar insufficiency is important for chiropractic and manual therapies.

Keywords: Arcuate foramen, C1 dorsal arch, Vertebral artery

Background

The Atlas, located at the cranio-cervical junction, is a ring-shaped vertebra. Normally, the vertebral artery glides easily with neck movements as it lies in the groove at the supero-lateral aspect of the C1 dorsal arch. The relationship of the VA to the dorsal arch of C1 has been well described. Cacciola, Ebraheim, and others have studied the course of the artery and the parameters relevant during surgery in the region [1–8]. Cacciola, et al. injected colored silicone into the arteries and veins of ten cadaveric specimen; and the microsurgical anatomy of the VAs were evaluated along its course from the C3 transverse process to its entrance into the vertebral foramen at the occipito-atlantal (C0-C1) level with

particularly close inspection of the relationship to the C2 vertebra [1]. The authors concluded that the intimate relationship makes the VA susceptible to injury during the surgical procedures in the region [1]. The multiple loops of the artery provide VA extra length which is probably essential to avoid any stretch during neck movements [1].

Certain anomalies of the Atlas vertebra may have clinical significance for surgery, chiropractic and other manual therapies [9–14]. Arcuate foramen have been shown to be commonly found anomalies with highly variable shapes and sizes [1–8, 15, 16]. A bony bridge is formed by ossification in the oblique part of the atlanto-occipital membrane above the passage of VA [15]. There are several names used for the bony bridge, among them: posterior ponticle, posticus ponticus, ponticulus posticus, kimmerle anomaly or arcuate foramen [15]. Of grave concern is whether the posterolateral bony bridge could

* Correspondence: salman.afsharpour@life.edu
[1]Basic Science Division, Department of Anatomy, Life University, College of Chiropractic, 1269 Barclay Circle, Marietta, GA 30060, USA
Full list of author information is available at the end of the article

involve VA compression and/or fixation (tethering). Cushing et al. reported that presence of arcuate foramen caused increased incidence of VA dissection because of tethering as it passed through the osseous bridges of arcuate foramina [9]. The number of patients treated with C1 lateral mass screws through the posterior arch has dramatically increased recently, therefore it is important to recognize the presence of arcuate foramen before performing the Goel procedure for placement of the screws [15–19].

A meta-analysis, by Elliot and Tanweer, demonstrated that arcuate foramen anomalies are not rare [15]. Their report described a systematic review of radiographic, cadaveric, and surgical data. They reported overall prevalence of arcuate foramina was 16.7 %; with 18.8 % in cadaver studies, 17.2 % in computed tomography studies, and 16.6 % in x-ray studies. Standard radiographs cannot demonstrate bilateral versus unilateral arcuate foramina. Elliot and Tanweer reported complete foramen in 9.3 % of patients and a partial or incomplete foramen in 8.7 %. In 5.4 % of cases, complete foramina were present bilaterally. In 7.6 % of cases, it was unilateral. They found no difference in prevalence between males and females [15].

Measurements of arcuate foramina are of interest because of the highly variable nature of the anomalies and their clinical implications. The arcuate foramina may possibly compress the VA. In a study by Krishnamurthy et al., 1044 complete undamaged dry human atlas vertebrae were examined [13]. These researchers found the trait was present in 13.8 % of their samples. They measured the mean length of the arcuate foramen at 7.16 mm on the left side and 9.99 mm on the right side in bilateral positive samples. It was 8.14 mm and 9.26 mm respectively in unilateral positive samples. They reported mean vertical height of arcuate foramen was 6.57 mm on the left side and 6.52 mm on the right side in bilateral positive samples. It was 4.91 mm and 5.38 mm respectively in unilateral positive samples. Besides genetic factors, the researchers discuss that mechanical external factors, such as carrying heavy objects on the head, could also play a role in the development of bridges [13]. It has been suggested that healthcare providers, including neurologists, neurosurgeons, and the medical community, in general, should have knowledge about the present variation and should try to look for it when dealing with the patients complaining of symptoms of vertebrobasilar insufficiency like headache, vertigo, and shoulder and arm pain [9–13, 14, 20–22].

This report describes an unusual finding during anatomy course instruction with cadavers provided by the Life University, College of Chiropractic. Anatomists generally recognized that skillful prosection leads to better visualization, demonstration and description for student learning [23, 24]. Anatomical descriptions of location, relation to neighboring structures, size and shape are often supported by drawings, but not often by photographic or radiographic images [23]. An increase in the use of computers for teaching anatomy has been reported [24]. Our study provided photography and x-rays of this clinically important anomaly for use in teaching. This report will discuss the anomalies of arcuate foramen found and clinical significance for surgery, as well as chiropractic and other manual therapies.

Case presentation
Methods and materials
Prosections are used primarily in the teaching of anatomy in disciplines as varied as human medicine, chiropractic, veterinary medicine, and physical therapy. There were 40 cadavers (20 males and 20 females) available for use in teaching anatomy in the university setting. Prosections of the suboccipital region were performed in routine teaching practices to allow students to investigate the passage of VA between foramen transversarium of the Atlas and penetration of the dura mater toward the cranial cavity. One male cadaver (Specimen A) presented with the anomalies of complete bilateral arcuate foramen, although two other cadavers had partial foramen (Specimens B and C). Visual observations were preserved with digital photography and dimension measurements were recorded (Figs. 1, 2, 3 and 4). Radiographic images were obtained in the frontal, bilateral oblique and neutral lateral (right and left) positions of the prosected suboccipital region of Specimen A to compare the visual effects of this variation (Figs. 5 and 6). These procedures were done between January 15, 2014 and August 25, 2014.

Results
Among the 40 cadavers, only one (Specimen A) showed the presence of almost symmetrical bilateral dorsal bony bridges and lateral osseo-fibrous rings. In this specimen, VAs were found passing through the lateral foramina but deep to the dorsal bony bridge, as shown in Fig. 1, and at higher magnification of the right side in Fig. 2. The detailed dissection showed only the sub-occipital nerve (C1 dorsal ramus) along with accompanying branch of the VA emerging through the oval opening between the dorsal and lateral arches (Figs. 1 and 2). VAs were found passing deep to the oval opening on both sides, they course from lateral to medial, toward the dural sheath at the C0-C1 level on their way to the cranial cavity. The opening on the left side measured 14 mm in length and 7.5 mm in height, and on the right measured 13 mm in length and 5 mm in height. Structurally, the dorsal aspect of lateral foramina, which made the lateral borders of each dorsally faced oval opening,

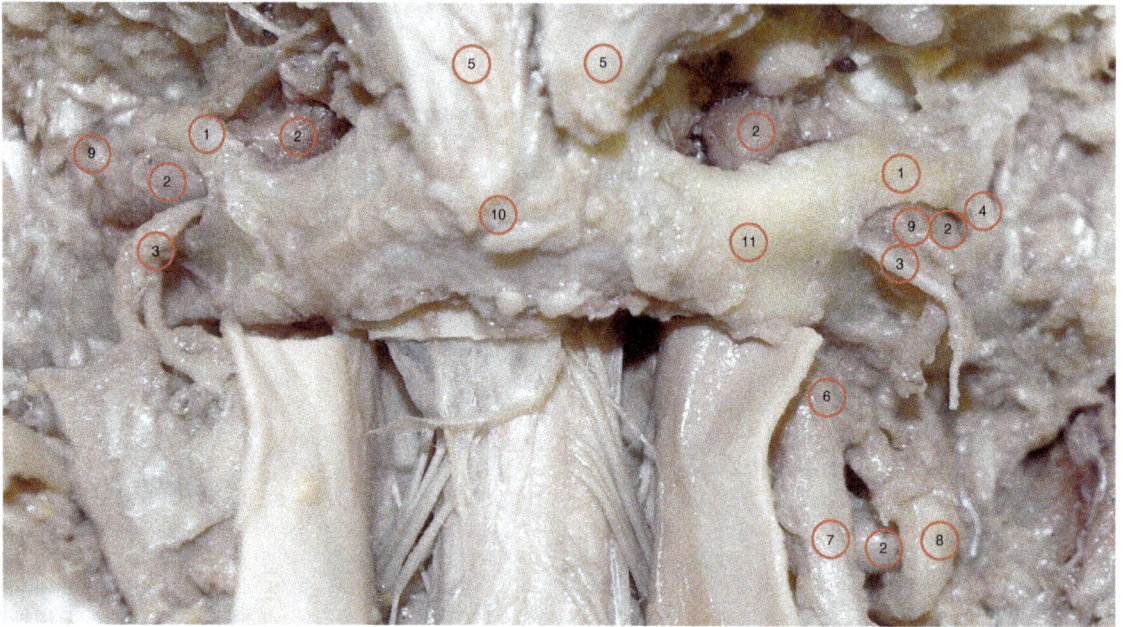

Fig. 1 Photograph of specimen A shows a posterior view of the sub-occipital region showing the atlas with symmetrical complete bilateral dorsal osseous bridges; the lateral osseofibrous bridge; and the oval opening between the two bridges. Also, the passage of VA through the tunnel formed by the dorsal and lateral bridges. The sub-occipitall nerve (C1 dorsal ramus) along with branches of vertebral artery emerging from the oval opening. 1. Dorsal bridge; 2. Vertebral artery; 3. C1 dorsal ramus; 4. Lateral bridge; 5. Rectus capitis posterior minor; 6. C2 dorsal root ganglion; 7. C2 dorsal ramus; 8. C2 ventral ramus; 9. Branches of VA; 10. Dorsal tubercle of atlas; 11. Dorsal arch of atlas

were osseo-fibrous i.e., they were not totally ossified. This border extended infero-laterally from the dorsolateral aspect of the C1 superior articular process to the dorsal root of the C1 transverse process. The oval windows' medial borders were bony. These bony bridges originated from the dorsal aspect of the C1 superior articular process and fused to the C1 dorsal arch (Figs. 1 and 2). The bony bridges were the same length on both sides, but twice as thick (5 mm) on the right side as the left side (2.5 mm). As a result, the dorsal opening on the right side (5 mm) was narrower than the left side (7.5 mm). Figure 3 demonstrates the anatomical relationship with dimension measurements of the dorsal and lateral foramina.

The photographic image of Specimen A showed the VAs were intimately attached to the ossified bridges as they passed deep to the lateral and medial borders of the oval opening on both sides. Branches of VAs along with sub-occipital nerves emerged through the oval openings (Figs. 1 and 2). For comparison, the normal membranes were demonstrated in Specimens B and C, except for a partial superior ossification of the inferior oblique part of the atlanto-occipital membrane (Specimen B is shown in Fig. 4, Specimen C is not shown).

The frontal radiographic image corresponded to an AP open mouth projection (Fig. 5). Radiographic findings included bilateral lateral ponticle formations which consist of ossification in the oblique part of the atlanto-occipital membrane passing laterally from the superolateral aspect of the atlas lateral mass to the transverse process. This appeared as a thicker ossific band on the right with a thinner, and possibly incomplete, ossific band on the left. The lateral image revealed arcuate foramen with complete ossification of the oblique portion of the atlanto-occipital membrane bridging the posterior lateral mass and the C1 dorsal arch bilaterally (Fig. 6).

Discussion

Specimen A showed a unique type of variation of the arcuate foramen anomaly related to the passage of the VA in the sub-occipital region. First, the VA passed from lateral to medial deep through a tunnel behind the oval windows bilaterally. Then, as it passed through the tunnel, the VA gave rise to branches which accompanied the sub-occipital nerve as it emerged dorsally through the oval window to supply the sub-occipital muscles. For comparison, the literature has provided other descriptions of VA passing through the arcuate foramina as well as a description of the normal course and position of VAs in the neck and sub-occipital region [1–8]. The two VAs, as commonly described, were found to originate from

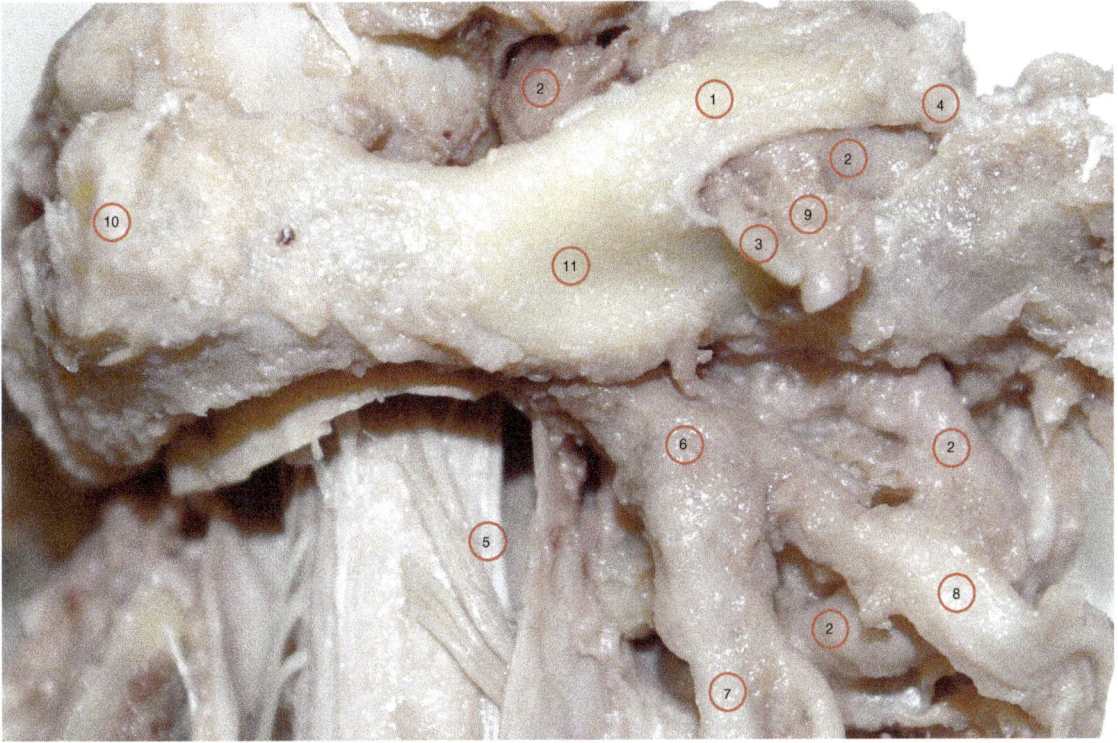

Fig. 2 A higher magnification of specimen A of the right posterolateral aspect of sub-occipital region showing the atlas with complete dorsal and lateral bridges; and the oval opening between the two bridges. Also, the passage of vertebral artery through the tunnel formed by the posterior and lateral bridges. The sub-occipital nerve (C1 dorsal ramus) along with branches of VA emerging from the oval opening. 1. Dorsal bridge; 2. Vertebral artery; 3. C1 dorsal ramus; 4. Lateral bridge; 5. Denticulate ligament; 6. C2 dorsal root ganglion; 7. C2 dorsal ramus; 8. C2 ventral ramus; 9. Branches of VA; 10. Dorsal tubercle of atlas; 11. Dorsal arch of atlas

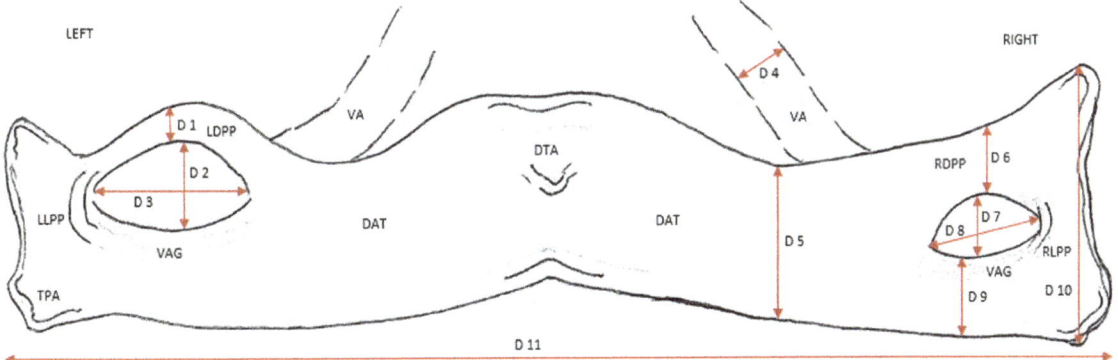

Fig. 3 Schematic drawing corresponding to Figs. 1 and 2 showing the dimension measurements associated with the dorsal arch of the atlas: D 1 = 2.5 mm, D 4 = 3.8 mm, D 7 = 5 mm, D 10 = 18 mm, D 2 = 7.5 mm, D 5 = 10 mm, D 8 = 13 mm, D 11 = 85 mm, D 3 = 14 mm, D 6 = 5 mm, D 9 = 6 mm. LDPP = Left dorsal ponticulus posticus; LLPP = Left lateral ponsiculus posticus; RDPP = Right dorsal ponticulus posticus; RLPP = Right lateral ponticulus posticus; DAT = Dorsal arch of atlas; DTA = Dorsal tubercle of atlas; VAG = Vertebral artery groove; VA = Vertebral artery

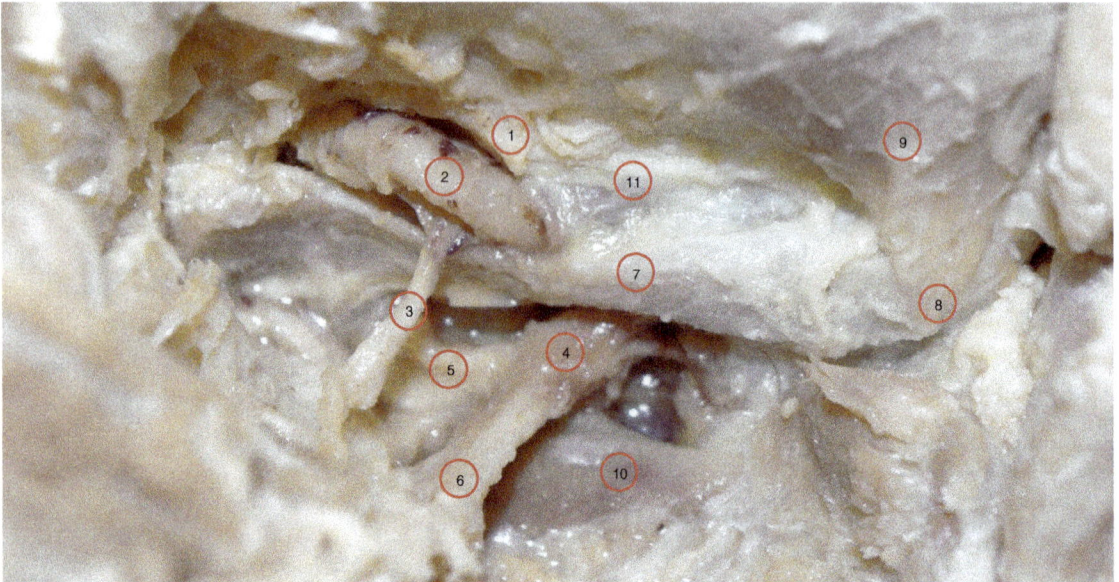

Fig. 4 A photograph of a specimen B shows a left posterolateral view of the sub-occipital region showing vertebral artery passage from lateral to medial under the oblique inferior boarder of the atlanto-occipital membrane. This part of atlanto-occipital membrane extends from the posteromedial aspect of the superior articular process of the atlas to the medial boarder of vertebral artery groove. It is this oblique ligament that ossifies and forms the posterior complete or incomplete arcuate foramen. Note this specimen has a partial ossification of the superior aspect of the atlanto-occipital membrane. 1. Oblique part of atlanto-occipital membrane with partial ossification superiorly; 2. Vertebral artery; 3. C1 dorsal ramus; 4. C2 Dorsal root ganglia; 5. C2 Ventral Ramus; 6. C2 dorsal ramus; 7. Dorsal arch of atlas; 8. Dorsal tubercle of atlas; 9. Rectus Capitis Posterior Minor; 10. Lamina of axis; 11. Atlanto-occipital membrane

the first part of the subclavian artery and then ascend through the transverse foramina of six cervical vertebrae (C6 to C1). In the sub-occipital region, they were found to wind posterior to the atlanto-occipital joint, laying on the groove located on the superior and lateral aspect of the dorsal arch of the atlas on their way to the cranium through the atlanto-occipital membrane then through the dorsolateral aspect of the spinal dural sheath at C0-C1 level and foramen magnum. Specimen B and C demonstrated similar partial

ossification of the superior aspect of the membrane. (Fig. 4 Specimen B, Specimen C is not shown)

The height and the length of the dorsal arcuate foramen in Specimen A were similar to previous studies. In our study, Specimen A measurements of the dorsal arcuate foramen included Length (14 mm Left, 13 mm Right) and Height (7.5 mm Left, 5 mm Right). In comparison, Krishnamurthy et al. found a Mean Vertical Height of 6.57 mm Left (range = 5.24 to 7.36 mm) and 6.52 mm Right (range = 6 - 6.90 mm).

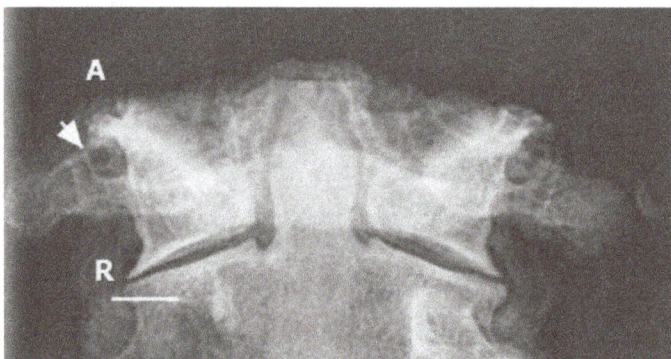

Fig. 5 Frontal radiographic view of C1 and C2 vertebrae demonstrating complete lateral ponticle (*arrow*) on right and incomplete on the left. Linear bar represent 10 mm

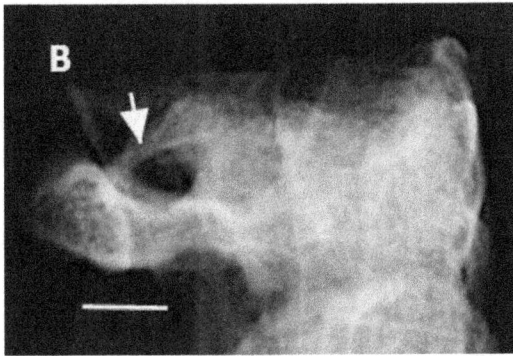

Fig. 6 Lateral radiographic view of C1 and C2 vertebrae demonstrating complete ossification of membrane (*arrow*) forming an arcuate foramen. Linear bar represent 10 mm

Krishnamurthy et al. also reported Mean Length was 7.16 mm Left (range = 5.28 - 9.56 mm) and 9.99 mm Right (range = 9.35 - 10.4 mm) [13]. Specimen A has longer length measurements because of the finding of the double foramina, similar to Tubbs et al. [5]. Tubbs et al. found both lateral and dorsal complete arcuate foramina of which the dorsal arch measured 12 mm in length. For surgeons, there is a discussion in the literature concerning surgical screw placement in the C1 lateral mass through the dorsal arch in the presence of arcuate foramen [15–19]. Of specific concern is how the false appearance of a widened dorsolateral arch would impact surgical decision for screw placement. We found the thickness of the dorsolateral aspect of the atlas arch in our specimen measured 6 mm on each side. Lee et al. reported that they found a measurement greater than 5 mm in only 13.7 % of their specimens with the average measurement only 4.13 mm. [19]. The significance of the measurement for surgical consideration is that 5 mm is the minimum requirement to safely pass a 3.5 mm screw via the C1 dorsolateral arch without injuring the VA, C2 dorsal root ganglion, C1 and C2 spinal nerves during surgical fixation of C1-C2 vertebrae (Figs. 1, 2 and 3).

There are clinical risks to consider with manual therapies with regard to whether arcuate foramina compresses the VA as it passes beneath the bony bridge which could lead to neurological conditions e.g. Vertebro Basilar Arterial Insufficiency (VBAI) [3, 25]. Mitchell and Vanitha concluded that VAs are in danger of compressive pressure resulting in stenosis from hyperextension of the head or manual pressure on the region, especially in the presence of arcuate foramen, during cervical manual manipulation [8, 25]. However Haynes, in 2005, found there was no risk of stenosis using a Doppler examination [26]. In 2001, Cushing et al. reported clinical findings that arcuate foramen caused increased incidence of VA dissection due to tethering within the arcuate foramina following traumatic events, especially with neck rotation [9]. Clinical assessment of classic signs and symptoms of VBAI should be evaluated in pre-screening procedures prior to manipulative therapies [20–22].

Our specimen showed the VAs have intimately adhered to the lateral and dorsal bridges as they passed through but were not compressed. In consideration of the risk of tethering and screw placement, it is important to include advanced imaging when the arcuate foramen is found on x-ray, especially in trauma cases. In 2014, Todd et al. reported on adverse events related to chiropractic care for children and infants but did not include arcuate foramen as an underlying pathology or increased risk for performing manual cervical manipulations [27].

In our radiographic study, we found that the arcuate foramen appeared as a ring-like structure on the lateral cervical view. However, when correlated with the true anatomical structure on the cadaveric specimen, it is not a simple ring-like foramen but it is instead an actual tunnel transmitting the vertebral vessels along with first cervical spinal nerve. No stenosis was found along the course of VAs on either side. Therefore, in such a variation of the anomaly, the vertebral artery is in a protected position rather than at risk of any physical pressures. The lateral ponticle has been reported as anatomically visible on 3 % of cervical radiographs and was present on this specimen, which identified the location of the artery on its course in a posterior - medial direction. According to Yocham and Rowe, no clinical relevance has been found to the radiographic finding of lateral ponticle [28].

Conclusion
Arcuate foramina have been shown to be commonly found highly variable anomalies, even in the same individual with a bilateral condition. It is possible for the VAs to be compressed by the arcuate foramina. However, based on our findings, the presence of such hard bridges over the VA may provide protection from compressive forces. Since the presence of these bridges may increase the incidence of VA dissection, it is therefore clinically significant for manual therapists and chiropractors. Pre-screening clinical assessment of classic signs and symptoms of VBAI is very important. For cervical manual manipulative therapy, evaluation for the presence of partial or complete arcuate foramen is recommended with radiographic imaging. In trauma cases, advanced imaging is highly recommended. For surgical cases, since arcuate foramen is not a rare anomaly, careful evaluation of

dorsal-lateral arch thickness is necessary for reducing the risk of VA, C2 dorsal root ganglion, C1 and C2 spinal nerve injuries from screw placement.

Consent

Cadavers are used in teaching and research with donor consent, which is kept on record in the anatomy department.

Competing interests

The authors declare that they have no competing interests.

Authors' contributions

SA carried out the prosection of cadavers for anatomy instruction and photography, conceived the study and participated in preparation of the manuscript. KH carried out the literature review and retrieval, participated in design of the study and in preparation of the manuscript. RBF provided radiographic expertise and written description of the radiographic images. SD participated in the study design, review of the literature and critical revision of the manuscript. All authors read and approved the final manuscript.

Authors' information

SA has a Ph.D. degree in anatomy and teaches all anatomy courses, including Central Nervous System and Peripheral Nervous System, at the college. He has been published in refereed journals and has presented at many neuroscience conferences. He recently presented a report at a chiropractic conference. KH has a Doctor of Chiropractic degree and has been involved in chiropractic research since 1989. She has many refereed publications in clinical research including practice–based research, case reports and a randomized clinical trial. She has presented various research reports at many chiropractic conferences. She has taught research methods and design for 12 years. RBF has a Doctor of Chiropractic degree and a Diplomate Certificate in Radiology. He teaches advanced radiology courses at the college. He has presented radiographic research reports at many chiropractic conferences and has several refereed publications. SD has a PhD. degree in anatomy and teaches histology as well as anatomy and osteology labs at the college.

Acknowledgements

We thank Dr. Mark Maiyer for his assistance in taking x-rays in the radiology laboratory and Mr. Adam Townsend for help in labelling the figures used in the manuscript.

Author details

[1]Basic Science Division, Department of Anatomy, Life University, College of Chiropractic, 1269 Barclay Circle, Marietta, GA 30060, USA. [2]Chiropractic Sciences Division, Life University, College of Chiropractic, 1269 Barclay Circle, Marietta, GA,   USA. [3]Clinical Sciences Division, Department of Radiology, Life University, College of Chiropractic, 1269 Barclay Circle, Marietta, GA, USA.

References

1. Cacciola F, Phalke U. Goel A vertebral artery in relationship to C1-C2 vertebrae: an anatomical study. Neurol India. 2004;52(2):178–84.
2. Ebraheim NA, Rongming X, Ahmad M, Heck B. The quantitative anatomy of the vertebral artery groove of the atlas and its relation to the posterior atlantoaxial approach. Spine. 1998;23(3):320–23.
3. Taitz C, Nathan H. Some observations on the posterior and lateral bridge of the atlas. Acta Anat. 1986;127(3):212–17.
4. Stubbs DM. The arcuate foramen. Variability in distribution related to race and sex. Spine. 1992;17(12):1502–04.
5. Tubbs RS, Shoja MM, Skokouhl G, Farahani RM, Loukas M, Oakes WJ. Simultaneous lateral and posterior ponticles resulting in the formation of a vertebral artery tunnel of the atlas: case report and review of the literature. Folia Neuropathol. 2007;45(1):43–6.
6. Tubbs RS, Johnson PC, Shoja MM, Loukas M, Oakes WJ. Foramen arcuale: anatomical study and review of the literature. J Neurosurg Spine. 2007;6:31–4.
7. Simsek N, Yigitkanli K, Comert A, Acar HI, Seckin H, Er U, et al. Neuroanatomical study: posterior osseous bridging of C1. J Clin Neurosci. 2008;15:686–8.
8. Mitchell J. The incidence of the lateral bridge of the atlas vertebra. Letter to the Editor. J Anat. 1998;193:283–5.
9. Cushing KE, Ramesh V, Gardner-Medwin D, Todd NV, Gholkar A, Baxter P, et al. Tethering of the vertebral artery in the congenital arcuate foramen of the atlas vertebra: a possible cause of vertebral artery dissection in children. Dev Med Child Neurol. 2001;43:491–6.
10. Wight S, Osborne N, Breen AC. Incidence of ponticulus posterior of the atlas in migraine and cervicogenic headache. J Manipulative Physiol Ther. 1999; 22(1):15–20.
11. Kuhta P, Hart J, Greene-Orndorff L, McDowell-Reizer B, Rush P. The prevalence of posticus ponticus: retrospective analysis of radiographs from a chiropractic health center. J Chiropr Med. 2010;9:162–5.
12. Beck RW, Holt KR, Fox MA, Hurtgen-Grace KL. Radiographic anomalies that may alter chiropractic intervention strategies found in a New Zealand population. J Manipulative Physiol Ther. 2004;27(9):554–9.
13. Krishnamurthy A, Nayak SR, Kahn S, Prabhu LV, Ramanathan LA, Kumar CG, et al. Arcuate foramen of atlas: incidence, phylogenetic and clinical significance. Rom J Morphol Embryol. 2007;48(3):263–6.
14. Chitroda PK, Katti G, Baba IA, Najmudin M, Ghali SR, Kalmath VJB. Ponticulus posticus on the posterior arch of atlas, prevalence analysis in symptomatic and asymptomatic patients of gulbarga population. J Clin Diagn Res. 2013; 7(12):3044–7.
15. Elliott RE, Tanweer O. The prevalence of the ponticulus posticus (arcuate foramen) and its importance in the Goel-Harms procedure: meta-analysis and review of the literature. World Neurosurg. 2014;82:e335–43.
16. Huang DG, Hao DJ, Fang XY, Zhang XL, He BR, Liu TJ. Ponticulus posticus. Spine J 2015. doi: 10.1016/j.spinee.2015.06.040. [Epub ahead of print]
17. Nakagawa H, Yagi K. Advancement in atlantoaxial fixation. World Neurosurg. 2014;82(1/2):e143–4. http://dx.doi.org/10.1016/j.wneu.2013.10.057.
18. Sonntag VKH. Beware of the arcuate foramen. World Neurosurg. 2014;82(1/2):e141–2. http://dx.doi.org/10.1016/j.wneu.2013.10.042.
19. Lee MJ, Cassinelli E, Riew KD. The feasibility of inserting atlas lateral mass screws via the posterior arch. Spine (Phila Pa 1976). 2006;31(24):2798–801.
20. Magareya ME, Rebbeck T, Coughlanc B, Grimmera K, Rivett DA, Refshaugee K. Pre-manipulative testing of the cervical spine review, revision and new clinical guidelines. Man Ther. 2004;9:95–108.
21. Futch D, Schneider MJ, Murphy D, Grayev A. Vertebral artery dissection in evolution found during chiropractic examination. BMJ Case Rep 2015. Published online 12 November 2015. doi: 10.113/bcr-2015-212568.
22. Cassidy JD, Boyle E, Cote P, He Y, Hogg-Johnson S, Silver FL, et al. Risk of vertebrobasilar stroke and chiropractic care. Results of a population-based case-control and case crossover study. J Manipulative Physiol Ther. 2009;32: S2010S208.
23. Vanitha TCG, Kadlimatti HS. Bilateral posterior and lateral ponticles resulting in the formation of vertebral artery canal for the atlas: case report. IOSR J Dental and Medical Sciences (IOSR-JDMS). 2014;13(5):82–4.
24. Haynes MJ, Cala LA, Melson A, Mastaglia FL, Milne N, McGeachie JK. Posterior ponticles and rotational stenosis of vertebral arteries. A pilot study using doppler ultrasound velocimetry and magnetic resonance angiography. J Manipulative Physiol Ther. 2005;28:323–9.
25. Todd AJ, Carroll MT, Robinson A, Mitchell EK. Adverse events due to chiropractic and other manual therapies for infants and children: a review of the literature. J Manipulative Physiol Ther. 2014. doi:10.1016/j.jmpt.2014. 09.008. [Epub ahead of print]
26. Yochum TR, Rowe LJ. Essentials of skeletal radiography. Philadelphia: Lippincott Williams & Wilkins; 2005. p. 269–70.
27. Senger M, Stoffels HJ, Angelova DN. Topography, syntopy and morphology of the human otic ganglion: a cadaver study. Ann Anat. 2014;196:327–35.
28. Berube D, Murray C, Schultze K. Cadaver and computer use in the teaching of gross anatomy in physical therapy education. J Phys Ther Educ Fall. 1999; 13(2):41–6.

13

Back pain in children surveyed with weekly text messages - a 2.5 year prospective school cohort study

Claudia Franz[1*], Niels Wedderkopp[1,2,3], Eva Jespersen[1], Christina T Rexen[1] and Charlotte Leboeuf-Yde[3]

Abstract

Background: Back pain is reported to occur already in childhood, but its development at that age is not well understood. The aims of this study were to describe BP in children aged 6–12 years, and to investigate any sex and age differences.

Methods: Data on back pain (defined as pain in the neck, mid back and/or lower back) were collected once a week from parents replying to automated text-messages over 2.5 school years from 2008 till 2011. The prevalence estimates were presented as percentages and 95% confidence intervals. Differences between estimates were considered significant if confidence intervals did not overlap. A test for trend, using a multi-level mixed-effects logistic regression extended to the longitudinal and multilevel setting, was performed to see whether back pain reporting increased with age.

Results: Depending on the age group, 13-38% children reported back pain at least once per survey year, and 5-23% at least twice per survey year. The average weekly prevalence estimate ranged between 1% and 5%. In the final survey year more girls than boys reported back pain at least twice. The prevalence estimates did not increase monotonically with age but showed a greater increase in children younger than 9/10, after which they remained relatively stable up to the age of 12 years.

Conclusions: We found that back pain was not a common problem in this age group and recommend health professionals be vigilant if a child presents with constant or recurring back pain. Our results need to be supplemented by a better understanding of the severity and consequences of back pain in childhood. It would be productive to study the circumstances surrounding the appearance of back pain in childhood, as well as, how various bio-psycho-social factors affect its onset and later recurrence. Knowledge about the causes of back pain in childhood might allow early prevention.

Keywords: Children, Back pain, Text messages

Background

Back pain (BP) is reported already in early childhood [1,2] and at least low back pain (LBP) accelerates in puberty [1,3,4]. However, little is known about the time of onset in childhood and the subsequent course of BP.

Epidemiologic studies of BP seldom include younger children and results are typically reported for age groups rather than for each year separately. Children are not easy to survey. They may find it difficult to answer a questionnaire due to insufficient language skills and problems in relating to pain and how to grade it, and also because of their limited understanding of the concept of time. It has, for example, been shown that children often have a limited memory of past or recurrent "ordinary" events, and can more easily remember unique and distinctive experiences [5]. As surveys on BP usually deal with recall periods beyond "today", this is a challenge, particularly when questions are asked about pain during the preceding year, a recall period often used in BP research.

* Correspondence: cfranz@health.sdu.dk
[1]Research in Childhood Health, Department of Sports Science and Clinical Biomechanics, University of Southern Denmark, Campusvej 55, 5230 Odense, Denmark
Full list of author information is available at the end of the article

Most studies on BP in the younger population thus concentrate on older children [6,7]. The paucity of valid data in younger children makes it difficult to determine the age at which BP starts to occur.

New research tools allow frequent data collection at low cost, thus removing much of the recall problem and enabling larger study samples that can distinguish between age groups in more detail and over longer periods of time.

The purpose of this study was to generate descriptive information on BP in children aged 6 to 10 years, who were surveyed weekly over 2.5 school years with automated text messages. We sought to obtain answers to the following questions:

1. What is the proportion of children reporting BP?
   i. at least once in a school year?
   ii. at least twice in a school year?
2. What is the average weekly proportion of children reporting BP during a school year?
3. Is there a difference in BP reporting between girls and boys?
4. Does BP reporting increase with age?

We expected the prevalence of BP to be fairly low, but that it would increase gradually with age or that there might be a cut-point when it would increase markedly. We also expected the vast majority of children who reported BP to do so only once, and that girls would have a higher prevalence of BP than boys.

Methods
Design
Longitudinal data from the Childhood Health, Activity and Motor Performance School Study Denmark (CHAMPS Study-DK) collected between October 2008 and July 2011 were used [8]. The CHAMPS study was a large prospective school-based project in the form of a natural experiment [9], which evaluated the effect of increased physical education on childhood health in general. The study was undertaken in Svendborg, Denmark, a municipality situated in a rural area with 59,000 inhabitants. The method of this study has been extensively described elsewhere [8]. The present study used only the CHAMPS data on BP (defined as pain in the neck, mid back and/or lower back) that were collected weekly with automated text messages.

Study population
The CHAMPS study included children in pre-school (grade 0) up to fourth grade in ten public schools. All the children also agreed to participate in the weekly registration of BP using automated mobile phone text messages. To allow for a phasing-in process, schools were included gradually between November 2008 and

August 2009. The study was kept open, with the possibility for new children to enter.

The text message data were collected over 2.5 school years ("survey years"). Thus, in the first survey year (2008/9), the children were in grades 0–4. In the second survey year (2009/10), these children were in grades 1–5 and in the third survey year (2010/11), they were in grades 2–6 (Table 1).

As Danish children rarely repeat their first school years, grade 0 pupils are typically 6/7 years old, grade 1 children are 7/8 years, grade 2 children are 8/9 years, grade 3 children are 9/10 years and grade 4 children are 10/11 years old. School-grade was thus considered a proxy for age.

The study results can be viewed in two different ways: i) The estimates of BP for each grade can be interpreted in relation to the other grades for each survey year (i.e. comparing different children) or ii) the estimates of BP can be followed longitudinally over the 2.5 survey years (i.e. following the same children over time).

Data collection from parents
As part of the CHAMPS study, weekly information on BP was collected using automated text messages (SMS-Track) each week from November 2008 until June 2011, except during the six weeks of summer holiday [8]. Every week on Sunday, the parents received the following question: "Has [NAME OF CHILD] during the last week had any pain in: 1. Neck, mid back and/or lower back, 2. Shoulder, arm or hand, 3. Hip, leg or foot and 4. No my child has not had any pain. The parents were asked to type the number in front of the correct answer in a return text message. Data used in this report related to items 1 and 4. Also information from a detailed questionnaire on the health of the child was available, as parents had filled in a questionnaire at baseline [8].

Quality of the SMS-Track data
The returned answers were automatically recorded and inserted into a database. A reminder was sent automatically if a response had not been received within 72 hours and, if necessary, again 120 hours after the initial text

Table 1 The distribution of school grades in the subsequent survey years

First survey year →	Second survey year →	Third survey year →
Grade 0	Grade 1	Grade 2
Grade 1	Grade 2	Grade 3
Grade 2	Grade 3	Grade 4
Grade 3	Grade 4	Grade 5
Grade 4	Grade 5	Grade 6

message was sent. The SMS-Track data were monitored and cleaned during data collection, and any inappropriate answers (e.g. a response in words) were checked through direct telephone contact with the parents.

The information was collected from parents to ensure continuity in data collection over several years. Proxy reports of children's BP were considered appropriate in this cohort, as self-report questionnaires in young children might be inaccurate [10-13]. A validation study was undertaken in order to determine the reproducibility of the SMS-Track reporting when comparing it with verbal reporting. The sensitivity for the SMS data was 0.98, specificity 0.87, positive predictive value 0.94 and the negative predictive value 0.95, indicating high validity of data [14].

Clinician-generated data

Parents who reported that their child had pain in the previous week were contacted by telephone at the beginning of the subsequent week by one of four clinicians. During the contact the specific location of pain (neck, mid back and/or lower back) and pain history were systematically recorded. If symptoms still persisted, the child was examined by a chiropractor, physiotherapist or a medical practitioner within the next fortnight.

Injuries were diagnosed according to the International Classification of Diseases (ICD-10) [15]. If necessary the child was referred for further para-clinical examination, such as X-ray, ultrasound or magnetic resonance imaging scan. If pathology was found the child was referred to relevant medical specialists for further examination and treatment. (Data on clinician-generated data and diagnosed back pain to be reported elsewhere).

Ethical approval

Ethics committee approval was obtained for the CHAMPS study (ID S20080047) and the study was registered with the Danish Data Protection Agency, as stipulated by the law J.nr. 2008-41-2240. Written informed consent was obtained from parents. Every parent and child also gave verbal acceptance prior to every clinical examination. All participation was voluntary with the option to withdraw at any time.

Data analysis

STATA 11.0 (StataCorp, College Station,Texas, USA) was used for data analyses. Some faulty answers were provided during the start-up-phase at each school, probably because of the novelty of the method. In the beginning it was therefore necessary to contact some of the parents in order to re-explain the correct use of the SMS-Track method. We thus considered the first 9 weeks of data collection at each school to be a pilot phase and data from that period were completely

excluded from analysis. The resulting data for analysis were thus collected over 22 weeks in the 1st survey year, 43 weeks in the 2nd survey year and 44 weeks in the 3rd survey year, giving a total of 109 weeks.

Prevalence estimates of BP at least once a survey year were based only on data from the 2nd and 3rd survey years (as the first survey year did not cover an entire school year). However, analysis of average weekly BP prevalence included data also from the first survey year.

BP reporting was determined for each grade in the survey years, first in relation to at least one BP report per individual and then for the number of BP reports per individual. All analyses were stratified by sex, but where there were no clear differences, results are reported for girls and boys together. Estimates were calculated using one decimal figure but are reported to the nearest whole figure, where 0.5 was rounded up. Differences between estimates were considered significantly different, if their 95% confidence intervals (CI) did not overlap.

Initially, weighted estimates were calculated to give more influence to the text messages from those parents who were consistently compliant, compared to those who only answered occasionally. The high response rate meant that the weighted and unweighted estimates were almost identical, however, and thus weighting of the data was abandoned.

A test for trend, using a multi-level mixed-effects logistic regression extended to the longitudinal and multilevel setting, was performed to see whether BP reporting was positively associated with age. Classes were grouped into three classes per survey year. In the first survey year, grade 0 was considered the first "class", grade 1 the second "class" and grades 2–4 the third "class". In the second survey year baseline grade 0, now grade 1, was defined as the first "class", grade 2 the second "class" and grades 3–5 the third "class". In the last survey year grade 2 was defined as the first "class", grade 3 the second "class" and grades 4–6 the third "class". Children, classes and schools were random effects and the explanatory variables were sex and the three classes. Potential patterns of missing values were analyzed using logistic regression analysis. Missing values because of practicalities concerning changed or wrong mobile numbers were dropped for analyses.

Results

Participants and text messages

Overall participation in the CHAMPS study was 1,218 children (81%) from ten schools. There were 113 dropouts due to children moving away from the municipality or changing to non-project schools. These dropouts were counterbalanced by 121 new children moving to project schools, due to normal demographic mobility [8]. Fifteen children dropped out for other reasons, mainly because answering text messages every week was considered too bothersome. Data from these dropouts were included in the analysis for as long as they participated in the study.

In principle all children were included in the study. However, four children had to be excluded from analysis as they had serious musculoskeletal pathologies at baseline. Thus there were 765, 1164 and 1171 children in the data analyses for the three survey years (Table 2). There were slightly more girls than boys in each survey year.

The average weekly response rate for SMS Track was 96.5% over the 109 weeks with a total of 108,283 observations recorded altogether. No pattern for missing values was found, thus these values were excluded from the analyses.

Proportion of children reporting BP at least once in a survey year

During the second or third survey years, three-quarters of children never reported any BP. The overall prevalence of BP was 25% [95% CI 23–28] in the second survey year for children in grades 1–5 and 24% [95% CI 22–27] in survey year three for children in grades 2–6. Prevalence of "BP at least once" was thus similar from one survey year to the next. Results on grade level ranged between 13% and 38%, when taking their confidence intervals into consideration (Figure 1).

No differences were seen in BP prevalence between girls and boys. However, as seen in Figure 1, BP became more common with age. This was confirmed with the test for trend on the data from the second survey year for grades 1–3, whereas the trend was not recognizable after third grade. Thus BP estimates increased from grades 0–3 and remained relatively stable after grade 3. Similar but less distinct findings were noted in the third survey year, when children were older.

Proportion of children reporting BP at least twice in a survey year

Overall mean prevalence of BP at least twice was 13% [95% CI 11.5-15.5] in the second survey year and 12% [95% CI 10.5-14] in survey year three. Overall prevalence rates were thus similar in the two survey years and were almost half the prevalence of BP reported at least once. Results on grade level ranged between 5% and 23%, when taking their confidence intervals into consideration (Figure 2).

Prevalence of BP at least twice was similar for girls and boys except in the 3rd survey year, where the overall prevalence was 15% [95% CI 13–18.5] for girls and 9% [95% CI 6.5-11] for boys (Additional file 1). As seen in Figures 3a-e., it was not common to report BP more than once but the prevalence increased with age. The test for trend on the data from the second survey year showed increased BP estimates from grades 1–3 and again, relatively stable estimates after grade 3.

Average weekly proportion of children reporting BP

Between 1% and 5% of children reported BP each week, with the lowest proportions in the lowest grades (Table 3).

Visual inspection revealed that estimates were 1-7% in girls and 1-6% in boys. The test for trend revealed increased BP estimates for grades 0–2 in the first survey year and for grades 1–3 in the second survey year, whereas the trend was not recognizable after grade 2 in the first survey year and grade 3 in the second survey year. Similar but less distinct findings were noted in the third survey year, when children were older.

Discussion

This is the first study assessing back pain in age-specific cohorts in childhood, where weekly follow-up was performed over a long period of time. We found that BP was relatively uncommon in childhood and occurred mainly as a single event, thus not as a recurring or chronic condition as often seen in adults. There was a tendency for the older age

Table 2 Number of participants and percentage of females in each grade and survey year

School grade in survey year 1	Participants in survey year 1		Participants in survey year 2		Participants in survey year 3	
	N	% girls	N	% girls	N	% girls
0	133	56%	207	53%	206	55%
1	160	55%	236	55%	237	54%
2	157	46%	251	46%	259	46%
3	155	51%	233	55%	233	55%
4	160	58%	237	62%	236	55%
Total/Mean	765	53%	1164	53%	1171	53%

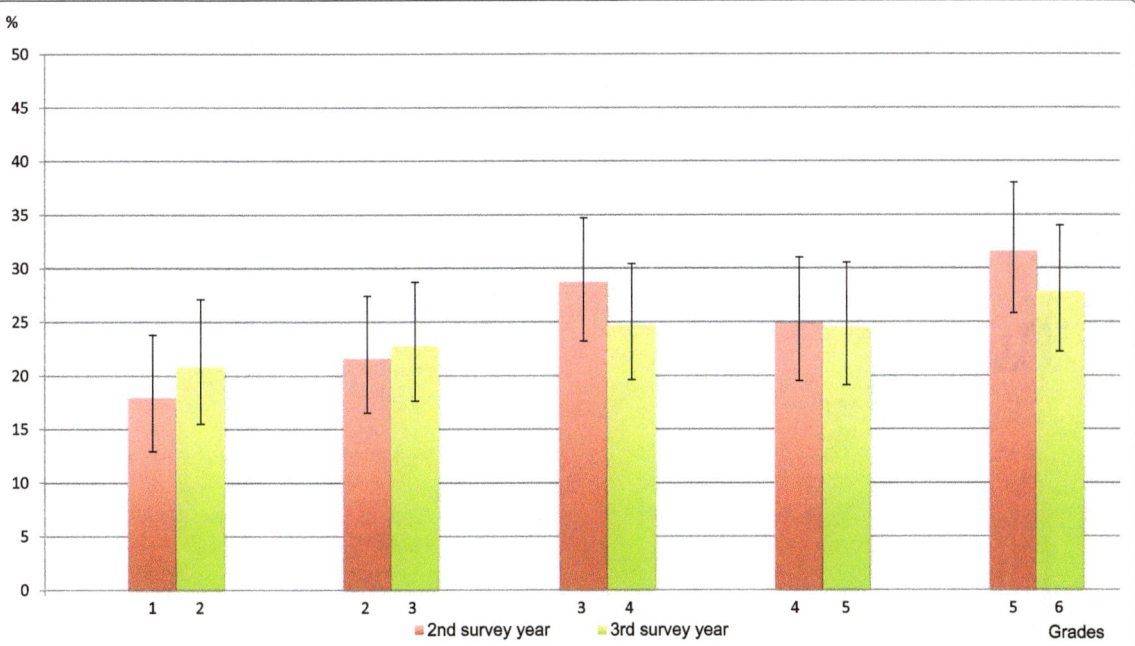

Figure 1 Percentage of children in each grade with BP at least once in a school year.

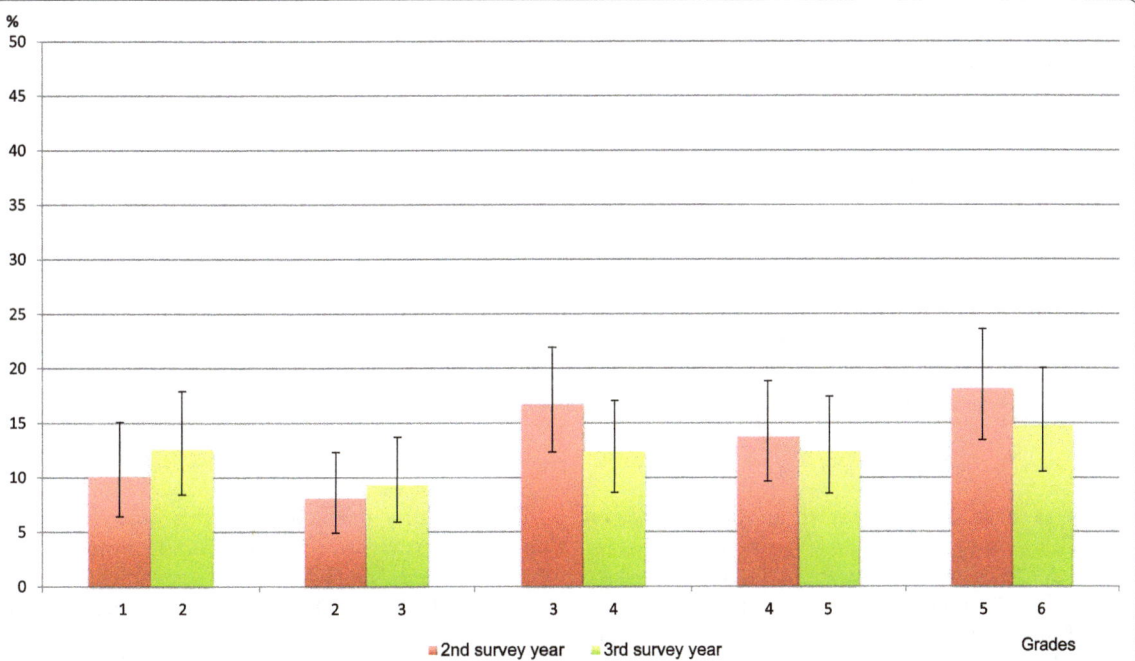

Figure 2 Percentage of children in each grade with BP at least twice in a school year.

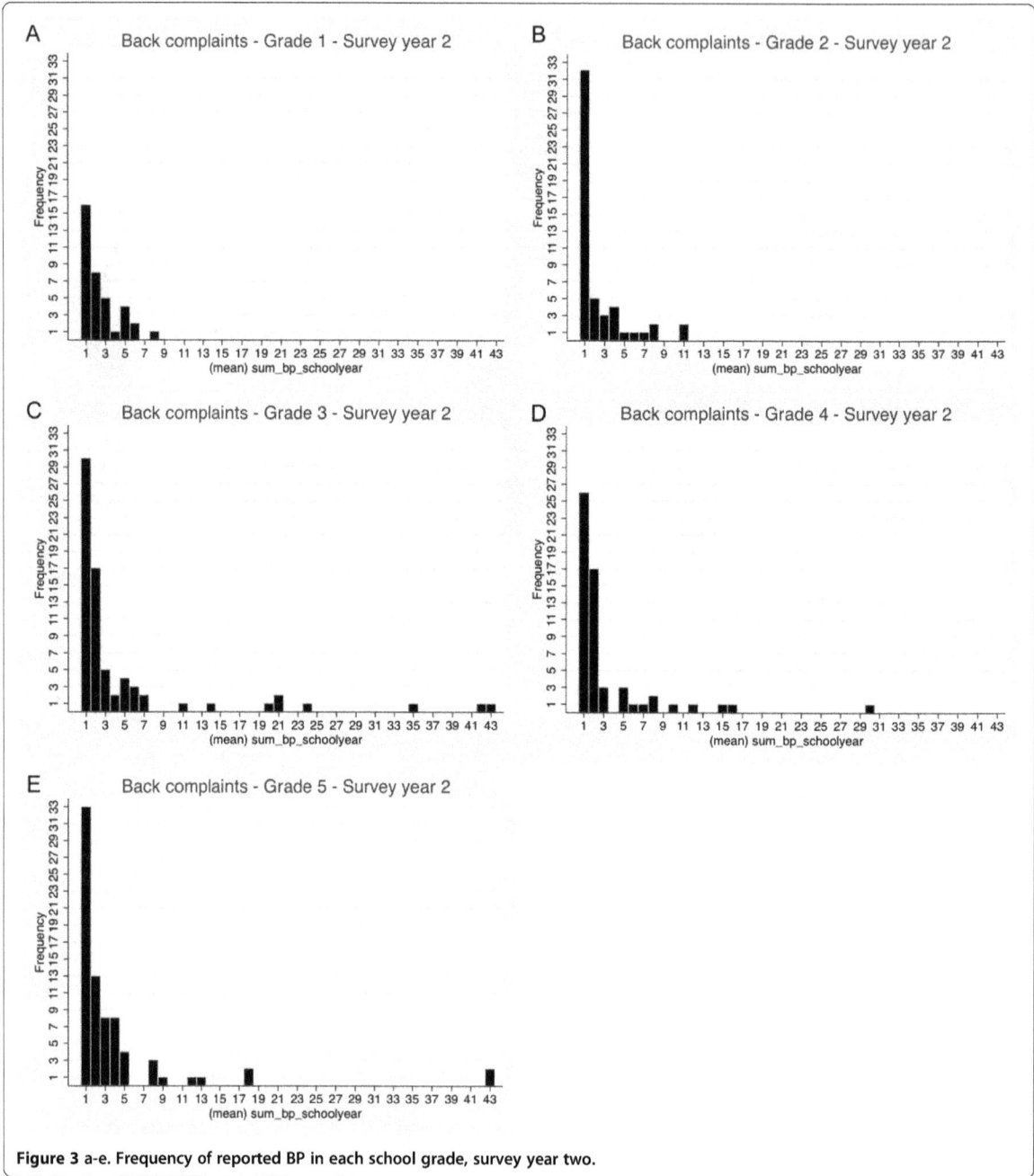

Figure 3 a-e. Frequency of reported BP in each school grade, survey year two.

groups to have a wider spread in the number of times BP was reported. More girls than boys reported BP at least twice in the 3rd survey year. An increase in BP reporting was seen in the first and second survey years, especially in children younger than 9/10 years and remained fairly stable up to the age of 12 years.

BP was fairly uncommon in this study group. In one full survey year, 75% of the 7–12 year-old children reported "no BP". Also a previous study reported that 78% of 11–14 year-olds belonged to the "no BP problem" cluster [16], where BP was defined as "pain in the past three months that lasted a whole day or more, or that had occurred several

Table 3 Average weekly percentage of children with back pain in each grade and survey year

School grade in survey year 1	Average weekly % (n) of children with back pain					
	Survey year 1		Survey year 2		Survey year 3	
0	1%	(n = 1)	1%	(n = 2)	2%	(n = 3)
1	1%	(n = 2)	1%	(n = 3)	1%	(n = 3)
2	5%	(n = 7)	3.5%	(n = 9)	3%	(n = 8)
3	3%	(n = 4)	2%	(n = 5)	2%	(n = 5)
4	3.5%	(n = 5)	3%	(n = 7)	3%	(n = 6)

times in a year" and follow-up was every 3rd month for 3 years.

Comparison to other studies – BP at least once

We identified one comparable article in which BP was reported as at least once over a certain recall period of some of the relevant age group (Table 4). As the recall period in that study was only one month it would be expected that the prevalence estimates were lower than ours. However, 33% of 9 year-olds and 28% of 13 year-olds reported BP [7]. This compared to 25% in our 9/10 year olds and 28% of those aged 12/13.

Comparison to other studies – BP at least twice

As only six of the children in our study reported BP every week for a whole school year, it is unlikely that many children experience "pain every week", a definition found in some previous research (Table 4).

We suspect that prevalence of BP as high as 14% and 17% in grades 5 and 6 [19] were artificially high due to using longer recall periods (e.g. 6 months). High estimates of pain every week for 6-16% of girls and 4-10% of boys aged 12 years [18] and of 18% in 12/13 year-old adolescents have also been reported [20].

Comparison to other studies – average weekly pain reporting

Our estimates for BP would be expected to be higher than results from two studies that asked children only about LBP using a recall period of one week [21,22]. This was not the case, however, as a Japanese study found point estimates for LBP in 9–12 year-olds of 3-6% [22], and a British study reported point estimates of LBP of 6-11% for boys and 9-13% for girls aged 10–13 years [21]. This compared to 1-5% in our 9–12 year-olds, 1-5% for boys and 2-5% for girls aged 10–13 years. A Swiss study reported that 16% of schoolchildren had complained of BP the previous week. However, this was an overall estimate of BP for students aged 7–17 years [1] (Table 5).

Comparison to others - do girls report BP more often than boys?

Girls appear to be more likely to express distress in response to pain than boys [23] and to give higher ratings of pain than boys [24]. Differential socialization or specific hormonal and biochemical mechanisms may contribute to these sex differences [20]. This has been seen also in other studies [1,18,20,25,26] from the age of 13, where girls were more likely to report BP than boys (Tables 6 and 7). However, below this age some studies reported no sex differences [7,19]. Our estimates of BP in boys and girls were similar when BP at least once a survey year was analyzed, but in the last survey year, girls were more likely than boys to report BP at least twice.

Comparison to others – does BP increase in this age group?

Our results showed increased reporting of BP up to the age of 9/10 years, after which reporting appeared to be fairly stable. Previous studies have also reported a significant increase before the age of 12/13 years [19,22,26], but even more after this age [1,6,7,12,18,22,26] (Tables 6 and 7). It would be interesting to follow children into puberty, a time that has previously been identified as the period of acceleration of spinal pain (Tables 6 and 7). As there is no clear step-wise increase in BP reporting, it is unlikely that BP is caused only by the mere "burden of living", i.e. it does not seem to be explained by the wear and tear of physical activities that accumulates over the childhood years.

Methodological considerations

The major strengths of this study are that the study sample was taken from the real world in a natural experiment, and that the sample size was fairly substantial. Memory decay would be unlikely, as data were collected weekly. Bias in reporting was also unlikely, as there was an exceptionally high response rate (96.5%) and data were collected consistently over 2.5 school years, which provided a unique opportunity to follow these children very closely over time. Parental reports

Table 4 Data from the epidemiologic literature on back pain at least once in children

	Mikkelsson et al. [17]	Hakala et al. [18]	Petersen et al. [19]	Stanford et al. [20]	Dunn et al. [16]	Kjær et al. [7]
Country	Finland	Finland	Sweden	Canada	USA	Denmark
Design	Cross sectional + follow up	Cross sect. + follow up	Cross sectional	Longitudinal (8 yrs)	Longitudinal (3 m/3 yrs)	Cross sectional + follow up
Study sample	Pupils from 19 primary schools	Population register. All Finns born on adjacent dates in summer	Randomized cluster sample of pupils	Non-institutionalized civilian population	Girls/boys initially 11 yrs randomly selected in GH database	Primary/secondary school. 38 state schools in one municipality
Response rate	83%	77%	97%	?	49%	62%, 57%, 58%
Valid sample size	1756	62677	1121	2488	1333	479, 439, 443
Data collection	Questionnaire	Questionnaire	Questionnaire	Computer ass. Interview + Questionnaire	Telephone survey + Questionnaire	Interview + Questionnaire
Age group	9, 12 (mean: 9.8, 11.8)	12,14,16,18 (mean: 12.6, 14.6, 16.6, 18.6)	6-13	10-18	11-14	9,13,15 (mean: 9.7, 13.1, 15.7)
Definition of back pain	Pain/ache in neck, upper back (UB), low back (LBP)	Back or neck pain the past half a year	Backache last 6 months	Backache past 6 months	Back pain a whole day or more in the past 3 months	Any spinal pain:
Recall period	3 months	6 months	6 months	6 months	3 months	1 month
Prevalence estimates never/ seldom	BP (UB, LBP)	BP + NP (12y)	BP (6-13y)	BP (12-13y)	BP (11-14y) 78%	BP (9y, 13y, 15y) 67%
Overall: monthly						33%, 28%, 48%
Frequency	Weekly	Weekly	≥ 1 Weekly:	Weekly	Low/high	
Once					10% (low prob.)	
Several/frequently/ continually	12.7% (Only mentioned in the discussion section)	Girls: 6-16% Boys: 4-10%	Grade 0: 2% Grade 1: 3% Grade 2: 3% Grade 3: 6% Grade 4: 7.5% Grade 5: 14% Grade 6: 17%	17.6%	1,3% (high prob.)	

Table 5 Data from the epidemiologic literature on "one week" prevalence of back pain (including LBP region)

	Balague et al. [1]	Jones et al. [21]	Sato et al. [22]
Country	Switzerland	England	Japan
Design	Cross sectional	Cross sectional	Cross sectional
Study sample	Schoolchildren in primary and secondary school (one school district)	Schoolchildren in three school districts	Elementary and junior high schoolchildren in Niigata City
Response rate	99%	93%	79,8%
Valid sample size	1666	500	34423
Data collection	Questionnaire	Questionnaire	Questionnaire
Age group	7-17 (mean 12)	10-16	9-15
Definition of back pain	BP (=all spinal pain)	LBP	Any LBP now
Recall period	Previous week	Previous week	Now
Overall - prevalence week/now	BP (7-17y)	LBP	LBP
	16%	10-13 y: Boys, Girls	9-10 y: 3%
		10-11y: 6%, 9%	10-11 y: 4%
		11-12 y: 9%, 10,5%	11-12 y: 6%
		12-13 y: 11%, 13%	12-13 y: 12%
		13-14 y: 13%, 17%	13-14 y: 17%
		14-15 y: 18%, 21%	14-15 y: 15%
		15-16 y: 23%, 21%	

were used as proxy measurements for their children's experiences of pain, which was both a potential strength and a weakness.

An earlier study [19] that used parental-assisted responses from children in grades 0–4 found rather low BP estimates, somewhat comparable to ours. However, in that study, when the children were aged 11/12 years, the data collection method changed so that the children completed the questionnaires themselves. At that time their prevalence estimates doubled, going from a weekly frequency of 7.5% to 14% [19]. It is uncertain which of the estimates (if any) was the most valid report. Parents are more likely to agree with their child on reporting LBP if disability levels are high [12] and on conditions that are common, visible, or diagnosed e.g. in longstanding illness [27]. However, we do not know how reliable the child–parent communication is on less severe pain and with frequent data collection. We hoped that the frequent text-message procedure would stimulate them to reflect and communicate appropriately. Asking children to report pain retrospectively over months or even a year will probably result in less valid answers and probably overestimation [3,28].

A potential weakness is that our study population lived in a medium-sized Danish rural municipality, which might have a different reporting pattern compared to a study population in larger cities or in other cultures. However, the comparison with the results in other studies reveals only logical differences, more related to the method of data collection than geographical or cultural differences. Other potential weaknesses were that we did not adjust for amount and type of physical activity. As half of the children received extra physical education lessons, this may have affected the estimates, although possibly in either direction. Other extrinsic or intrinsic factors will be taken into account in future studies. Furthermore, data gathered from the clinicians were not included in the manuscript. Also the latter topic will be dealt with in other reports.

Conclusion

BP does not appear to be a major problem in childhood. Knowledge about the causes of BP in childhood might allow early prevention, however, and the topic is therefore important from a public health viewpoint.

It would be productive for further research to study the circumstances surrounding the appearance of back pain in childhood, as well as how various bio-psychosocial factors affect its onset and later recurrence. A better understanding of the severity and consequences of back pain in childhood is also needed.

From a clinical viewpoint, health professionals should be vigilant if children present with constant or recurring back pain, as such a pattern appears to be unusual in this population group.

Table 6 Data from the epidemiologic literature on back pain in boys and girls (age included)

	Balague et al. [1]	Brattberg et al. [25]	Taimela et al. [6]	Hakala et al. [18]	Watson et al. [12]
Country	Switzerland	Sweden	Finland	Finland	England
Design	Cross Sectional	Cross sectional + follow up	Cross sectional	Cross sect. + follow up	Cross sectional
Study sample	Schoolchildren in primary and secondary school- one school district	Pupils from 26 urban schools	Pupils from 45 different public schools	Population register. All Finns born on adjacent dates in summer (1985–9, 1993–7)	Pupils from secondary schools; state + private, urban + rural
Response rate	99%	87%	82%	77%	92% (LBP)
Valid sample size	1666	1245/ 471	1171	62677	1376 (LBP)
Data collection	Questionnaire	Questionnaire	Questionnaire	Questionnaire	Questionnaire
Age group	7-17(mean 12)	8, 11, 13, 17	7, 10, 14, 16	12,14,16,18(12.6, 14.6, 16.6, 18.6)	11-14
Definition of back pain	LBP, BP (=all spinal pain)	Do you often have back pain?	LBP interfering with school/leisure activities + recurrent LBP past 12 months	Back or neck pain during the past half a year	LBP for one day or longer in the past month
Gender	Girls > Boys (+BP ++LBP)	Girls > Boys all age groups. Significant among the 13 and 17-year-old pupils	No general difference. Girls > boys in recurrent LBP reporting	Girls > boys No interaction between sex but increasing trend was seen in girls – boys U shaped curve	Girls > Boys
Age (prevalence increase)	>13	Trend of more long-lasting BP in older age groups. Especially among girls	Recurrent LBP increases > 14, 16	Prevalence increased with age	Increase with age in girls and boys

Table 7 Data from the epidemiologic literature on back pain in boys and girls (age included)

	Petersen et al. [19]	Grøholt et al. [26]	Sato et al. [22]	Stanford et al. [20]	Kjær et al. [7]
Country	Sweden	Nordic countries	Japan	Canada	Denmark
Design	Cross sectional	Cross sectional	Cross sectional	Longitudinal – 8 yrs	Cross sectional + follow up
Study sample	Randomized cluster sample of pupils	Population registries children survey	Elementary and junior high school-children in Niigata City	Non-institutionalized civilian population (1994–5, 1996–7, 1998–9, 2002–3)	Primary/secondary school. 38 state schools in one municipality
Response rate	97%	64.5-69%	79.8%	?	62%, 57%, 58%
Valid sample size	1121	5911 (BP)	34423	2488	479, 439, 443
Data collection	Questionnaire	Questionnaire	Questionnaire	Computer ass. Interview + Questionnaire	Interview + Questionnaire
Age group	6-13	7-9, 10–12, 13–15, 16-17	9-15	10-18	9, 13, 15 (mean 9.7, 13.1, 15.7)
Definition of back pain	Backache the last 6 months	Has the child had any of the following complaints? (BP, headache e.g.)	Any LBP now	Backache past 6 months	Any spinal pain
Gender	No gender difference	Girls > boys in all pain categories	11-12y girls > boys	Girls > boys	No difference in overall back (spinal) pain reporting at age 9 and 13 yrs.
Age (prevalence increase)	Prevalence of bachache higher from grades 4–6 than in grades 0–3 (Method change)	BP + headache most prevalent in the oldest age groups compared to the youngest	Increasing prevalence with grade levels until age 14 (LBP: Point prevalence)	Girls 12–18 yrs > boys 12–18 yrs	> 13 yrs

Additional file

Additional file 1: Table S1. Number of children with back pain at least
once in a survey year. **Table S2.** Number of children with back pain at
least twice in a survey year. **Table S3.** Number of girls with back pain
at least twice in a survey year. **Table S4.** Number of boys with back
pain at least twice in a survey year.

Competing interests
The authors declare that they have no competing interests.

Authors' contributions
NW was responsible for the overall study concept and design. CF, EJ, CTR
and NW were responsible for the acquisition of text messaging data. CF and
NW were responsible for the analysis and interpretation of data. CF and
CY drafted the manuscript. All authors took part in a critical revision of the
manuscript. All authors read and approved the final manuscript. NW
obtained the funding. The study was supported by grants from the Danish
Chiropractors' Foundation, The IMK Foundation, The Nordea Foundation, The
Tryg Foundation – all private, non-profit organisations, which support research
in health prevention and treatment. TEAM Denmark, the elite sport organisation
in Denmark, provided the grant for the text messaging system.

Acknowledgements
The authors would like to thank the participants, their parents and the
participating schools, The Svendborg Project and the municipality of
Svendborg. The authors wish to acknowledge the members of the CHAMPS
Study-DK not listed as coauthors of this paper: H. Klakk and T. Junge. Finally,
the authors would like to acknowledge K Froberg and LB Andersen, Research
in Childhood Health, Department of Sports Science and Clinical Biomechanics,
University of Southern Denmark.

Author details
[1]Research in Childhood Health, Department of Sports Science and Clinical
Biomechanics, University of Southern Denmark, Campusvej 55, 5230 Odense,
Denmark. [2]The Sport Medicine Clinic, Orthopaedic Department, Hospital of
Lillebaelt, Lillebaelt, Denmark. [3]Research Department, Spine Center of
Southern Denmark, Hospital Lillebaelt, Middelfart and Institute of Regional
Health Services Research, University of Southern Denmark, Denmark.

References
1. Balague F, Dutoit G, Waldburger M: **Low back pain in schoolchildren.
   An epidemiological study.** *Scand J Rehabil Med* 1988, **20:**175–179.
2. Troussier B, Davoine P, de Gaudemaris R, Fauconnier J, Phelip X: **Back pain
   in school children. A study among 1178 pupils.** *Scand J Rehabil Med* 1994,
   26:143–146.
3. Burton AK, Clarke RD, McClune TD, Tillotson KM: **The natural history of low
   back pain in adolescents.** *Spine (Phila Pa 1976)* 1996, **21:**2323–2328.
4. LeResche L, Mancl LA, Drangsholt MT, Saunders K, Korff MV: **Relationship of
   pain and symptoms to pubertal development in adolescents.** *Pain* 2005,
   118:201–209.
5. von Baeyer CL, Marche TA, Rocha EM, Salmon K: **Children's memory for
   pain: overview and implications for practice.** *J Pain* 2004, **5:**241–249.
6. Taimela S, Kujala UM, Salminen JJ, Viljanen T: **The prevalence of low back
   pain among children and adolescents. A nationwide, cohort-based
   questionnaire survey in Finland.** *Spine (Phila Pa 1976)* 1997, **22:**1132–1136.
7. Kjaer P, Wedderkopp N, Korsholm L, Leboeuf-Yde C: **Prevalence and
   tracking of back pain from childhood to adolescence.** *BMC Musculoskelet
   Disord* 2011, **12:**98.
8. Wedderkopp N, Jespersen E, Franz C, Klakk H, Heidemann M, Christiansen C,
   Moller NC, Leboeuf-Yde C: **Study protocol. The Childhood Health, Activity,
   and Motor Performance School Study Denmark (The CHAMPS-study DK).**
   BMC Pediatr 2012, **12:**128.
9. Craig P, Cooper C, Gunnell D, Haw S, Lawson K, Macintyre S, Ogilvie D,
   Petticrew M, Reeves B, Sutton M, Thompson S: **Using natural experiments
   to evaluate population health interventions: new Medical Research
   Council guidance.** *J Epidemiol Community Health* 2012, **66:**1182–1186.
10. Baranowski T, Smith M, Baranowski J, Wang DT, Doyle C, Lin LS, Hearn MD,
    Resnicow K: **Low validity of a seven-item fruit and vegetable food frequency
    questionnaire among third-grade students.** *J Am Diet Assoc* 1997, **97:**66–68.
11. Peterson L, Harbeck C, Moreno A: **Measures of children's injuries: self-reported
    versus maternal-reported events with temporally proximal versus delayed
    reporting.** *J Pediatr Psychol* 1993, **18:**133–147.
12. Watson KD, Papageorgiou AC, Jones GT, Taylor S, Symmons DP, Silman AJ,
    Macfarlane GJ: **Low back pain in schoolchildren: occurrence and
    characteristics.** *Pain* 2002, **97:**87–92.
13. Szpalski M, Gunzburg R, Balague F, Nordin M, Melot C: **A 2-year prospective
    longitudinal study on low back pain in primary school children.** *Eur Spine
    J* 2002, **11:**459–464.
14. Kaalstad C: **TA: Ryggproblemer hos barn og kvaliteten av datainnsamling
    i et epidemiologisk studie.** In *Master thesis.* University of Southern
    Denmark: Sports Science and Clinical Biomechanics Department; 2011.
15. World Health Organization: *International statistical classification of diseases
    and related health problems. ICD-10. Tenth revision, Volume 1.* Geneva; 1992.
16. Dunn KM, Jordan KP, Mancl L, Drangsholt MT, Le Resche L: **Trajectories of
    pain in adolescents: a prospective cohort study.** *Pain* 2011, **152:**66–73.
17. Mikkelsson M, Salminen JJ, Kautiainen H: **Non-specific musculoskeletal
    pain in preadolescents. Prevalence and 1-year persistence.** *Pain* 1997,
    73:29–35.
18. Hakala P, Rimpela A, Salminen JJ, Virtanen SM, Rimpela M: **Back, neck, and
    shoulder pain in Finnish adolescents: national cross sectional surveys.**
    BMJ 2002, **325:**743.
19. Petersen S, Bergstrom E, Brulin C: **High prevalence of tiredness and pain
    in young schoolchildren.** *Scand J Public Health* 2003, **31:**367–374.
20. Stanford EA, Chambers CT, Biesanz JC, Chen E: **The frequency, trajectories
    and predictors of adolescent recurrent pain: a population-based
    approach.** *Pain* 2008, **138:**11–21.
21. Jones MA, Stratton G, Reilly T, Unnithan VB: **A school-based survey of
    recurrent non-specific low-back pain prevalence and consequences in
    children.** *Health Educ Res* 2004, **19:**284–289.
22. Sato T, Ito T, Hirano T, Morita O, Kikuchi R, Endo N, Tanabe N: **Low back
    pain in childhood and adolescence: a cross-sectional study in Niigata
    City.** *Eur Spine J* 2008, **17:**1441–1447.
23. Fearon I, McGrath PJ, Achat H: **'Booboos': the study of everyday pain
    among young children.** *Pain* 1996, **68:**55–62.
24. Chambers CT, Giesbrecht K, Craig KD, Bennett SM, Huntsman E: **A comparison
    of faces scales for the measurement of pediatric pain: children's and
    parents' ratings.** *Pain* 1999, **83:**25–35.
25. Brattberg G: **The incidence of back pain and headache among Swedish
    school children.** *Qual Life Res* 1994, **3**(Suppl 1):S27–S31.
26. Groholt EK, Stigum H, Nordhagen R, Kohler L: **Recurrent pain in children,
    socio-economic factors and accumulation in families.** *Eur J Epidemiol*
    2003, **18:**965–975.
27. Sweeting H, West P: **Health at age 11: reports from schoolchildren and
    their parents.** *Arch Dis Child* 1998, **78:**427–434.
28. van den Brink M, Bandell-Hoekstra EN, Abu-Saad HH: **The occurrence of
    recall bias in pediatric headache: a comparison of questionnaire and
    diary data.** *Headache* 2001, **41:**11–20.

14

A non-randomised experimental feasibility study into the immediate effect of three different spinal manipulative protocols on kicking speed performance in soccer players

Kyle Colin Deutschmann[1], Andrew Douglas Jones[2] and Charmaine Maria Korporaal[3*]

Abstract

Background: The most utilized soccer kicking method is the instep kicking technique. Decreased motion in spinal joint segments results in adverse biomechanical changes within in the kinematic chain. These changes may be linked to a negative impact on soccer performance. This study tested the immediate effect of lumbar spine and sacroiliac manipulation alone and in combination on the kicking speed of uninjured soccer players.

Methods: This 2010 prospective, pre-post experimental, single-blinded (subject) required forty asymptomatic soccer players, from regional premier league teams, who were purposely allocated to one of four groups (based on the evaluation of the players by two blinded motion palpators). Segment dysfunction was either localized to the lumbar spine (Group 1), sacroiliac joint (Group 2), the lumbar spine and sacroiliac joint (Group 3) or not present in the sham laser group (Group 4). All players underwent a standardized warm-up before the pre-measurements. Manipulative intervention followed after which post-measurements were completed. Measurement outcomes included range of motion changes (digital inclinometer); kicking speed (Speed Trac™ Speed Sport Radar) and the subjects' perception of a change in kicking speed. SPSS version 15.0 was used to analyse the data, with repeated measures ANOVA and a p-value <0.05 (CI 95%).

Results: Lumbar spine manipulation resulted in significant range of motion increases in left and right rotation. Sacroiliac manipulation resulted in no significant changes in the lumbar range of motion. Combination manipulative interventions resulted in significant range of motion increases in lumbar extension, right rotation and right SI joint flexion. There was a significant increase in kicking speed post intervention for all three manipulative intervention groups (when compared to sham). A significant correlation was seen between Likert based-scale subjects' perception of change in kicking speed post intervention and the objective results obtained.

Conclusions: This pilot study showed that lumbar spine manipulation combined with SI joint manipulation, resulted in an effective intervention for short-term increases in kicking speed/performance. However, the lack of an *a priori* analysis, a larger sample size and an unblinded outcome measures assessor requires that this study be repeated, addressing these concerns and for these outcomes to be validated.

Keywords: Chiropractic, Manipulation, Athletic performance, Soccer

* Correspondence: charmak@dut.ac.za
[3]Department of Chiropractic and Somatology, Chiropractic Programme, M. Tech:Chiropractic, CCFC, CCSP, ICSSD, Durban University of Technology, Durban, South Africa
Full list of author information is available at the end of the article

Introduction

The instep kicking technique is the most commonly used kicking technique in soccer, which allows the development of an optimum kicking speed [1-3]. This kicking technique requires that the power is generated through the co-ordinated effort of the muscles and the motion of all the joints involved (viz. lumbar spine, sacroiliac joint, hip, knee and foot and ankle) [4,5]. Thus, this kicking technique's biomechanics are seen as a segmented motion pattern sequence which initiates from the at the spine and moves distally down the open biomechanical chain [4-7]. As, the lumbar spine and sacroiliac joint are both proximal parts of this biomechanical chain, they form the basis for motion which follows the open chain movement pattern, and thus initiate the forward motion during kicking [2,5]. Thus musculoskeletal co-ordination forms the basis for the kicking action and closely controls the compression forces being transferred towards the spine, stabilising and keeping the upper body balanced and upright, whilst transmitting the requires forces down the kinematic chain [8].

To achieve the above, the player's approach or backswing phase of the kicking technique requires that the lumbar spine rotates posteriorly and extends allowing the trunk to rotate towards the kicking leg [2,9,10]. At the end of the swing limb loading phase the lumbar spine is rotated and extended, in accordance with soccer technique, in order to appropriately load the thoracolumbar fascia for recoil and wind up prior to the kick. This increase in musculo-ligamentous torque during in the wind up, allows for maximum distance to be achieved when striking the ball. Once, the swing phase is initiated by the trunk, the lumbar spine rotates towards the supporting leg to transfer momentum from the larger proximal segments to the distal smaller ones, in order to accelerate the kicking limb into flexion at the hip [2,9,10], as it speeds towards the ball.

At this point Cohan [11] and Gilchrist et al., [8], concur that the hip and sacroiliac musculature are required to work together to effect movement of the pelvis (for example hip joint extension causes anterior pelvic tilt and extending the SI joint). Similarly, hip flexion is associated with posterior pelvic tilt and allows the SI joint to assume a flexed position [2]. By contrast, during the foot planting phase, the SI joint is active in absorbing and controlling the force being transmitted through the body and down the biomechanical chain, as a result of the ground reactive force acting on the limb [2].

It is therefore evident that the instep soccer kick is a complex maneuver, on which the outcome of a soccer game depends [12,13]. Thus, players are expected to perform this "routine action" at their maximum potential every time they kick the ball to score. This co-ordination of this components of this complex maneuver impacts

on the kicking speed [direct result of a summation of forces created by the musculoskeletal basis of the kick and its generated momentum down the biomechanical chain] [2,4,5,8]. In addition, an increase in the distance over which the open kinematic chain can move, it is hypothesized that there will be an increase in the potential to achieve a higher foot speed at the point of impact [2,9,10,14].

This hypothesis concurs with the literature, which indicates that when immobilization or restricted motion exists within any of these joint segments, it results in adverse changes in the surrounding ligaments, tendons, muscular tissue and vascular elements [15-17]. It is through these functional impairments with a loss of tensile strength of ligaments, adhesions formation [15,16,18,19], loss of muscular or ligamentous flexibility and joint range of motion (ROM) decreases [17,19-22], that performance may be decreased . Therefore it is the opinion of several authors that improved spinal joint mobility and muscle flexibility can be achieved through the use of manipulation [15,16,22-25].

Thus the restoration of normal biomechanics and neurological input [26-29], increased flexibility and mobility of joints and surrounding tissues resulting from manipulation [23,30,31] may result in increased speed of the biomechanical chain during the kicking motion.

There is however, limited published literature on the immediate post manipulation effect of manipulation on the ROM of the low back joints in asymptomatic subjects. Therefore, this study determined whether manipulation of the lumbar spine and the sacroiliac joints increased the ROM at within these anatomical regions (measured goniometrically) and whether this was associated with changes in kicking speed and the subjective perception of the kicking ability.

Method

Recruitment and informed consent

On Institutional Research and Ethics Committee of the Durban University of Technology (034/10) approval of this study in 2010, the subjects were recruited after permission was received from the Highway Action Center. Players were informed of the study by the placement of advertisements at the arena and through word of mouth. In addition players in the regional premier league teams were approached by the researcher in order to request participation (convenience sampling) [32]. Subsequent interaction with the potential subjects required that the soccer players read and understood the letter of information and informed consent as approved by the IRB and agreed to participate by voluntarily signing the informed consent.

On agreement to participate the subjects were then required to undergo a clinical assessment (case history, physical and orthopedic examinations), which was administered at the Chiropractic Day Clinic, to ensure that the subjects complied with the inclusion criteria.

Sample size and allocation
A sample size of 40, asymptomatic subjects was required for this study, resulting in ten subjects in each of four intervention groups. Due to the lack of access to national league teams, the researcher was limited to regional premier league teams. This resulted in a relatively small sample pool (approximately 75 soccer players) from which to draw subjects for this study. As a result the sample size was based on a pragmatic decision rather than a statistical evaluation of sample size (viz. *a prior* analysis).

The subjects were purposively assigned to one of four intervention groups, based on the level of the motion segment dysfunction. This was based on a standardised motion palpation protocol developed from Bergmann and Peterson [21], Schafer and Faye [33] and Bergmann, Peterson and Lawrence [34], of the lumbar spine and sacroiliac joints. This procedure was performed independently by both the researcher and the clinical supervisor [35]. The subjects were allocated to their respective group - lumbar spine (Group 1), sacroiliac joint (Group 2), the lumbar spine and sacroiliac joint (Group 3) - by those joint dysfunctions that were commonly agreed to by the researcher and the clinical supervisor. Those subjects with no joint dysfunction in the palpated joints were placed into Group 4.

Sample characteristics
Subjects were required to be males, between the ages of 18 to 35 and had to be soccer athletes (no distinction was made with regard to player position), as all players must be able to kick and due to the small numbers that were available. Subjects were required to have clinical signs of joint dysfunction (asymptomatic, e.g. pain) [21,34] in either the lumbar spine or the sacroiliac joints or both. Exclusion criteria included subjects who presented with contraindications to spinal manipulations [21,34].

Procedure
After subjects signed informed consent, inclusion into the study (at the initial consultation) and allocation to a group (at the data collection arena/subsequent consultation) was determined. All players were instructed through a standardized warm-up procedure prior to measurements being taken. Each player was taken through a standardized procedure required which included a warm up run around the outside of an indoor court, a seated self stretch of the hamstrings, a prone self stretch for the quadriceps femoris, a seated stretch for the adductor muscles, a supine stretch for the quadratus lumborum and a standing gastrocnemius and soleus [36].

After the completion of the warm up procedure the pre-intervention measurements were taken: lumbar (flexion, extension, lateral flexion, and rotation) and sacroiliac (flexion and extension) range of motion parameters. The player was then required to complete a maximum run-up distance of 3 meters (the angle of the run-up was not specified so as to not interrupt the subjects natural kicking technique [6]); whilst completing an instep kick performed at maximum power. All three kicks were required to be taken with the preferred foot only.

This was then followed by the group-appropriate intervention:

- For lumbar SI, the lumbar roll technique was used as described by Szaraz [37].
- For the sacroiliac manipulation, a side lying technique was used with pisiform, posterior superior iliac spine contact as described by Bergmann, Peterson, and Lawrence [34].
- A combination of the above for the combination group.
- Laser intervention for the sham group.

Manipulation of a dysfunctional joint was considered successful if on reassessment after the manipulation, the motion palpation of that joint [33,34] showed improvement post manipulation and there was agreement between the researcher and the clinical supervisor (blinded to manipulation).

After the intervention the post-intervention measures were administered immediately (in order of lumbar and sacroiliac range of motion, repeated kicking outcomes and the subjective perception of the kick (improved, the same or worse)).

Outcome measures
The range of motion was measured using a Saunders digital inclinometer [38]. Mayer, Kondraske, Beals and Gatchel [39], found that there was minimal error when using an inclinometer, however where error might be seen is on the examiners ability to locate bony anatomical landmarks (which was overcome in this study by marking the appropriate landmarks).

Lumbar range of motion: flexion, extension, lateral flexion and rotation motion was assessed according to the outlines provided in the manual by the Saunders Group [38] and Mayer, Kondraske, Beals and Gatchel [39].

Sacroiliac Range of Motion (only flexion motion was assessed), was assessed as outlined by Schafer and Faye [33], Bergmann, Peterson and Lawrence [34] and Saunders [38]. Calculations were done according to Arab et al., [40].

Performance was measured using the SpeedTrac™ Speed Sport Radar, which measured the kicking speed of the subjects. This device (EMG Companies, Wisconsin, USA) utilized Doppler signal processing to measure speeds of small projectiles. An internal antenna sends out radio waves at a specific frequency, so when a moving object, such as a kicked ball, enters the range of this signal it alters the frequency. The frequency of the reflected signal off the ball changes the frequency in proportion to the ball's speed. The radar then displays the speed in the units of choice, in this case km/h. The signal transmitted is able to pass through netting without being affected. Therefore, a protective barrier can be placed between the moving object and the radar without affecting the accuracy of the measurements in any way. The speed range of the radar is 10-199 km/h, and the distance range is approximately nine meters. The accuracy of the radar is within 2-3 km/h

[EMG Companies, Wisconsin, USA]. The SpeedTrac™ Speed Sport Radar was set up (specifically for this study), in the indoor arena behind the netting of the goal, so as to protect the unit; give the most accurate readings (7.5 meters away from the kicking point) and to give the subjects a target to assist aim.

In terms of the subjective outcomes of the study, subjects were all required to answer the following question post intervention, "Did you feel that your kicking speed increased or decreased or remained the same following the treatment?" (3 point Likert Scale).

Statistics

SPSS version 15.0 was used to analyse the data. A p value < 0.05 indicated statistical significance. Demographic characteristics were compared between the groups using ANOVA tests. Intra-group comparisons of outcomes

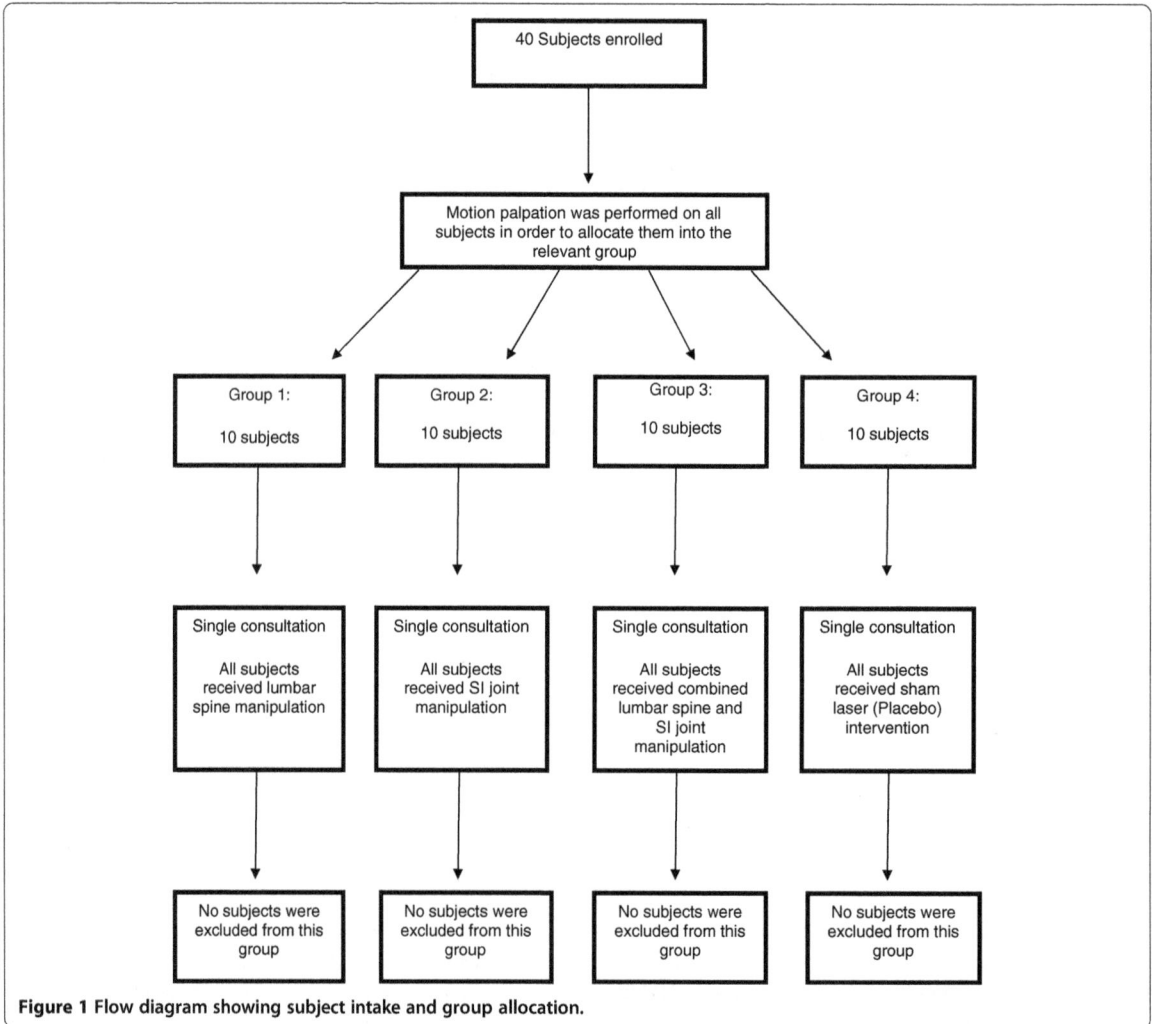

Figure 1 Flow diagram showing subject intake and group allocation.

Table 1 Baseline measures between the groups

	Lumbar spine manipulation		SI joint manipulation		Combined		Sham		p-value
	Mean	S.D	Mean	S.D	Mean	S.D	Mean	S.D	
Height (cm)	175.3	4.3	175.6	6.6	180.6	8.5	177.3	3.9	0.209
Weight (kg)	75.6	5.6	75.8	11.1	81.9	8.0	75.3	7.1	0.234
Age (years)	23.5	3.4	24.1	4.0	23.1	3.4	23.0	2.9	0.890

There was no distinction of gender, all participants were male.

over time were achieved using within-subjects repeated measures ANOVA. A significant time effect indicated a significant effect of the intervention where each subject was used as their own control. Intra and inter-group comparison of interventions was achieved using between and within groups repeated measures ANOVA. A significant time verses group effect indicated that the interventions produced different results over time. Comparison of subjective and objective change in kicking speed was assessed using cross tabulations and Pearson's chi square tests [41]. Normalcy of data were computed utilizing the Kolmogorov's Smirnov test and normal probability plots.

Table 2 The statistically significant ROM p values post intervention

Group	Intervention	Movement	Mean pre readings (degrees)	Mean post readings (degrees)	p value
Group 1	Lumbar spine manipulation	Lumbar Left Rotation	**4.95**	**5.33**	**0.026**
		Lumbar Right Rotation	**4.88**	**5.34**	**0.005**
		Lumbar Flexion	56.73	57.14	0.173
		Lumbar Extension	24.24	24.73	0.121
		Lumbar Right Lateral Flexion	25.45	25.73	0.107
		Lumbar Left Lateral Flexion	25.01	25.78	0.130
		Sacro-iliac motion (all)			>0.05
Group 2	SI joint manipulation	Lumbar Left Rotation	5.78	5.83	0.224
		Lumbar Right Rotation	5.88	5.98	0.343
		Lumbar Flexion	57.34	57.34	No change
		Lumbar Extension	24.83	24.93	0.343
		Lumbar Right Lateral Flexion	26.69	26.69	No change
		Lumbar Left Lateral Flexion	26.61	26.61	No change
		Sacro-iliac motion (all)			>0.05
Group 3	Lumbar spine and SI joint manipulation	Lumbar Extension	**24.6**	**25.81**	**0.014**
		Lumbar Flexion	56.49	56.69	0.162
		Lumbar Left Rotation	**4.89**	**5.59**	**0.001**
		Lumbar Right Rotation	**4.95**	**5.62**	**0.005**
		Lumbar Right Lateral Flexion	25.9	26.11	0.094
		Lumbar Left Lateral Flexion	25.61	26.13	0.125
		Right SI joint flexion	**7.305**	**7.98**	**0.024**
		All other SI motion			>0.05
Group 4	Sham laser	Lumbar Extension	24.7	24.7	No change
		Lumbar Flexion	58.68	58.68	No change
		Lumbar Left Rotation	5.26	5.49	0.269
		Lumbar Right Rotation	5.43	5.57	0.150
		Lumbar Right Lateral Flexion	26.24	26.24	No change
		Lumbar Left Lateral Flexion	26.16	26.16	No change
		Sacro-iliac motion (all)			>0.05

Analysis: Wilk's lambda, with a 95% confidence interval.

Results

Figure 1 outlines the flow of subjects through the study, based on the procedure outlined in the methodology. In terms of the baseline (pre-intervention) measurements between the groups there was no significant differences in terms of the subjects age, height and weight (demographic data) (Table 1).

In terms of the pre-post intervention measures (using the Wilks Lambda tests), statistically significant increases in right and left lumbar spine rotation ranges of motion (Group 1) and lumbar spine extension, right and left lumbar spine rotation and sacroiliac joint flexion range of motion (Group3) were reflected. No significant changes were seen with Group 2 and Group 4 (Table 2).

Table 3 Intergroup comparisons

	Effect	Statistic	p value
Inter-group Lumbar Flexion Comparison	Time	0.785	**0.015**
	Time*Group	0.782	0.183
	Group	0.515	0.675
Inter-group Lumbar Extension Comparison	Time	0.603	**<0.001**
	Time*Group	0.571	**0.003**
	Group	0.291	0.832
Inter-group Lumbar Left Lateral Flexion Comparison	Time	0.804	**0.022**
	Time*Group	0.757	0.124
	Group	0.588	0.627
Inter-group Lumbar Right Lateral Flexion Comparison	Time	0.733	**0.004**
	Time*Group	0.714	0.059
	Group	0.453	0.717
Inter-group Lumbar Left Rotation Comparison	Time	0.421	**<0.001**
	Time*Group	0.518	**0.001**
	Group	1.918	0.144
Inter-group Lumbar Right Rotation Comparison	Time	0.458	**<0.001**
	Time*Group	0.633	**0.012**
	Group	2.688	0.061
Inter-group Left SI Flexion 1 Comparison	Time	0.810	**0.025**
	Time*Group	0.768	0.148
	Group	0.269	0.847
Inter-group Left SI Flexion 2 Comparison	Time	0.862	**0.022**
	Time*Group	0.799	**0.042**
	Group	0.231	0.874
Inter-group Right SI Flexion 1 Comparison	Time	0.777	**0.012**
	Time*Group	0.729	0.078
	Group	0.941	0.431
Inter-group Right SI Flexion 2 Comparison	Time	0.760	**0.008**
	Time*Group	0.652	**0.017**
	Group	0.677	0.572
Inter-group average kicking speed comparison	Time	0.417	**<0.001**
	Time*Group	0.485	**<0.001**
	Group	0.349	0.790
Inter-group maximum kicking speed comparison	Time	0.592	<0.001
	Time*Group	0.586	< 0.001
	Group	0.330	0.804

Analysis: Wilk's lambda, with a 95% confidence interval.

In the intergroup comparisons Table 3 reflects the outcomes between the groups. This Table agrees with the outcomes of Table 2, where the significant differences seen pre-post for the individual groups are also the same reasons for the significant differences between the groups. Additionally all three manipulative Groups showed statistically significant increases in kicking speeds (Table 4) with the sham laser intervention no effect post intervention for kicking speed. Further, a significant relationship between perception of improved performance and the improvement in kicking speed was noted (Table 5 (average kicking speed)/Table 6 (maximum kicking speed)), but there was no correlation between in the improved kicking speed and range of motion of either the lumbar spine or the sacroiliac joints.

Discussion

Due to the fact that in all four Groups the subjects were aware that they were being studied, it was considered that the full effects of the Hawthorne principles were negated as each group would have had a similar exposure to these effects and thus they would have been negated in the inter-group comparisons [32,42].

In light of the above, the results seem to suggest that, manipulation of the lumbar spine alone or in conjunction with the sacroiliac joint, seems to result in the most significant results in soccer players, with regards to kicking speed. This outcome may be attributed to the nature of the lumbar spine manipulation (rotation) used, coupled with slight extension [29], which lends itself to the recorded results where the only statistically significant differences were noted in the rotation and extension motions during inter-group comparisons (Table 2).

Additionally, the lumbar spine and sacroiliac joint combination manipulation group achieved the highest rate of improvement followed by the sacroiliac joint manipulation and then lumbar spine manipulation groups. This outcome concurs with the results obtained by Sood [43], where it was found that combination groups (thoracic and lumbar manipulation) resulted in the greatest

degree of improvement and significant (p < 0.000) improvement for action cricket fast bowlers' bowling speed. This is however in contrast to the findings of Le Roux [44] in amateur golfers where no significant improvements were seen in participants that received combination manipulation interventions. The difference may lie in the fact that Sood [43] and this study utilized athletes specialized roles as opposed to the amateur athletes in the study by Le Roux [44]. This is supported by Gowan et al. [45], Shrier et al. [46] and Lauro and Mouch [47].

It may however also need to be considered that athletes respond differently to manipulation when combined with another modality, as found in the study by Costa et al. [48], where a combination of manipulation and stretching improved the overall outcome for the athletes. This concept of muscle stretch may have adversely affected the outcomes of this study as athletes were placed in the lumbar roll position for the sacro-iliac and lumbar spine manipulation procedures and not for the sham laser intervention. This would have predisposed the intervention groups to muscle stimulation that may not have been present in the sham laser intervention group. Further, different responses to manipulation may be sport specific, position specific or perception specific in terms of the athlete, but may also be related to the definition of the musculoskeletal dysfunction and the intervention combinations/chiropractic care utilized [49], as well as the known neurophysiological effects of manipulation [50].

In this study, the performance results can only be due to the fact that athletes responded biomechanically (only range of motion was measured) to manipulation due to the effect of the manipulation on the joints and surrounding anatomical structures [26]. These outcomes therefore support and suggest that the biomechanical [2] role of the lumbar spine and sacroiliac joint manipulation does affect the instep kicking technique, through mechanisms suggested by Herzog, [23] and Pickar, [26]. Additionally, this concurs with results found in sports related research [30,51,52], indicating that increased movement of the

Table 4 The statistically significant kicking speed p values post intervention

Group	Intervention	Average/maximum	Mean pre value	Mean post value	Average change	p value
Group 1	Lumbar spine manipulation	Average	93.67	97.19	3.52 km/h	0.009
		Maximum	97.2	100.9	3.70 km/h	0.029
Group 2	SI joint manipulation	Average	94.19	99.62	5.43 km/h	0.001
		Maximum	97	103.5	6.50 km/h	0.001
Group 3	Lumbar spine and SI joint manipulation	Average	96.03	102.6	6.57 km/h	< 0.001
		Maximum	101	105.6	4.60 km/h	0.002
Group 4	Sham	Average	100.02	98.58	-1.44 km/h	0.070
		Maximum	102.5	100.4	-2.10 km/h	0.096

Analysis: Wilk's lambda, with a 95% confidence interval.

Table 5 Cross tabulation of subjective change and objective change in average kicking speed

			Objective change in kicking speed (avg.)		
			Decrease	Same	Increase
Subjective change in kicking speed	Decrease	Count	1	0	0
		Percentage	100.0%	.0%	.0%
	Same	Count	6	2	6
		Percentage	42.9%	14.3%	42.9%
	Increase	Count	1	0	24
		Percentage	4.0%	.0%	96.0%
Total		Count	8	2	30
$p = 0.001$		Percentage	20.0%	5.0%	75.0%

biomechanical chain could increase the ball speed following foot-ball impact. Studies show that manipulative interventions (with controlled external conditions) resulted in players acquiring appropriate balance [2] between the musculoskeletal structures [20] leading to the improvements in performance.

Although the neurological effect of the manipulation was not measured in this study, it may have played a role in attaining the positive outcomes (increased kicking performance and increased range of motion). This possibility is supported by Pickar [26], Murphy [27]; Herzog [28], Symons [29] and Suter et al. [30], whose collective literature suggests that the outcome of a complex motion is most likely related to improved neurological co-ordination. This would suggest that an increased limb swinging speed and thus resultant kicking speed would result in improved performance.

The majority of the subjects' perception was that the kicking speed had increased following the intervention. The perception of increase was matched with 96% of the subjects actually increasing the average kicking speeds and 92% increasing the maximum kicking speeds post intervention. There was, therefore, a statistically significant association between changes in kicking speeds immediately post intervention and the subjects' perception of change in kicking speed.

Limitations
One of the major limitations in this study was that of sample size.

Future research
Future research needs to measure the neurological effect of manipulation and its impact in all forms of sport, but particularly soccer players to substantiate the outcomes of this study. Outcomes measures should include of measures neurological function, as it has been shown that manipulation results in neurological change in the cervical spine [52,53], which may also impact on biomechanical outcomes achieved.

Further research could also explore the effects of ipsilateral and contra lateral manipulation of the lumbar spine in combination with sacroiliac joint manipulation and how this would alter outcomes on kicking speed. Also, research on the effect of manipulation of the joints both lower down and higher up the kinematic chain be considered – either in isolation or in combination. Both of the above studies would benefit from utilizing professional players that have position specific training, which may increase the ability to detect smaller variances in range of motion and other outcome measures, as their kicking performance would be more consistent.

Table 6 Cross tabulation of subjective change and objective change in maximum kicking speed

			Objective change in kicking speed (max)		
			Decrease	Same	Increase
Subjective change in kicking speed	Decrease	Count	1	0	0
		Percentage	100.0%	.0%	.0%
	Same	Count	7	0	7
		Percentage	50.0%	.0%	50.0%
	Increase	Count	1	1	23
		Percentage	4.0%	4.0%	92.0%
Total		Count	9	1	30
$p = 0.005$		Percentage	22.5%	2.5%	75.0%

Conclusions

This pilot study has demonstrated that lumbar spine and SI joint manipulation, when combined are an effective intervention for a short-term increase in kicking speed after one intervention. These outcomes are however only generalizable to those subjects that had improved motion of the dysfunctional motion segment on motion palpation after manipulation. Additionally, the use of a larger sample calculated on an *a priori* analysis would assist in validating the outcomes of this study and reduce the risk of type II error. This along with improved measures, obtained by utilizing a blinded assessor for the outcome measures; increase frequency of the intervention may assist in conclusively supporting or refuting the results obtained in this study.

Competing interests
The authors declare that they have no competing interests.

Authors' contributions
KCD principle researcher, who obtained his Master in Technology of Chiropractic degree. ADJ supervisor of the masters study. CMK presenter of study at Federation Internationale de Chiropractique du Sport symposium as well as manuscript preparation, co-ordination and update. All authors read and approved the final manuscript.

Funding
The study was funded through a grant from the Durban University of Technology.

Author details
[1]M.Tech:Chiropractic, Durban, South Africa. [2]M.Dip:Chiropractic, MMedSci (Sports Science), CCSP, Durban, South Africa. [3]Department of Chiropractic and Somatology, Chiropractic Programme, M.Tech:Chiropractic, CCFC, CCSP, ICSSD, Durban University of Technology, Durban, South Africa.

References
1. Ingley B, Harris B. Soccer kick biomechanics [online]. Available at: http://www.ultimatesoccercoaching.com/soccer-kick/soccer-kick-biomechanics.html. 2001. Accessed 18 November 2009.
2. Kellis E, Katis A. Biomechanical characteristics and determinants of instep soccer kick. J Sports Sci Med. 2007;6:154–65.
3. Nunome H, Georgakis A, Shinkai H, Suito H, Tsujimoto N and Ikegami Y. Impact phase kinematics of side-foot and instep soccer kick. J Biomech 2007;40(S2).
4. Lees A. Biomechanics applied to soccer skills. In: Reilly T, editor. Science and soccer. London: E and FN Spon; 1996.
5. Lees A, Nolan L. The biomechanics of soccer: a review. J Sports Sci. 1998;16:211–34.
6. Dørge H, Bull Andeersen T, Sørensen H, Simonsen T. Biomechanical differences in soccer kicking with the preferred and the non-preferred leg. J Sports Sci. 2002;20:293–9.
7. Luhtanen P. Kinematics and kinetics of maximal instep kicking in junior soccer players. In: Reilly T, Lees A, Davids K, Murphy W, editors. Science and football. London: E and FN Spon; 1998.
8. Gilchrist R, Frey M, Nadler S. Muscular control of the lumbar spine. Pain Physician. 2003;6:361–8.
9. Barfield W, Kirkendall D, Yu B. Kinematic instep kicking differences between elite female and male soccer players. J Sports Sci Med. 2002;1:72–9.
10. Ishmail A, Mansor M, Ali M, Jaafar S, Johar M. Biomechanics analysis for right leg instep kick. J Appl Sci. 2010;10(13):1286–92.
11. Cohan S. Sacroiliac joint pain: a comprehensive review of anatomy, diagnosis, and treatment. Anaesth Analg. 2005;101:1440–53.
12. Sterzing T, Henning E. The influence of friction properties of shoe upper materials on kicking velocity in soccer. J Biomech. 2007;40(2):195.
13. Bir C, Cassatta J, Janda D. An analysis and comparison of soccer shin guards. Clin J Sports Med. 1995;5(2):95–9.
14. Young W, Clothier P, Otago L, Bruce L, Liddell D. Acute effects of static stretching on hip flexor and quadriceps flexibility, range of motion and foot speed in kicking a football. J Sci Med Sport. 2004;7(1):23–31.
15. Cramer GD, Tuck NR, Knudsen JT, Fonda SD, Schliesser JS, Fournier JT, et al. Effects of side posture positioning and side posture adjusting on the lumbar zygopophyseal joints as evaluated by magnetic resonance imaging: a before and after study with randomisation. J Manipulative Physiol Ther. 2000;23:380–94.
16. Cramer CG, Gregerson DM, Knudsen JT, Hubbard BB, Ustas JA, Cantu JA. The effects of side posture positioning and spinal adjusting on the lumbar Z joints: a randomised controlled trial with sixty four subjects. Spine. 2002;27(22):2459–66.
17. Mooney V, Robertson J. The facet syndrome. Clin Orthop Relat Res. 1976;115:149–56.
18. Paris S. Anatomy as related to function and pain. symposium on evaluation and care of lumbar spine problems. Orthop Clin North Am. 1983;14:476–89.
19. Jortikka MO, Inkinen RI, Tammi MI, Parkkinen JJ, Haapala J, Kiviranta I, et al. Immobilisation causes longlasting matrix changes both in the immobilised and contralateral joint cartilage. Ann Rheum Dis Suppl. 1997;56(4):255–61.
20. Appell HJ. Muscular trophy following immobilisation. A review. Sports Med. 1990;10(1):42–58.
21. Redwood D. Spinal adjustment for low back pain. Semin Integr Med. 2003;1(1):42–52.
22. Bergmann TF, Peterson DH. Chiropractic technique: 3rd ed. St. Louis, Missouri, United States of America: Elsevier Health Science; 2010.
23. Herzog W. The mechanical, neuromuscular and physiologic effects produced by the spinal manipulation. In: Herzog W, editor. Clinical biomechanics of spinal manipulation. New York: Churchill Livingstone; 2000.
24. Gatterman MI, Cooperstein R, Lantz C, Perle SM, Schneider MJ. Rating specific chiropractic technique procedures for common low back conditions. J Manipulative Physiol Ther. 2001;24(7):449–56.
25. Ianuzzi A, Khalsa PS. Comparison of human lumbar facet joint capsule strains during simulated high velocity, low amplitude spinal manipulation versus physiological motions. Spine J. 2005;5:277–90.
26. Pickar J. Neurophysiological effects of spinal manipulation. Spinal J. 2002;2(5):357–71.
27. Murphy BA, Dawson NJ, Slack JR. Sacroiliac joint manipulation decreases the h-reflex. Electroencephalogr Clin Neuro Physiol. 1995;35:87–94.
28. Herzog W, Scheele D, Conway PJ. Electromyographic responses of back and limb muscles associated with spinal manipulative therapy. Spine. 1999;24:146–53.
29. Symons BP, Herzog W, Leonard T, Nguyen H. Reflex responses associated with activator treatment. J Manipulative Physiol Ther. 2000;23:155–9.
30. Suter E, McMorland G, Herzog W, Bray R. Conservative lower back treatment reduces inhibition in knee-extensor muscles: a randomized controlled trial. J Manipulative Physiol Ther. 2000;25(2):76–80.
31. Fox M. Effect on hamstring flexibility of hamstring stretching compared to hamstring stretching and sacroiliac joint manipulation. Clin Chiropractic. 2006;9:21–32.
32. Mouton J. Understanding social research. 3rd ed. Pretoria: Van Shaik Publishers; 1996.
33. Schafer R, Faye J. Motion palpation and chiropractic technique. 2nd ed. Huntington Beach, California, United States of America: The Motion Palpation Institute; 1989.
34. Bergmann T, Peterson D, Lawrence D. Chiropractic Technique. New York, New York, United States of America: Churchill Livingstone Inc; 1993.
35. Marcotte J, Normand MC, Black P. Kinematics of motion palpation and its effect on the reliability for cervical spine rotation. J Manipulative Physiol Ther. 2002;25(7):E7.
36. Travell JG, Simons DG. Myofascial pain and dysfunction: the trigger point manual. Baltimore: Williams and Wilkins; 1983.
37. Szaraz ZT. Compendium of chiropractic technique. 2nd ed. Toronto: Vivian L.R. Associates Ltd. Technical Publications; 1990.
38. Saunders H. Saunders digital inclinometer users guide. 4250 Norex Dr, Chaska, Minnesota, 55318-3047: The Saunders Group, Inc; 1998.
39. Mayer TG, Kondraske G, Beals SB, Gatchel RJ. Spinal range of motion. Accuracy and sources of error with inclinometric measurement. Spine. 1997;22(17):1976–84.

40. Arab A, Abdollahi I, Joghataei M, Golafshani Z, Kazemnejad A. Inter- and intra-examiner reliability of single and composites of selected motion palpation and pain provocation tests for sacroiliac joint. Man Ther. 2009;14:213–21.

41. Esterhuizen T. (Private communications), 16 August 2010, 14:06 PM.

42. McCarney R, Warner J, Iliffe S, Van Haselen R, Griffin M, Fisher P. The hawthorne effect: a randomised, controlled trial. BMC Med Res Methodol. 2007;7:30.

43. Sood K. The immediate effect of lumbar spine manipulation, thoracic spine manipulation, combination lumbar and thoracic spine manipulation and sham laser on bowling speed in action cricket fast bowlers. Durban: Master's Degree in Chiropractic, Durban University of Technology; 2008.

44. Le Roux S. The immediate and short term effect of spinal manipulative therapy (SMT) on asymptomatic amateur golfers in terms of performance indicators. Durban: Master's Degree in Chiropractic, Durban University of Technology; 2008.

45. Gowan ID, Jobe FW, Tibone JE, Perry J, Moynes DR. A comparative electromyographic analysis of the shoulder during pitching: professional versus amateur pitchers. Am J Sports Med. 1987;15(6):586–90.

46. Shrier I, MacDonald D, Uchacz G. A pilot study on the effects of pre-event manipulation on jump height and running velocity. Br J Sports Med. 2006;40:947–9.

47. Lauro A, Mouch B. Chiropractic effects on athletic ability. J Chiropractic Res Invest. 1991;6(4):84–7.

48. Costa SMV, Chibana YET, Giavarotti L, Compagnoni DS, Shiono AH, Satie J, et al. Effect of spinal manipulative therapy with stretching compared with stretching alone on full-swing performance of golf players: a randomised pilot trial. J Chiropractic Med. 2009;8:165–70.

49. Greenstein JS. Chiropractic enhancement of sports performance. Adv Chiropractic. 1997;4:295–320.

50. Leach R. The chiropractic theories: a textbook of scientific research. 4th ed. Philadelphia, Pennsylvania: Lippincott Williams and Wilkins. ISBN 978-0683307474

51. Bicalho E, Setti J, Macagnan J, Cano J, Manffra E. Immediate effects of a high-velocity spine manipulation in paraspinal muscles activity of nonspecific chronic low-back pain subjects. Man Ther. 2010;15:469–75.

52. Botelho MB, Andrade BB. Effect of cervical spine manipulative therapy on judo athletes' grip strength. J Manipulative Physiol Ther. 2012;35(1):38–44.

53. Cramer G, Brudgell B, Henderson C, Khalsa P, Pickar J. Basic science research related to chiropractic spinal adjusting: the state of the art and recommendations revisited. J Manipulative Physiol Ther. 2006;29(9):726–60.

15

Reliability of diagnostic ultrasound in measuring the multifidus muscle

Eirik Johan Skeie[1*], Jan Arve Borge[2], Charlotte Leboeuf-Yde[3], Jenni Bolton[4] and Niels Wedderkopp[5]

Abstract

Background: Ultrasound is frequently used to measure activity in the lumbar multifidus muscle (LMM). However previous reliability studies on diagnostic ultrasound and LMM have included a limited number of subjects and few have used Bland-Altman's Limits of Agreement (LOA). Further one does not know if activity affects the subjects' ability to contract the LMM.

Methods: From January 2012 to December 2012 an inter- and intra-examiner reliability study was carried out in a clinical setting. It consisted of a total of four experiments with 30 subjects in each study. Two experienced examiners performed all measurements. Ultrasound measurements were made of: 1. the LMM in the resting state, 2. during a contracted state, 3. on subsequent days, and, before and after walking. Reliability and agreement was tested for 1. resting LMM, 2. contracted LMM, and 3. thickness change in the LMM. Mean values of three measurements were used for statistical analysis for each spinal level. The intra-class correlation coefficient (ICC) 3.1 and 3.2 was used to test for reliability, and Bland-Altman's LOA method to test for agreement.

Results: All of the studies indicate high levels of reliability, but as the LMM thickness increased (increasing contraction) the agreement between examiners was poorer than for low levels of contraction.

Conclusions: The use of diagnostic ultrasound to measure the LMM seems to be reliable in subjects who have little or no change in thickness of the LMM with contraction.

Keywords: Diagnostic ultrasound, Measurement, Lumbar multifidus, Agreement, Reliability, Limits of agreement, Intraclass correlation coefficient

Introduction

The lumbar multifidus muscle and low back pain

It is well known that non-specific low back pain (LBP) is a prevalent disorder often with numerous recurring episodes [1]. Currently there is no objective clinical test that is able to differentiate subjects with nonspecific LBP from pain free subjects, nor is there any clinical test than can predict the occurrence or recurrence of LBP. Even though the exact cause of LBP remains unknown, some studies indicate that fat infiltrations in the multifidus musculature (LMM) are associated with back pain [2]. Numerous studies have been carried out on the LMM in relation to the presence of LBP with and without radiculopathy [3-9], as well as LMM size and function as a prognostic factor for LBP [10,11], predictive effects of changes in the LMM in LBP patients [12,13] and LMM changes in relation to treatment of LBP [14-16]. Changes of the LMM function have also been noted in people who previously had LBP [17] and even in those with experimentally induced LBP [18]. Therefore it seems possible that there may be a link between the function and/or morphology of the LMM and LBP. Hence function of the LMM may be easily altered by pain and slow to recover.

Evaluating the LMM with diagnostic ultrasound

When evaluating the LMM with ultrasound, this is done by comparing the thickness of resting muscle with that of activated muscle. The reason for this is findings in prior studies that have demonstrated reduced ability to contract the LMM in low back pain patients [7,9] as well as in patients who have previously suffered from LBP [17]. Hodges et al. [19] investigated the use of ultrasound to measure muscle contraction on several muscles

* Correspondence: eirikjs@online.no
[1]MChiro, MSc, Ulriksdal 2, 5009 Bergen, Norway
Full list of author information is available at the end of the article

other than the LMM. The study found the architectural parameters measured by ultrasound and EMG showed a nonlinear relationship, and the majority of muscle thickness change took place in the range up to 30% of maximal voluntary contraction [19]. For the LMM a close correlation was found between values measured by ultrasound and activity measured by EMG when the contractions were in the range of 19 to 34% of maximum contraction [20].

Earlier studies on diagnostic ultrasound and the LMM differed greatly on methodology, procedures, equipment, muscles tested, sample size, LBP presentation, and levels of physical fitness of participants. A systematic review by Hebert et al. [21] reported poor methodological quality of previous studies on diagnostic ultrasound and LMM, only 6 of the 24 studies included in the systematic review were considered high quality studies.

When measuring the thickness of the LMM, earlier studies have shown that averaging the thickness of three measurements optimizes reproducibility [22,23]. Very good inter-rater agreements between novice and experienced examiners have been found when measuring LMM thickness [24]. Good inter- and intra-rater reliability has also been reported between experienced examiners [25] and novice examiners [23,26,27]. In order to activate the LMM one can lift either the contralateral arm or leg. An earlier study found only marginal difference in contraction when lifting the contralateral arm or leg: The same study also noted that transducer position has little effect on intra and inter-rater reliability of diagnostic ultrasound and the LMM [23]. The systematic review by Hebert et al. [21] highlights that reliability increases with more experienced examiners, and that only a minority of studies have reported low levels of reliability.

Need for further studies on diagnostic ultrasound
Criticism has been raised against several of the studies on inter- and intra-rater reliability of the LMM when measured with diagnostic ultrasound. Hebert et al. [21] highlighted different methods in measuring the LMM in previous studies, and several of these had small sample sizes (<15), asymptomatic subjects, and only some of the studies looked at the measurement of contraction. None of the previous studies investigated how general activity, such as gait might affect measurements of the LMM using diagnostic ultrasound. The reason for investigating gait, is the suggestion that the spine is the key to locomotion of the lower limbs [28]. More recent studies have shown increased electromyographic activity in the LMM during walking [29].

Methodological considerations
Previous studies that investigated reproducibility of measurements of LMM with diagnostic ultrasound have

done so by examining reliability of measurements. To test this statistically, the intra-class correlation coefficient (ICC) is commonly used. However, the concept of reproducibility consists also of agreement. Agreement is best illustrated with Bland-Altman's Limits of Agreement (LOA) method [30-33] because it helps detect any systematic differences between the individual measurements (i.e., fixed bias) and is able to identify possible outliers. However only rarely in previous studies on diagnostic ultrasound and the LMM have both these methods been used [26].

Aim and objectives of the present study
In order to bring forth a coherent picture on the issue of the potential usefulness of ultrasound diagnosis on the LMM in people with LBP, a number of projects were carried out. We started with the most basic aspects, moving towards the more advanced ones, using both the ICC and LOA methods for our statistical analyses. Specifically, the study had the four following objectives in relation to the ultrasound diagnostic procedure on the LMM:

1. To study the inter-examiner reliability of diagnostic ultrasound when measuring LMM thickness on one still image.
2. To study the inter-examiner reliability of diagnostic ultrasound when measuring LMM contraction on two sets of still images.
3. To study the intra-examiner reliability of diagnostic ultrasound when measuring LMM contraction on two different occasions.
4. To study the stability of measurements of LMM contraction with diagnostic ultrasound by comparing these before and after the subjects exercised.

Methods
Examiners
Inter and intra-examiner reliability was tested between two chiropractors who were both experienced in diagnostic ultrasound for the musculoskeletal system. Examiner 1 had four years of experience in diagnostic ultrasound and examiner 2 had eight years of experience. At the time of the study both the examiners held a postgraduate diploma in diagnostic ultrasound. Before the study, both examiners agreed upon and developed the protocol of diagnostic ultrasound that was applied in this study.

Study subjects
An a priori decision was made to include 30 study subjects to test each of the four study objectives. These subjects were recruited consecutively from a chiropractic practice

from January 2012 to December 2012. The sample size was considered a convenience sample as the study was conducted in a routine clinical practice setting. The majority of these subjects were LBP patients although patients with other spinal complaints such as mid back pain, neck pain, and/or extremity pain were also included. In addition some pain-free subjects were recruited from outside the clinic. This case mix was to include subjects with the potential ability to produce a contraction of the LMM as well as those with the potential not to. Subjects were recruited during the clinic's opening hours, normally around the end of the day and during lunch hours when both examiners were available. Each of the total 120 subjects took part in only one of the projects outlined above. All subjects gave verbal and written consent to inclusion in the study. Application for ethics approval was sent to the Regional Committees for Medical and Health Research Ethics (REC) in Norway. REC considered the project a quality assurance project and therefore no special permission from REC was needed to complete the project.

Procedures
Ultrasound measurements
In this study all the measurements of the LMM were taken with the subjects in a prone position with a pillow placed under the abdomen to flatten the lumbar lordosis as this provides better contact for the transducer. A Medison Accuvix V10 ultrasound scanner with a 3–7 MHz curvilinear probe was used. To identify the level of the LMM in the lumbar spine, the transducer was placed longitudinally along the spine with the midpoint over the spinous processes of interest. The sacrum was recognized as a longitudinal structure in contrast to the shorter curved spinous processes. The probe was then moved laterally and angled slightly medially until the facet joint in question could be visualized as described by Kiesel [20]. At this point the probe was directly overlying the LMM, and a measurement was taken from the apex of the facet joint to the plane between the thoracolumbar fascia and the subcutaneous fat. The reason for utilizing the on-screen callipers was to make the study as clinically relevant as possible. Previous studies have analysed the images offline. However, this is not common in a clinical setting. Care was taken not to move too far laterally as this would lead to imaging of the erector spinae muscles and not the LMM. Figure 1 illustrates placement of the calipers.

Objective 1: Inter-examiner reliability of LMM thickness on the same still image
For all study subjects in objective 1, a single image was generated of the LMM by one of the examiners. The first examiner then placed a marker on the image on the mammillary process of the level to be measured. Examiner 1 subsequently measured the distance three times with the calliper software on the ultrasound machine, saving each image onto the ultrasound machine's hard drive. The callipers and saved images were removed before examiner 2 entered the room, leaving only the still image with the marker in place on the screen. Examiner 2 then performed the same measurement procedure. Thereafter the data were transferred to a separate paper by examiner 1 who calculated mean values.

Objective 2: Inter-examiner reliability of LMM contraction on separate still images
For all subjects, images of the LMM in the resting and contracted states were generated independently by each of the examiners. The spinal level to be measured was chosen from predetermined criteria (a total of thirty average measurements, fifteen from the left and fifteen from the right, and evenly distributed between L3-L5). Examiner 1 generated an image of the LMM in the resting state with the subject in prone position (Figure 1). Thereafter a split screen was utilized and the subject performed the contralateral arm lifting task as described by Kiesel [20] but with no hand held load. Then a second image (Figure 1: Image 2) was captured of the contracted LMM with the arm in the elevated position, and the thickness of the LMM was measured on screen of the two images (Figure 1: Image 1: resting thickness, Figure 1: Image 2: contracted thickness). This procedure was performed three times by both examiners for each subject, giving three sets of measurements of the LMM in the resting and contracted states for each level for each examiner. The three sets of images with the measurements in place were saved onto the ultrasound machine's hard drive. Examiner 1 removed the saved images from the screen before examiner 2 entered the room. Examiner 2 then repeated the same procedure. After examiner 2 left the room, the data were then transferred to two separate sheets of paper by examiner 1. Examiner 1 calculated mean measurements for the individual measurements by both examiners (mean resting and contraction values). In addition contraction of the LMM was expressed as raw change in thickness (contracted LMM minus resting LMM). Contraction was expressed as an exact change in thickness and not in a relative percentage because there is missing evidence to support that the LMM contracts as a unit.

Objective 3: Intra-examiner reliability of LMM contraction using two sets of still images on two different days
For all subjects, three sets of measurements were generated on two different days giving a total of six sets of measurements per subject. Examiner 1 performed all measurements. To reduce the risk of recall, a minimum of five days

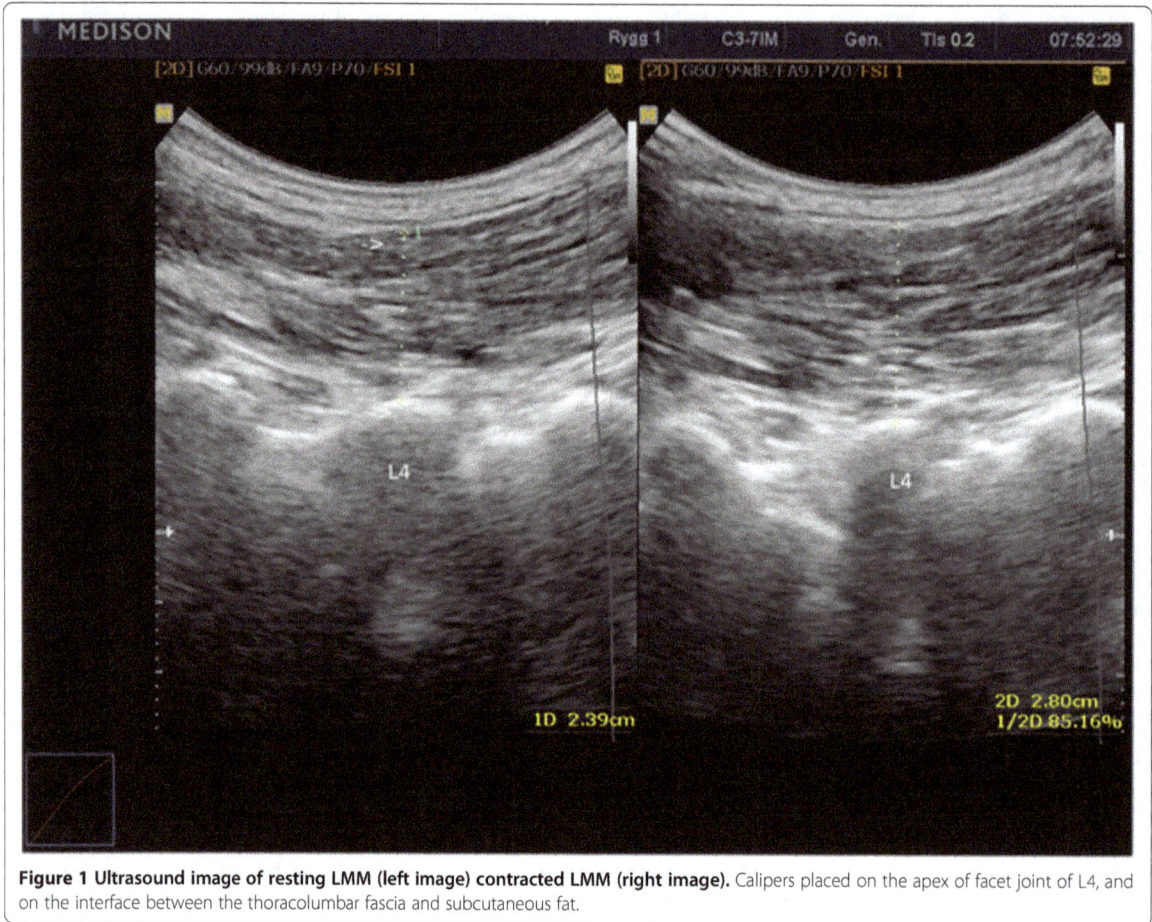

Figure 1 Ultrasound image of resting LMM (left image) contracted LMM (right image). Calipers placed on the apex of facet joint of L4, and on the interface between the thoracolumbar fascia and subcutaneous fat.

elapsed between measurements during which a large number of patients had been examined, making recall of previous measurements unlikely. The procedure for obtaining the images was the same as for objective 2. The measurements obtained by the examiner were saved onto the ultrasound machine, and recorded on two different sets of paper that were kept separate until all measurements had been obtained. The first sets of measurements were deleted off the ultrasound machines hard drive on the same day as they were generated. This was done to avoid examiner 1 being able to read the first set of measurements when performing measurements on the second day. Examiner 2 then calculated the mean of resting and contracting LMM values for day 1 and day 2.

Objective 4: Repeatability of measurements of LMM contraction with diagnostic ultrasound before and after the subjects walked around the table

For all subjects examiner 1 generated two sets of images. Again, examiner 1 performed all measurements. The procedure for obtaining resting and contraction measurements

of LMM were the same as in objectives 2 and 3. For each subject three sets of measurements were taken both before and after the subject walked around the table (exercised). When recording the measurements, examiner 1 first saved the first three sets of measurements on the ultrasound machine's hard drive, after which the subject exercised. During the exercise the first sets of measurements had been cleared from the screen. The second three sets of measurements taken were saved on the same subject file but annotated as "after". The reason for clearing the images from the screen was to prevent examiner 1 from reading the measurements from the "before" measurements when recording the second sets of measurements. After the measurements were completed, examiner 2 transferred the data onto a separate sheet of paper and calculated mean values for the individual measurements by examiner 1 (mean resting thickness and contraction thickness before the patient had walked, and mean resting and contraction values after the subject had walked around the table). The contraction was expressed as raw change in thickness (contracted LMM – resting LMM).

Statistical analyses

Correlation between examiners was measured in three ways:

1. For study objectives 1 to 4, ICC were determined in two ways, both as two way mixed single measures (3.1) and as two way mixed average measures (3.2) in order to evaluate inter- and intra-rater reliability. ICC 3.1 and 3.2 are the correct forms of ICC to use when the subjects are randomly selected but the examiners are not [34]. In this analysis, both subjects and examiners are seen as potential sources of systematic variability.

There is no consensus of what constitutes a good ICC value [35]. According to the guidelines by Kottner et al. [33] the ICC values should be at least 0.90 or 0.95 if individual and important decisions should be made based on ICC statistics. A systematic review by Hebert et al. [21] on the reliability of diagnostic ultrasound on the abdominal and lumbar trunk muscles used ICC values above 0.75 to indicate good reliability and below 0.75 to indicate poor reliability.

2. LOA were also calculated for study objectives 1, 2 and 4 and shown in order to determine differences between the means of the measurements. The LOA is shown as a graph in which the individual measurements are plotted making it possible to observe if the results vary as a function of the size of the measurements.

3. In addition to the ICC values for study objective 3, a linear plot was constructed in order to evaluate the level of LMM contraction in the subjects on two different days.

The analyses were carried out by an independent person (NW) using STATA version 12.1.

Results

Descriptive data

A detailed description of the study subjects is shown in Table 1. Each experiment consisted of a different sample of 30 subjects.

Objective 1. To study the inter-examiner reliability of diagnostic ultrasound when measuring LMM thickness on one still image

Good inter-examiner reliability was found between examiners (Table 2). The mean difference between examiners was low and the LOA narrow in range (Figure 2, Table 3). The greatest difference on an individual measurement between the two examiners, gave a measurement difference of approximately 2% when applied to the average LMM thickness.

Objective 2. To study the inter-examiner reliability of diagnostic ultrasound when measuring LMM contraction on two sets of still images

Good inter-examiner reliability was also found between examiners when measuring resting and contracted LMM (Table 2). The LOA plots (Figures 3 and 4, and Table 3) for resting and contracted LMM showed a small average difference between examiner 1 and 2. However the LOA plots (Figures 3 and 4, and Table 3) were substantially wider than in study 1. The average difference between examiners measuring resting LMM was very low (Table 3), but the greatest difference on an individual measurement equated to a difference of as much as 21% between examiners (Figure 3). For the contracted LMM the average difference between examiners measuring resting LMM was very low (Table 3). But the greatest difference on an individual measurement of the LMM resulted in a 19% difference between examiners (Figure 4).

When LMM contraction was expressed as contracted LMM minus relaxed LMM good inter-examiner reliability was found (Table 2). The LOA plot (Figure 5, Table 3) demonstrated a low average difference between the examiners. But compared with the LOA plots (Figures 3 and 4) for measurements of contracted and relaxed LMM, the average difference between examiners increased when expressing contraction as LMM

Table 1 Descriptive data on subjects

Subjects, total.									
Total (N)	Male (N)	Female (N)	Mean age (Yrs.)	Age range (Yrs.)	SD (Yrs.)	LBP (N)	Neck/Midback pain (N)	Extremity pain (N)	Pain free (N)
120	64	56	38	20-69	±12	88	23	4	5
Study objective 1									
30	18	12	38	20-69	±13	25	5	0	0
Study objective 2									
30	14	16	37	20-65	±12	20	5	1	4
Study objective 3									
30	15	15	38	20-59	±11	23	7	0	0
Study objective 4									
30	17	13	40	20-68	±11	20	6	3	1

Table 2 Mean measurements for LMM and ICC values for study objective 1–4

Objective 1 Interexaminer reliability of measuring LMM thickness using one still image			
Mean LLM thickness examiner 1	Mean LLM thickness examiner 2	ICC average	ICC individual
27.9 mm ± 3.2 mm	27.9 mm ± 3.2 mm	0.999 (0.997-0.999)	0.997 (0.994-0.999)
Objective 2 Interexaminer reliability of measuring LMM contraction using two sets of still images.			
Mean relaxed LLM thickness examiner 1 (distance 1)	Mean relaxed LLM thickness examiner 2 (distance 1)	ICC average	ICC individual
28.9 mm ± 6.4 mm	29.0 mm ± 6.1 mm	0.97 (0.94-0.99)	0.95 (0.89-0.98)
Mean contracted LLM thickness examiner 1 (distance 2)	Mean contracted LLM thickness examiner 2 (distance 2)	ICC average	ICC individual
32.1 mm ± 7.0 mm	32.0 mm ± 6.7 mm	0.97 (0.94-0.99)	0.95 (0.90-0.98)
Distance 2–1 examiner 1	Distance 2–1 examiner 1	ICC average	ICC individual
3.1 mm ± 2.2 mm	3.0 mm ± 2.0 mm	0.98 (0.96-0.99)	0.97 (0.92-0.98)
Objective 3 Intraexaminer reliabilty of measuring LMM contraction using 2 sets of still images taken on 2 different days.			
Mean relaxed LLM thickness (distance 1 day 1)	Mean relaxed LLM thickness (distance 1 day 2)	ICC average	ICC individual
28.4 mm ± 5.3 mm	28.4 mm ± 4.8 mm	0.99 (0.97-0.99)	0.97 (0.94-0-99)
Mean contracted LLM thickness (distance 2 day 1)	Mean contracted LLM thickness (distance 2 day 2)	ICC average	ICC individual
29.7 mm ± 6.0 mm	29.6 mm ± 5.5 mm	0.97 (0.93-0.99)	0.94 (0.88-0.97)
Distance 2–1 day 1	Distance 2–1 day 2	ICC average	ICC individual
1.4 mm ± 1.7 mm	1.3 mm ± 1.7 mm	0.97 (0.93-0.99)	0.94 (0.88-0.97)
Objective 4 Measuring LMM contraction before and after a motor task on two sets of still images.			
Mean relaxed LLM thickness (distance 1 before task)	Mean contracted LLM thickness (distance 2 before task)	Mean relaxed LLM thickness (distance 1 after task)	Mean contracted LLM thickness (distance 2 after task)
30.6 mm ± 5.5 mm	34.1 mm ± 6.6 mm	29.9 mm ± 5.3 mm	34.6 mm ± 6.4 mm
Distance 2–1 before	Distance 2–1 after	ICC average	ICC individual
3.5 mm ± 2.6 mm	3.5 mm ± 2.5 mm	0.98 (0.97-0.99)	0.97 (0.94-0.99)

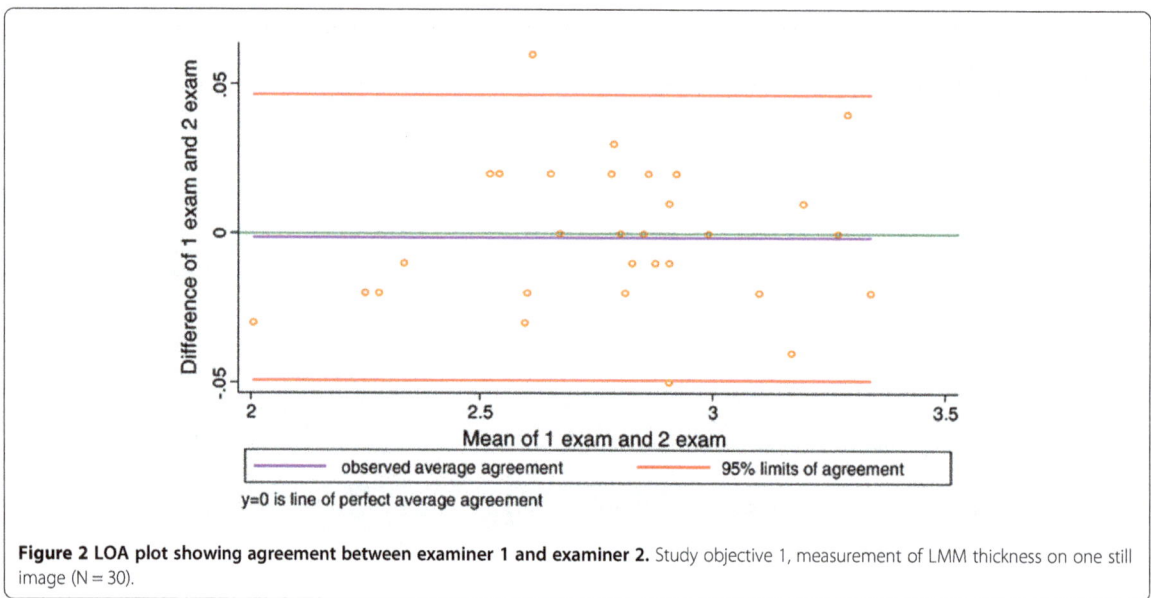

Figure 2 LOA plot showing agreement between examiner 1 and examiner 2. Study objective 1, measurement of LMM thickness on one still image (N = 30).

Table 3 Mean difference and LOA range study 1, 2, and 4

Objective 1		
	Mean difference	LOA range
Relaxed LMM	0.01 mm ± 0.24 mm	[−0.48; 0.47 mm]
Objective 2		
Relaxed LMM	0.08 mm ± 2.0 mm	[−4.07; 3.92 mm]
Contracted LMM	0.06 mm ±2.0 mm	[−3.93; 4.06 mm]
Contracted-Relaxed LMM	0.14 mm ±0.55 mm	[−0.94; 1.22 mm]
Objective 4		
Relaxed LMM	0.7 mm ± 0.9 mm	[−1.09; 2.49 mm]
Contracted LMM	0.7 mm ± 0.9 mm	[−1.18; 2.51 mm]
Contracted-Relaxed LMM	0.04 mm ± 0.65 mm	[−1.32; 1.25 mm]

minus relaxed LMM. The greatest difference on an individual measurement equated to a 45% difference in measurements between the two examiners. The LOA (Figure 5) demonstrated a funnel shape with the opening to the right. On the x-axis the volume increased towards the right suggesting poorer agreement with increasing muscle thickness.

It is also possible to express contraction as a relative percentage change and not as a raw measurement. This was performed as a separate analysis to see if it changed the LOA plot. Figure 6 shows contraction expressed this way. This resulted in a change in the funnel shape of the LOA plot into a more linear increase indicating that the examiners agreed less as the muscle thickness increased.

Objective 3. To study the intra-examiner reliability of diagnostic ultrasound when measuring LMM contraction on two different days

Again, there was good intra-examiner reliability both for relaxed and contracted LMM (Table 2). ICC values for contraction expressed as contracted LMM minus relaxed LMM (Table 2) also demonstrated excellent intra-examiner reliability.

The linear plot in Figure 7 shows little change in measurements from day to day, and that the vast majority of the subjects had little or no ability to contract their LMM. Only five subjects are seen on the right end of the scale demonstrating a volume change representing contraction. Four of the subjects had around 4 mm volume increase of the LMM and one subject had around 6 mm volume change. On average this equates to a relative thickness change between 14 and 20%. This study did not attempt to correlate the level of pain with contraction, so it is not possible to determine whether these subjects suffered from LBP.

Objective 4. To study the repeatability of measurements of LMM contraction with diagnostic ultrasound before and after the subjects walked around the table

There was good intra-examiner reliability for relaxed and contracted LMM on days 1 and 2 (Table 2). Good intra-examiner agreement was also seen for contraction expressed as contracted minus relaxed LMM (Table 2). The LOA plots for relaxed and contracted LMM (Figures 8 and 9) were very similar to those in study objective 2

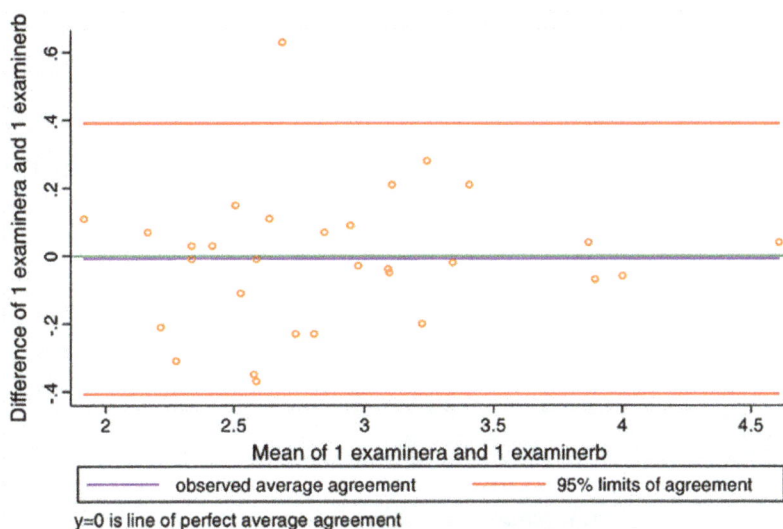

Figure 3 LOA plot showing agreement between examiner 1 and examiner 2. Study objective 2, measurement of resting LMM on two sets of images (N = 30).

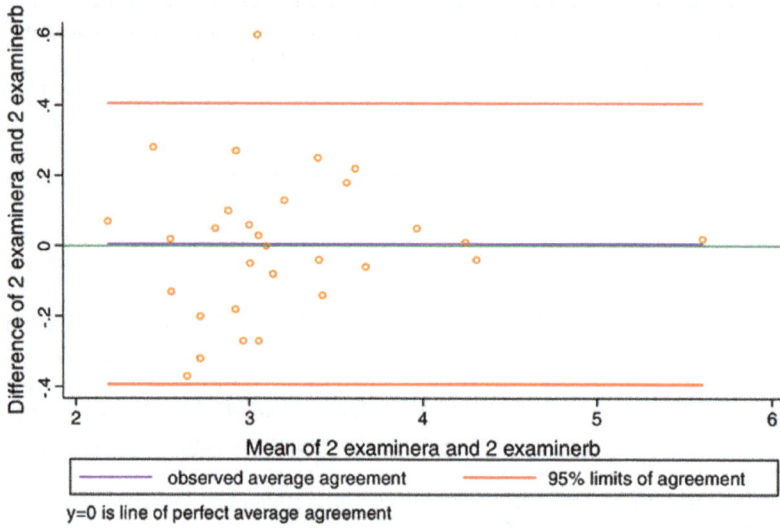

Figure 4 LOA plot showing agreement between examiner 1 and examiner 2. Study objective 2, measurement of contracted LMM on two sets of images (N = 30).

(Figures 3 and 4). The average difference for relaxed and contracted LMM was still low although greater than those found in study 2 (Table 3). Nonetheless the standard deviation for resting and contracted LMM is lower than that seen in study objective 2. The greatest difference for an individual measurement was equal to 6% measurement difference before and after the subject exercised. For contracted LMM the greatest difference on an individual measurement was equal to 5% measurement difference. When expressing contraction as (contracted LMM minus relaxed LMM) a similar plot to Figure 5 is seen in Figure 10. Again a moderate funnel shape can be seen, indicating less agreement as the LMM thickness increases. The average difference is also very low (Table 3). The greatest difference in LMM contraction on an individual measurement gave a measurement difference in muscle thickness as high as 7% before and after the subject exercised.

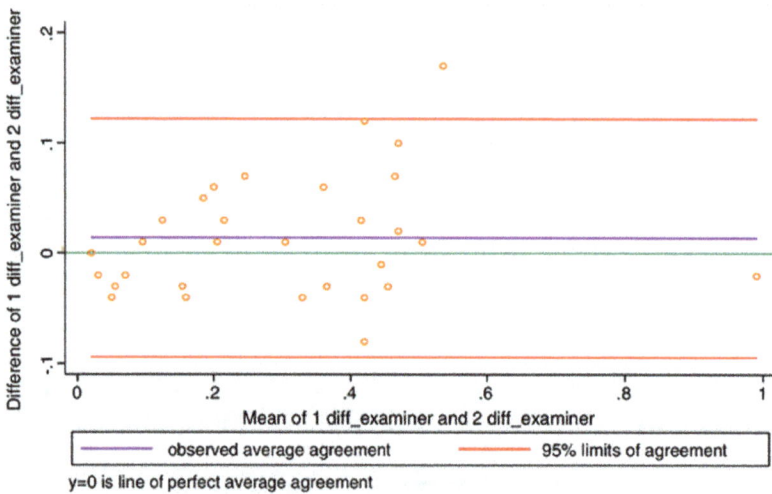

Figure 5 LOA plot showing agreement between examiner 1 and examiner 2. Study objective 2, measurement of contraction (distance 2 – distance 1) LMM on two sets of images (N = 30).

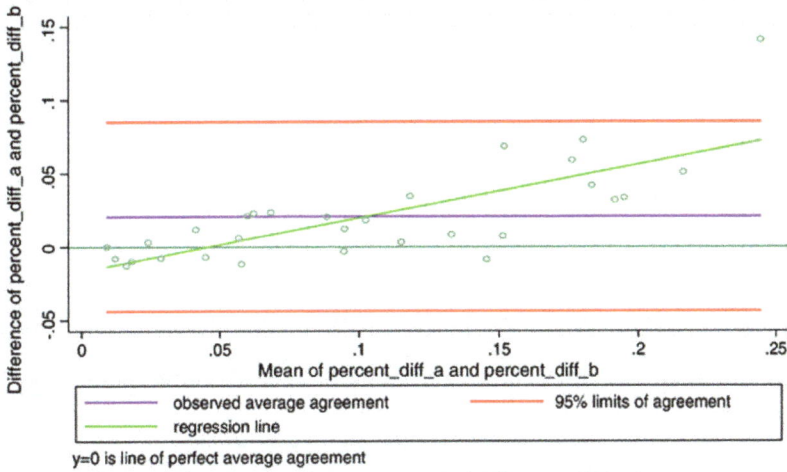

Figure 6 LOA plot showing agreement between examiner 1 and examiner 2. Study objective 2, measurement of LMM contraction expressed as relative % (distance 2 – distance 1)/distance 1) on two sets of images (N = 30).

Discussion

We performed four independent studies to test if diagnostic ultrasound can be used to reliably examine the thickness of the LMM in situations that relate to the various stages of examination. To analyse our data, we used both ICC and LOA. Our results were encouraging. Average measurements were used for analysis. The reliability of the measurements of LMM thickness was good in all four studies. This was the case when two examiners used the same still image, when they used two sets of still images, when one examiner measured the same person on two different days, and before/after the study-subject had walked around for a while.

However, it was noted that good agreement was mainly present in subjects who had little or no change in muscle thickness (contraction), probably making this method less reliable to measure thickness change as seen with contraction. Because this study sample consisted mainly of people with chronic back problems, it was not possible to study further the cut-points for good and less good reliability.

Limitations and weaknesses

Another weakness was that the examiners in these four experiments were clinicians in the clinic where the study subjects were treated. This meant that they would have met and/or treated several of these subjects. Nevertheless, many patients come through this clinic over time, a large proportion of which would be examined with diagnostic ultrasound. It would be impossible for the clinicians to remember individual values to a larger extent, and none

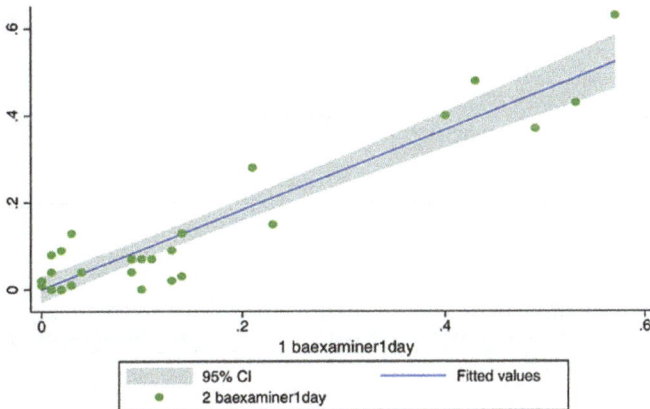

Figure 7 Scatter plot of subjects in study objective 3. Day to day scatter, x-axis shows day 1, y axis day 2.

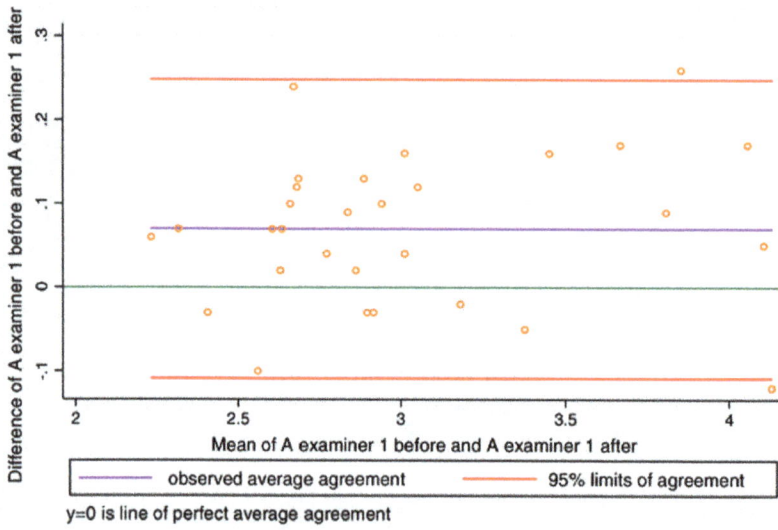

Figure 8 LOA plot showing agreement between examiner 1 before and after the subject performed a motor task. Study objective 4, measuring resting LMM before and after a simple motor task on two sets of images (N = 30).

of them had a special need to "prove" anything, but performed this study with an open and curious mind. It is unlikely that the results would be biased for this reason.

The subjects in this study were recruited from a clinical setting, the majority of which had LBP. This can be seen as both a strength and a weakness. It would have been preferable with a more mixed study sample, but the presence of people with LBP made it possible to study the usefulness of diagnostic ultrasound in a typical setting. The negative aspect is that the results cannot necessarily be generalized to other populations.

Comparison with other studies

When comparing our results to others one can only look at the ICC values. Our results, are all similar to previous

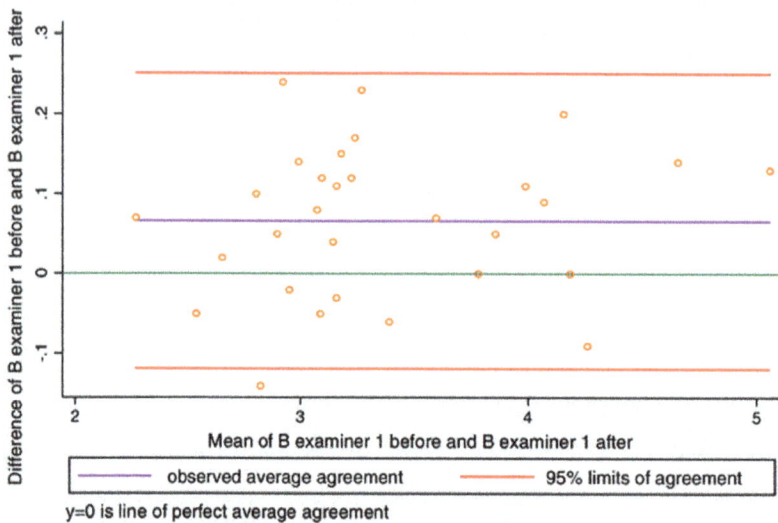

Figure 9 LOA plot showing agreement between examiner 1 before and after the subject performed a motor task. Study objective 4, measuring contracted LMM before and after a simple motor task on two sets of images (N = 30).

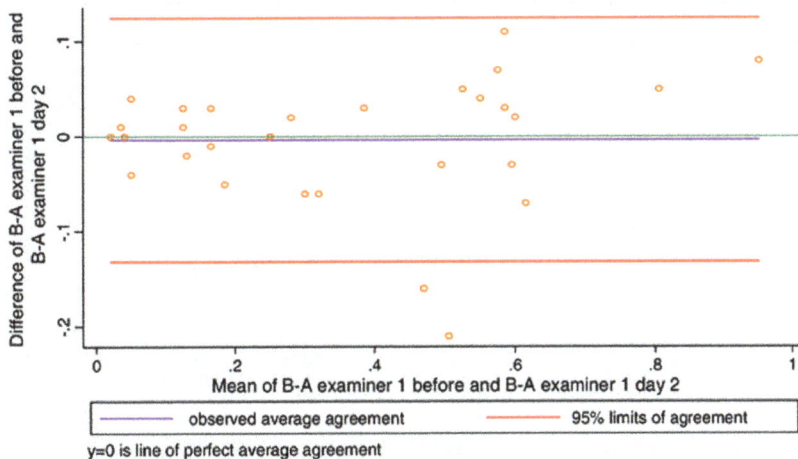

Figure 10 LOA plot showing agreement between examiner 1 before and after the subject performed a motor task. Study objective 4, measurement of contraction (distance 2 – distance 1) LMM on two sets of images (N = 30).

studies [21-23,26,27]. The main difference from our study to others is that we have demonstrated through the LOA analysis, a poorer agreement between two examiners who measure LMM thickness on two different sets of images. We also found less agreement between two examiners who measure contraction of the LMM. The agreement does seem to diminish when the thickness of the LMM is increasing more than 4 mm (relative increase of approximately 14%).

It has previously been shown that it is difficult for subjects with LBP to contract the LMM [18]. Our study did not aim to correlate LBP and ability to contract the LMM, however the majority of the subjects were LBP sufferers and this might be the reason why the majority of subjects had little or no ability to contract the LMM. We also included subjects without LBP, which may be reflected in the measurements that indicate a thickness increase in the LMM. As we only wanted to investigate the measurements this needs to be explored further in other studies.

Recommendations for further studies

Further exploration of utilization of diagnostic ultrasound on the LMM is needed. The examiners showed a low level of agreement when measuring LMM thickness change in the subjects who were able to contract of the LMM, but a good level of agreement when measuring LMM thickness change in the subjects who were not capable of contracting the LMM. It could be possible to categorize the contraction in groups to see if this increases the agreement. However this would be easier if one could use relative contraction measured in % as a scale. But if one were to use relative contraction as a measurement, further studies need to be conducted to

see if different parts of the LMM contracts as a unit. From a more clinical perspective correlation between pain and LMM contraction measured with diagnostic ultrasound needs to be performed, as well as studies that examine subjects who never had low back pain to obtain more knowledge of how the LMM normally would contract. The clinical utilization of diagnostic ultrasound in measuring the muscle contraction of the LMM is not clear, as normal ranges are not fully established [36]. However, diagnostic ultrasound could possibly be used for identifying subjects who are not capable of contracting the LMM.

Conclusion

Our results indicate that ultrasound examination of the lumbar multifidus muscle is a reliable method when used by experienced examiners in people with chronic LBP, with poor contracting ability of their multifidus muscles and the average of three measurements is utilized.

Competing interests
The authors have no financial or non-financial competing interests to declare. The foundation Et Liv i Bevegelse (ELiB) partly funded the study.

Authors' contributions
EJS, JAB, and CLY formed the study idea. All authors were involved in the design of the study, interpretation of data, revision of the manuscript, and all gave final approval of the manuscript. NW performed the data analysis. JB revised the manuscript and was also supervisor for the projects part of the MSc at the Anglo European College of Chiropractic and Bournemouth University. Parts of this study was used for an MSc degree in diagnostic ultrasound at the Anglo- European College of Chiropractic. EJS, JAB, CLY and JB set up the study. EJS and JAB conducted all intra and inter-rater measurements. NW performed the statistical analysis. EJS drafted the manuscript. CLY, JB and NW reviewed the manuscript. All authors reviewed and approved the manuscript in its final form.

Acknowledgements

The authors want to thank participating subjects, and especially Jeffrey Hebert for his input on reviewing this article. The authors would also thank the Norwegian Chiropractic Association for financial support towards the MSc degree in musculoskeletal ultrasound for EJS and JAB.

Funding

This study recieved funding from the Norwegian independant research foundation Et liv i bevegelse (ELIB).

Author details

[1]MChiro, MSc, Ulriksdal 2, 5009 Bergen, Norway. [2]DC, MSc, Ulriksdal 2, 5009 Bergen, Norway. [3]Department Spincenter of Southern Denmark Hospital Lillebælt, Østre Hougvej 55, DK-5500 Middelfart, Denmark. [4]Anglo European College of Chiropractic. Research Department, 13-15 Parkwood Road, Bournemouth BH5 2DF England, UK. [5]Orthopaedic Department, Center for Spine Surgery, Hospital of Lillebaelt, Institute of Regional Health Service Research and Center for Research in Childhood Health, University of Southern Denmark, Østre Hougvej 55, DK5500 Middelfart, Denmark.

References

1. Donelson R, McIntosh G, Hall H. Is it time to rethink the typical course of low back pain? PMR. 2012;4(6):394–401.
2. Kjaer P, Bendix T, Sorensen JS, Korsholm L, Leboeuf-Yde C. Are MRI-defined fat infiltrations in the multifidus muscles associated with low back pain? BMC Med. 2007;5:2. doi:10.1186/1741-7015-5-2.
3. Zhao WP, Kawaguchi Y, Matsui H, Kanamori M, Kimura T. Histochemistry and morphology of the multifidus muscle in lumbar disc herniation: comparative study between diseased and normal sides. Spine. 2000;25 (17):2191–9.
4. Yoshihara K, Nakayama Y, Fujii N, Aoki T, Ito H. Atrophy of the multifidus muscle in patients with lumbar disk herniation: histochemical and electromyographic study. Orthopedics. 2003;26(5):493–5.
5. Kader DF, Wardlaw D, Smith FW. Correlation between the MRI changes in the lumbar multifidus muscles and leg pain. Clin Radiol. 2000;55(2):145–9.
6. Hides J, Gilmore C, Stanton W, Bohlscheid E. Multifidus size and symmetry among chronic LBP and healthy asymptomatic subjects. Man Ther. 2008;13(1):43–9.
7. Danneels L, Coorevits P, Cools A, Vanderstraeten G, Cambier D, Witvrouw E, et al. Differences in electromyographic activity in the multifidus muscle and the iliocostalis lumborum between healthy subjects and patients with sub-acute and chronic low back pain. Eur Spine J. 2002;11(1):13–9.
8. Parkkola RR, Rytökoski UU, Kormano MM. Magnetic resonance imaging of the discs and trunk muscles in patients with chronic low back pain and healthy control subjects. Spine. 1993;18(7):830–6.
9. Wallwork TL, Stanton WR, Freke M, Hides JA. The effect of chronic low back pain on size and contraction of the lumbar multifidus muscle. Man Ther. 2008;14(5):496–500.
10. Lee HI, Song J, Lee HS, Kang JY, Kim M, Ryu JS. Association between cross-sectional areas of lumbar muscles on magnetic resonance imaging and chronicity of low back pain. Ann Rehabil Med. 2011;35(6):852–9.
11. Heydari A, Nargol AVF, Jones APC, Humphrey AR, Greenough CG. EMG analysis of lumbar paraspinal muscles as a predictor of the risk of low-back pain. Eur Spine J. 2010;19(7):1145–52.
12. Wong AYL, Parent EC, Funabashi M, Stanton TR, Kawchuk GN. Do various baseline characteristics of transversus abdominis and lumbar multifidus predict clinical outcomes in non-specific low back pain? A systematic review. Pain. 2013;154(12):2589–602.
13. Zielinski KA, Henry SM, Ouellette-Morton RH, DeSarno MJ. Lumbar multifidus muscle thickness does not predict patients with low back pain who improve with trunk stabilization exercises. Arch Phys Med Rehabil. 2013;94(6):1132–8.
14. Danneels L, Vanderstraeten G, Cambier D, Witvrouw E, Bourgois J, Dankaerts W, et al. Effects of three different training modalities on the cross sectional area of the lumbar multifidus muscle in patients with chronic low back pain. Br J Sports Med. 2001;35(3):186–91.
15. Weber BRB, Grob DD, Dvorák JJ, Müntener MM. Posterior surgical approach to the lumbar spine and its effect on the multifidus muscle. Spine. 1997;22(15):1765–72.
16. Hides JA, Jull GA, Richardson CA. Long-term effects of specific stabilizing exercises for first-episode low back pain. Spine. 2001;26(11):E243–8.
17. Macdonald D, Moseley GL, Hodges PW. Why do some patients keep hurting their back? Evidence of ongoing back muscle dysfunction during remission from recurrent back pain. Pain. 2009;142(3):183–8.
18. Kiesel KB, Uhl T, Underwood FB, Nitz AJ. Rehabilitative ultrasound measurement of select trunk muscle activation during induced pain. Man Ther. 2008;13(2):132–8.
19. Hodges PW, Pengel LHM, Herbert RD, Gandevia SC. Measurement of muscle contraction with ultrasound imaging. Muscle Nerve. 2003;27(6):682–92.
20. Kiesel KB, Uhl TL, Underwood FB, Rodd DW, Nitz AJ. Measurement of lumbar multifidus muscle contraction with rehabilitative ultrasound imaging. Man Ther. 2007;12(2):161–6.
21. Hebert JJ, Koppenhaver SL, Parent EC, Fritz JM. A systematic review of the reliability of rehabilitative ultrasound imaging for the quantitative assessment of the abdominal and lumbar trunk muscles. Spine. 2009;34 (23):E848–56.
22. Koppenhaver SL, Parent EC, Teyhen DS, Hebert JJ, Fritz JM. The effect of averaging multiple trials on measurement error during ultrasound imaging of transversus abdominis and lumbar multifidus muscles in individuals with low back pain. J Orthop Sports Phys Ther. 2009;39(8):604–11.
23. Larivière C, Gagnon D, De Oliveira E, Henry SM, Mecheri H, Dumas J-P. Ultrasound measures of the lumbar multifidus: effect of task and transducer position on reliability. PMR. 2013;5(8):678–87.
24. Wallwork TL, Hides JA, Stanton WR. Intrarater and interrater reliability of assessment of lumbar multifidus muscle thickness using rehabilitative ultrasound imaging. J Orthop Sports Phys Ther. 2007;37(10):608–12.
25. Van K, Hides JA, Richardson CA. The use of real-time ultrasound imaging for biofeedback of lumbar multifidus muscle contraction in healthy subjects. J Orthop Sports Phys Ther. 2006;36(12):920–5.
26. Koppenhaver SL, Hebert JJ, Fritz JM, Parent EC, Teyhen DS, Magel JS. Reliability of rehabilitative ultrasound imaging of the transversus abdominis and lumbar multifidus muscles. Arch Phys Med Rehabil. 2009;90(1):87–94.
27. Wong AYL, Parent EC, Kawchuk GN. Reliability of two ultrasonic imaging analysis methods in quantifying lumbar multifidus thickness. J Orthop Sports Phys Ther. 2012;43(4):251–62.
28. Gracovetsky S. An hypothesis for the role of the spine in human locomotion: a challenge to current thinking. J Biomed Eng. 1985;7(3):205–16.
29. Saunders SW, Schache A, Rath D, Hodges PW. Changes in three dimensional lumbo-pelvic kinematics and trunk muscle activity with speed and mode of locomotion. Clin Biomech. 2005;20(8):784–93.
30. Zaki R, Bulgiba A, Ismail R, Ismail NA. Statistical methods used to test for agreement of medical instruments measuring continuous variables in method comparison studies: a systematic review. PLoS One. 2011;7(5): e37908. doi:10.1371/journal.pone.0037908.
31. Hanneman SK. Design, analysis, and interpretation of method-comparison studies. Adv Crit Care. 2008;19(2):223–34.
32. Bland JMJ, Altman DGD. Statistical methods for assessing agreement between two methods of clinical measurement. Lancet. 1986;1(8476):307–10.
33. Kottner JJ, Audige LL, Brorson SS, Donner AA, Gajewski BJB, Hróbjartsson AA, et al. Guidelines for reporting reliability and agreement studies (GRRAS) were proposed. Int J Nurs Stud. 2011;48(6):661–71.
34. Rankin G, Stokes M. Reliability of assessment tools in rehabilitation: an illustration of appropriate statistical analyses. Clin Rehabil. 1998;12(3):187–99.
35. Shrout PE. Measurement reliability and agreement in psychiatry. Stat Methods Med Res. 1998;7(3):301–17.
36. Teyhen DS, Childs JD, Stokes MJ, Wright AC, Dugan JL, George SZ. Abdominal and lumbar multifidus muscle size and symmetry at rest and during contracted states normative reference ranges. J Ultrasound Med. 2012;31(7):1099–110.

16

A biopsychosocial approach to primary hypothyroidism: treatment and harms data from a randomized controlled trial

Benjamin T. Brown[1*], Petra L. Graham[2], Rod Bonello[3] and Henry Pollard[4]

Abstract

Background: Hypothyroidism is a common endocrine condition. There is evidence to suggest that, for a proportion of sufferers, the standard medical treatment does not completely reverse the constitutional and neuropsychiatric symptoms brought about by this condition. The management of hypothyroidism follows a biomedical model with little consideration given to alternative management approaches. There exists anecdotal evidence and case reports supporting the use of a biopsychosocial-based intervention called Neuro-Emotional Technique (NET) for this population. The aim of this study was to explore the potential short-medium term clinical efficacy and safety of NET for individuals with primary hypothyroidism.
Design
Placebo-controlled, blinded, parallel groups, randomized trial.

Methods: Ninety adults with a diagnosis of primary hypothyroidism were recruited from Sydney, Australia. Blinded participants were randomized to either the NET or placebo group and received ten intervention sessions over a six week period. The primary outcome involved the measurement of states of depression using the DASS-42 questionnaire. Secondary outcomes included thyroid function, thyroid autoimmunity testing, SF-36v2 questionnaire, resting heart rate and temperature measurement. Outcomes were obtained at baseline, seven weeks and six months. Questionnaires were completed at the private clinics, and serum measures were obtained and analysed at commercial pathology company locations. Heart rate and temperature were also measured daily by participants. Linear mixed-effects models were used to analyse the continuous outcomes. Unadjusted odds ratios with 95% confidence intervals were calculated for the binary outcomes.

Results: Participants were randomly allocated to the NET (n=44) and placebo (n=46) groups. A proportion of the sample displayed neuropsychiatric disturbances and alterations in quality of life measures at baseline. There were no statistically significant or clinically relevant changes in the primary or secondary outcomes between the NET and placebo groups at time seven weeks or six months. There were a few short-lived minor adverse events reported in both the NET and placebo groups that coincided with the application of the intervention.

Conclusions: The application of the NET intervention appears to be safe, but did not confer any clinical benefit to the participants in this study and is unlikely to be of therapeutic use in a hypothyroid population.

Clinical trials registration number: Australian and New Zealand Clinical Trials Registry Number: 12607000040460.

Keywords: Chiropractic, Hypothyroidism, Randomized controlled trial, Therapeutics, Neuro-emotional technique

* Correspondence: benjamin.brown@mq.edu.au
[1]Department of Chiropractic, Macquarie University, Balaclava Road, North Ryde 2109NSW, Australia
Full list of author information is available at the end of the article

Background

Hypothyroidism is a common endocrine condition that affects a significant proportion of individuals worldwide. Using data from a community-based sample from an iodine-replete region in Western Australia, it is estimated 0.54 % of Australians suffer from this condition [1]. Females are more likely to develop hypothyroidism compared to males (Prevalence - women 1–2 % and men 0.1 %) [1–3]. The primary variant of this disease accounts for the vast majority (99 %) of cases. Primary hypothyroidism is due to a failure of the thyroid gland and results in a deficient concentration of thyroid hormones in the serum. The most common cause of this glandular failure is an autoimmune condition called Hashimoto's thyroiditis [4, 5]. The symptoms of overt hypothyroidism are based on deficits in energy metabolism and thermogenesis. Consequently, patients present with a constellation of physical and neuropsychiatric findings (i.e. musculoskeletal complaints, depression, free-floating anxiety, memory deficits) [6, 7], and in cases of thyroid autoimmunity, formation of antibodies to thyroglobulin (Tg) and thyroid peroxidase (TPO) [4]. The gold-standard treatment for primary hypothyroidism is relatively straightforward and involves supplementation of one of the deficient hormones using a synthetic version of the thyroid hormone - thyroxine. This synthetic analogue is called levothyroxine (LT4). The treatment dosage of thyroid hormone is gradually titrated upwards until an individual displays normal physiological concentrations of free-thyroxine (FT4) and thyroid stimulating hormone (TSH) in the serum. Put simply, the product of the dysfunctional gland is 'topped up' using an exogenous source of thyroid hormone, with the required dose being modified according to the patient's FT4 and TSH assay results. The patient continues with this program, combined with regular check-ups, either for the rest of their lives or until some event occurs (e.g. pregnancy) that warrants a change in the patient's thyroxine dosage. The normal reference range for TSH is 0.4–3.5 mIU/L. Patients receiving thyroid hormone replacement are given sufficient quantities of thyroxine to maintain their serum TSH concentrations within an ideal range (0.5–2.0 mIU/L) [8].

While the treatment regimen for primary hypothyroidism is regarded by many as one of the major 'success stories' of medicine [9], there is evidence to suggest that a small proportion of individuals with managed-hypothyroidism continue to display the overt manifestations of the disease despite normalised blood test results - indicating a euthyroid state [10–12]. Furthermore, the decreased quality of life (QOL) that is observed in hypothyroid individuals does not always improve with the appropriate treatment [10, 13–15]. Large community-based studies [14, 16, 17] demonstrate that there is neurocognitive and psychological impairment in individuals with hypothyroidism. Unfortunately, in some patients, the restoration of normal thyroid hormone levels through thyroxine supplementation only partially ameliorates these impairments.

One of the main reasons for the persistence of symptoms in euthyroid patients with hypothyroidism is the underlying autoimmune process. Patients with Hashimoto's thyroiditis are more likely to experience higher symptom loads with reference to mood and quality of life, despite being euthyroid [18]. Furthermore, it is not uncommon for patients with Hashimoto's thyroiditis to have other comorbid autoimmune conditions e.g. rheumatoid arthritis [19]. The presence of these additional conditions contributes to an increased symptom load that is unaltered by the restoration of normal thyroid hormone concentrations in the serum. McDermott [20] suggests that a complete blood count, serum 25-hydroxyvitamin D, erythyrocyte sedimentation rate, sleep apnoea testing, celiac disease testing as well as a metabolic, hormonal, psychological, and lifestyle assessment should be performed in euthyroid patients with persistent symptoms. This strategy can be used to rule out comorbid medical conditions and/or to identify modifiable risk factors.

Researchers [21, 22] have identified polymorphisms in genes that encode for the deiodinase enzymes in patients with hypothyroidism. There is preliminary evidence to suggest [23] that patients with polymorphisms in the Deiodinase Type II gene may display poorer outcomes on levothyroxine therapy compared with patients receiving preparations containing both levothyroxine and liothyronine (synthetic T3). However, this combination therapy has not proven superior to standard monotherapy [24–27].

With respect to therapeutic intervention, very little attention has been given to the main cause of primary hypothyroidism – thyroid autoimmunity [28]. The main reason for this is that the pathogenesis of thyroid autoimmunity is not fully understood [28]. Current research suggests that autoimmune thyroid disease may result from complex interactions between environmental triggers and genetic susceptibilities [29–32]. The purported environmental triggers include: iodine excess [33, 34], selenium deficiency [35], fetal microchimerism [36, 37], infections [38, 39], and stress [40]. With regard to stress as an environmental trigger, associations have been reported most frequently with Graves' disease [41–46].

Psychological stress, via alterations in the sympathetic-adrenal-medullary (SAM) axis and the hypothalamic-pituitary-adrenal (HPA) axis, can have deleterious effects on the endocrine and immune systems [47–49]. With respect to the immune system, chronic stress shifts the balance of the cell-mediated immune response, specifically suppressing the subset of T-helper lymphocytes called the Th1 cells [49]. This suppression has a permissive effect on the production of another subset of T-helper cells called Th2 cells [50]. This shift in the Th1/Th2 balance has been observed in certain autoimmune diseases such as Systemic Lupus Erythematosus and Graves' disease [50, 51]. As a hyperactivation of the HPA axis is a common response to most forms of stress [52], it would be logical to expect a shift to Th2 dominance and a resultant increase in cases of Graves' disease in genetically susceptible individuals who are stressed. The contribution of stress to Hashimoto's thyroiditis however is less intuitive. There is some research to suggest that there is HPA axis hypoactivation in patients with hypothyroidism [53, 54]. While hyperactivation of the HPA axis leads to a suppression of Th1 dominant states, a hypoactivation of the HPA axis promotes Th1 dominant states [50]. Autoimmune conditions such as rheumatoid arthritis, Hashimoto's thyroiditis, multiple sclerosis and diabetes type I are T-cell mediated diseases, however they are thought to occur due to these Th1 dominant states [50, 55, 56]. Hypoactivation of the HPA axis has also been observed in patients with a history of childhood abuse [57] and post-traumatic stress disorder [58], which may be an adaptive response to intense or prolonged psychological stress. The role of stress in Hashimoto's thyroiditis has received far less attention compared to the role of stress in Graves' disease [59]. While it is biologically plausible that stress could play an etiological role in genetically susceptible individuals, there are no reported positive associations between stress and autoimmune induced hypothyroidism in the current literature [60–62].

Anecdotal evidence and case reports [63, 64] exist that suggest that a biopsychosocial-based intervention called Neuro-Emotional Technique (NET), which is described as a mind-body stress reduction intervention [65, 66], may be useful in the treatment of hypothyroidism. This technique has been taught and used by practitioners of varying backgrounds since the late 1980s [66], however there is very little quality evidence regarding its therapeutic utility and safety in a primary care setting.

The aim of this manuscript is to outline and discuss the results from a randomized controlled trial of the biopsychosocial-based intervention, NET, for individuals with primary hypothyroidism. This document has been prepared using the CONSORT 2010 guide for the reporting of parallel group randomized trials [67, 68], as well as the associated documents for randomized trials of non-pharmacological treatments [69], and the guide to harms reporting [70].

Methods

The research presented in this manuscript was approved by the Macquarie University Ethics Review Committee (Reference no.: HE-27AUG2004-MO3136).

Design

Parallel, blinded, multi-centre (11 sites), randomized, placebo-controlled, trial conducted from August 2006 –

March 2010. The study was designed to align with quality recommendations set out in the PEDro scale [71] and The Delphi list [72] as well as with the relevant CONSORT guidelines available at the time of trial design [67, 69, 70, 73, 74].

Participants

The study team sought to recruit participants from the Sydney Metropolitan area of Australia using advertisements in a variety of hardcopy and electronic media. Participants were randomized into either the NET group or the placebo group after being screened for eligibility by the chief investigator.

Inclusion criteria - participants

For inclusion, participants had to be ≥18 years of age and have received a diagnosis of primary overt hypothyroidism from a qualified medical practitioner or specialist. In long-standing hypothyroidism there is pituitary thyrotroph hyperplasia [75]. For this reason, it can take up to six months for TSH levels to fall into normal ranges after the initiation of LT4 therapy [76]. Based on this information, if a respondent was taking medication, e.g. levothyroxine, it was stipulated that they be on a stable dose of this medication for at least six months before enrolment into the trial. Acknowledging that treatment is commonly initiated promptly after diagnosis, participants were only included in the trial if they had received their diagnosis more than six months prior to enrolment. Participants were not asked by the research team to alter or cease their thyroid medication at any point during the trial as this would be deemed unethical given the experimental nature of the intervention. However, participants were asked to immediately report any such changes to the chief investigator so that this information could be incorporated into the interpretation of the final results.

Exclusion criteria – participants

Participants who were <18 years of age were excluded. Individuals with variants of hypothyroidism other than primary overt hypothyroidism, such as hypopituitarism, were excluded. This also included iatrogenic forms of hypothyroidism. Individuals who were on medications that could potentially impair thyroid function e.g. Lithium were excluded. Participants who reported a history of significant head or neck trauma/surgery/radiotherapy were excluded, as were individuals with diagnosed serious psychological or physical co-morbidities. Females who were pregnant or looking to conceive within the trial period were excluded. As participants were required to interact mentally and physically with the practitioner during the intervention phase of the trial, those with cognitive or physical disabilities e.g. individuals who are hard of hearing were excluded from the trial.

Inclusion criteria – practitioners

It was necessary that the practitioners applying the intervention were well-versed with the NET procedure. Consequently, practitioners were only included if they had attained the maximum qualification available at the time ('Certification' in NET) [77] and a minimum experience of two years with the procedure. This ensured a high degree of competency and also acted as a means of standardising the intervention. Practitioners were required to be available for the full duration of the intervention phase for each participant. Practitioners had to agree to treat within the confines of the research methodology and comply with the study protocol, which included the application of a placebo intervention to the relevant participants. The treating practitioners were asked to make times available in their normal practice hours for the treatment of the trial participants. There was no remuneration offered to the practitioners involved in the trial.

Inclusion criteria – research centres

The research was conducted at 11 private practices. To be included as a research venue, the practice had to fulfil several criteria: be located in the Sydney Metropolitan area, have practitioners with the relevant training and clinical expertise in NET, and be open at least two days per week with capacity for both during and after-hours business operations.

Intervention

The NET and placebo procedures have been described in depth by several authors [63, 64, 78–84] and it is not within the scope of this article to replicate this discussion. A detailed version of the NET and placebo protocols used in this trial was published in an open-access journal in 2010 [85]. The treatment protocol used in this study was also similar to that employed by Karpouzis *et al.* [78] and Karpouzis [79].

The placebo treatment was developed by a panel that included experts in NET and members of the research team. The placebo intervention was designed to closely mimic the NET intervention protocol but with the purported therapeutic components removed and replaced with innocuous steps.

Participants who were randomized to the intervention group received ten NET treatments over a six week period. Similarly, participants in the placebo group received ten placebo treatments over the same period. Two treatments per week were scheduled in the initial four weeks and one treatment per week in the final two weeks of the intervention phase. There was no further intervention after this point. Each treatment, NET or placebo, went

for 5–20 min in duration. Participants attended the same clinic and saw the same practitioner for all of their treatments, all participants attended clinics that were closest to their place of work or residence.

All practitioners involved in the trial were given a training session by the chief investigator, and issued with an information booklet detailing the steps involved with the application of each individual arm of the intervention (NET and Placebo). Practitioners were instructed to deliver the placebo treatment with the same vigour and enthusiasm as the NET treatment. Both practitioners and participants had 24-hour access to the chief investigator at all times during the trial via a toll-free telephone number.

Outcomes

Several outcome variables were used to capture potential psychological and/or physiological changes that may have coincided with the application of therapy.

Primary outcome

The primary outcome was the change in depressive states at 7 weeks and 6 months using the Depression, Anxiety, Stress Scale (DASS-42) [86]. The normal range for states of depression is between zero and nine points, with scores greater than nine indicating high states of depression. States of depression was chosen as the primary outcome as it is one of the most common neuropsychiatric symptoms observed in primary overt hypothyroidism, and it is a commonly reported symptom in individuals with continued symptomatology despite normalised thyroid function tests.

Secondary outcomes

Although it was anticipated that many of the participants would be entering into the trial with pre-existing management plans, i.e. thyroid hormone replacement schedules, it was prudent that thyroid function tests be added to the list of outcomes. The thyroid function tests included the serum measurement of thyroid stimulating hormone (TSH), free-thyroxine (FT4) and free-triiodothyronine (FT3) concentrations. The normal reference range used in this research for TSH was 0.40–3.50 mIU/L and the assay calibration range was 0.00–100.00 mIU/L [87]. The normal reference range used in this research for FT4 and FT3 was 9.0–19.0 pmol/L and 2.6–6.0 pmol/L respectively. The calibration range for the FT3 and FT4 assays was 0.000–9.216 pmol/L and 0.00–77.22 pmol/L respectively [88, 89].

In addition to the thyroid function tests, serum concentrations of antibodies to thyroid peroxidase (TPO-Ab) and thyroglobulin (Tg-Ab) were also measured. The normal reference range for TPO-Ab was 0–35 mIU/L, and the normal reference range for Tg-Ab was 0–40 mIU/L. The calibration range for the TPO-Ab and the TG-Ab assays was 0.0–1000.0 mIU/L and 0.0–3000.0 mIU/L respectively [90, 91].

The remaining items on the DASS-42 questionnaire, states of anxiety and stress, were assessed (Normal Range: Anxiety 0–7, and Stress 0–14). Scores outside of the normal reference range indicate abnormal states.

The Short Form-36 version two (SF-36v2) questionnaire [92] was also included in the list of secondary outcomes. The mean score for a normal population for the domains and component summary scores is 50 norm-based scoring points with a standard deviation of 10 points. High scores on the SF-36v2 represent high functioning whereas scores below the normal mean indicate poorer function.

In addition to the DASS and SF-36v2 questionnaires, participants were instructed to measure their resting heart rate (RHR) (radial pulse method) and resting temperature (RT) at a set time each day and record this data in a diary provided by the researchers. The normal ranges for RHR used for this trial were 75–85 bpm. Participants measured their RT by placing a digital thermometer in their axilla for approximately one minute. The normal reference range for resting temperature used in this research was 35.5–37 °C.

The aim with each of these primary and secondary outcomes measures was to examine the change in each measure at 7 weeks and 6 months to determine whether there was evidence that NET was different (efficacious) compared to placebo. This schedule would allow for the detection of any slow adaptations of the Hypothalamic Pituitary Thyroid axis in response to any short term (7 weeks) and medium term (6 months) benefit derived from the NET intervention.

Schedule of assessments

Baseline measurements were taken for both the primary and secondary outcomes. Thyroid function tests and thyroid auto-antibody measurements were performed at commercial pathology facilities approximately one week before the commencement of the intervention. The DASS, SF-36v2, and a demographic questionnaire were issued and completed by participants at the respective clinic just prior to the initial treatment. The first follow-up assessment was performed at seven weeks which included; a thyroid function test, serum thyroid auto-antibody measurements, and the DASS and SF-36v2 questionnaires. A second follow-up assessment was performed at six months which was identical to the one performed at seven weeks only with the addition of a health update questionnaire (HUQ) (Appendix). The HUQ was designed by the research team to capture any changes in a participant's health status, i.e. changes in medication, lifestyle, or major life events in the previous six months that may have influenced the final results and the associated interpretation. The daily home recording

of RT and RHR commenced one week before the intervention phase and continued for the full duration of a participant's enrolment in the trial.

Blinding survey

The chief investigator contacted each participant by phone after the participant's final results had been received. The chief investigator thanked the participant for their involvement in the trial and asked them to identify which group, NET or placebo, they felt that they had been allocated to. The participant's response was recorded and used to assess the adequacy of the blinding process.

Harms data

A combination of active and passive harms surveillance was used in this study. Practitioners were required to maintain clinical records for each participant visit during the intervention phase. At the beginning of each intervention session participants were asked by the treating practitioner if they had experienced any adverse events in the period that followed the last intervention. Participants were also asked how they felt directly after each intervention. Any responses to these questions were detailed in the participants' records. In addition to the active harms surveillance participants were also asked to contact the chief investigator if any problems or difficulties arose using the toll free telephone number. These two strategies, combined with information from the HUQ, were used to capture any adverse events that may have coincided with the application of the intervention. These data were compiled and used in the final interpretation of technique safety by the chief investigator. *Adverse events* were defined as an adverse consequence of the intervention (placebo or NET) that occurred any time after the first intervention. Classification of the event as being an 'adverse event' was determined by either the participant and/or members of the research team.

Modifications to the trial protocol

There were several modifications made to the trial protocol between August 2006 and March 2010. In 2007, the pathology company commissioned to analyse the serum measures changed the methodology for analysing the thyroid auto-antibody concentrations. This resulted in the early auto-antibody measures being incompatible/non-comparable to the newer measures. This change prompted the research team to change the TPO-Ab and the Tg-Ab from being continuous variables to dichotomous variables (i.e. either 'within' the normal reference range or 'outside' of normal reference range) in the final analysis. This resulted in a loss of sensitivity with respect to the minimal clinically important difference detectable for this particular measure.

As the measurement of TSH and FT4 is the standard 'first-line' test for individuals with thyroid dysfunction, there were several instances in which the pathology company, due to internal protocols, did not measure the FT3 or thyroid auto-antibody concentrations. Many of these cases were picked up by the chief investigator, however there were instances in which the participant's sample was destroyed before the chief investigator was able to notify the pathology company of the omission. This resulted in six participants having only partial data for certain variables. This remains a limitation of the study.

As the trial was run over a four year period, there were several changes in the line-up of treating practitioners. Four practitioners started out in 2006. Eight more practitioners were recruited between 2006 and 2010, and four practitioners ceased their involvement in the study during this period due to personal reasons. Despite these changes, each participant received their intervention from a single practitioner.

Sample size

A two-sided, power-analysis indicated that 51 participants per group would yield a greater than 80 % chance of detecting a difference in depression scores of at least four points in the NET group compared to placebo group using a standard deviation of 6.97 based on normative data [86, 93]. A four point reduction in depression scores, as defined by the DASS-42, would represent a clinically meaningful reduction in states of depression. The ranges for the depression scale are: normal 0–4, mild 5–6, moderate 7–10, severe 11–13 and extremely severe 14+ [86].

Stopping guidelines

Guidelines were set that dictated that the trial would be stopped in the event of serious adverse events occurring in participants during their participation in the trial.

Randomization

A simple randomization technique was employed. A random sequence generator [94] was used to produce a random sequence with no repeats. These numbers were then recorded on individual pieces of paper and placed into opaque envelopes which were then sealed. After each consenting participant completed their initial blood test an envelope was selected for that participant by the chief investigator. Participants allocated an even number were assigned to the NET group, and those receiving an odd number were assigned to the placebo group. The chief investigator, practitioners and other researchers remained naive to a participant's group allocation until just before the application of the intervention.

Blinding

Pathology company staff and any primary care provider/s involved in the participant's non-trial management (e.g. the participant's general practitioner or endocrinologist) were blinded to the group allocations. The allocation of individual participants to treatment groups was concealed to the chief investigator up until the point of a participant commencing treatment. Practitioners were notified of each participant's group allocation prior to performing the intervention and were instructed not to reveal the allocation to the participant. Individual participants were not told their group allocation until the end of their involvement in the trial and after the completion of the blinding survey (Table 1).

Statistical procedures

The R software program [95] was used to conduct all the analyses. Linear mixed-effects (LME) models were employed for all continuous outcome measures except for the thyroid antibody concentrations. Linear mixed-effects models utilise all available data to provide unbiased estimates of the mean difference between groups in the presence of missing at random data and hence form an intention to treat (ITT) analysis [96]. Since these are more widely used methods, the imputation techniques and statistical methods described in the original protocol were not conducted. The thyroid antibody measures had been dichotomised and logistic mixed-effects models were the planned analysis technique. However model convergence issues meant that it was necessary to calculate unadjusted odds ratios with 95 % confidence intervals for each time point instead. The final data set was screened for errors prior to all analyses. P-values for the interaction and pairwise difference at each time point have been presented for each outcome measure together with 95 % confidence intervals (CI). All participants were analysed according to their initial group allocation. A sensitivity analysis was conducted by adjusting for baseline differences between groups by using baseline data as a covariate in the mixed-effects model. However, the effect of this was that

Table 1 Trial timeline. The trial timeline depicts the timing of all interventions and outcomes measured during the trial

Event	Week 1	Weeks 2-7	Week 8	Week 26	Week 27
Intervention					
Thyroid function tests					
DASS questionnaire					
SF-36v2 questionnaire					
Demographic questionnaire					
Basal temperature recording					
Basal heart rate recording					
Health update questionnaire					
Blinding survey					

Shaded Area = Event occurrence, *DASS* depression anxiety stress scale, *SF-36v2* short form 36 version 2 cases with missing baseline data were excluded from the analysis and the analysis may no longer be considered ITT. Demographic characteristics of participants were summarised using frequency tables. Summary values (mean, median, minimum, maximum, and standard deviation) for each group were used for the discussion of baseline group equivalence. Fisher's exact test was used to analyse the results of the blinding survey. Two-sided tests with a significance level of 5 % were used throughout all analyses. No corrections (e.g. Bonferroni method) were made to the significance level to adjust for multiple testing due to the exploratory nature of the secondary analyses.

Results

Post-randomization losses to follow-Up and protocol deviations

The dropouts and protocol deviations that occurred at various phases of the trial are detailed in Fig. 1.

Not all participants in the NET group received the full ten treatments. The reasons for these protocol deviations were either: personal reasons (1/44), administrative error (5/44), the deterioration of a pre-existing medical condition (1/44), minor reaction to treatment (1/44), other time commitments (1/44), and undisclosed reason/s (2/44). With regards to outcome measures, the main reasons for missing data were administrative errors at the private clinics or the pathology company. Several participants in the NET and placebo groups found the daily recording of heart rate and temperature inconvenient and cumbersome. As a result, there was incomplete compliance with the recording of these outcomes.

Not all participants in the placebo group received the full schedule of interventions or completed the full complement of outcomes. The reasons for these deviations were: work issues (1/46), expenses associated with travel to the clinic location (1/46), undisclosed reason/s (5/46), dissatisfaction with the placebo intervention (3/46), other time commitments (1/46), non-compliance with the trial protocol (5/46), and administrative error (4/46).

Dates of recruitment

Recruitment for the clinical trial took place between August 2006 and March 2010. Two hundred and forty five individuals responded to the advertisements for participation. Eligible consenting participants were followed for six months after randomization.

Trial closure

A strict external schedule (stopping rule) was imposed that meant that the trial must be commenced and completed between August 2006 and October 2010 due to the length of the chief investigator's PhD

candidature. No interim analyses were performed and hence the decision to close the trial was independent of the trial outcomes. The prescribed schedule meant that no further participants could be recruited after March 2010 despite needing additional participants to fulfil the sample size target.

Baseline participant data

The demographic information and the mean baseline clinical characteristics for participants are presented in Tables 2 and 3 respectively. The two groups were very similar with respect to demographic data. A comparison of the baseline clinical data is presented below.

Primary outcome - baseline

Boxplots of baseline depression scores are depicted in Fig. 2. The mean and median depression scores for the placebo group were within normal range, however the mean score for the NET group fell just outside of the normal range. A large proportion (19/44) of participants in the NET group and 15/46 participants in the placebo group reported states of depression that fell outside of the normal range at the time of initial testing.

Secondary outcomes and clinical data - baseline

With respect to baseline clinical data, the mean TSH scores for the NET group were skewed by one individual with an extremely high TSH value that remained high at the subsequent seven week and six month reassessments. With reference to thyroid autoimmunity, 30/44 participants in the NET group demonstrated higher than the normal concentrations of TPO-Ab and 12/44 demonstrated higher than normal concentrations of Tg-Ab. Similar results were seen in the placebo group with 30/46 and 14/46 of participants demonstrating abnormally high TPO-Ab and Tg-Ab concentrations respectively.

With respect to the additional DASS items, 17/44 of the NET group and 10/44 of the placebo group reported anxiety scores in the mild to severe range. A considerable proportion of the trial participants also reported mild to extremely severe stress scores (NET 19/44, Placebo 13/44).

The mean baseline scores for the SF-36v2 questionnaire revealed that the trial participants had lower mean self-reported general health (NET 11/44, Placebo 9/46), vitality (NET = 21/44, Placebo 23/46) social functioning (NET 9/44, Placebo 11/46) and mental health (NET 8/44, Placebo 10/46) compared to normative data.

Resting temperature was comparable and within normal range at baseline for both the NET and placebo groups. The data regarding heart rate highlight that the majority of participants in both the NET and placebo groups had

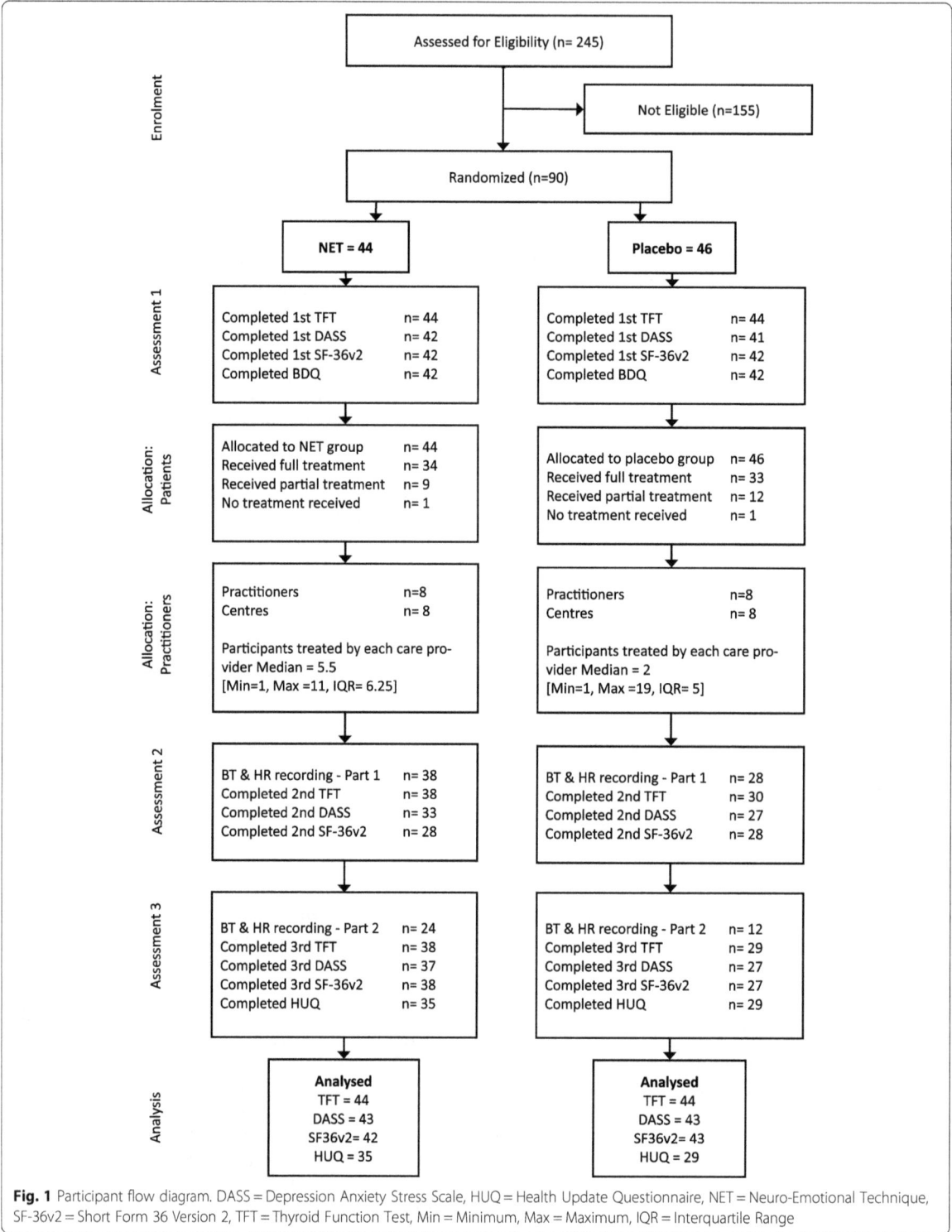

Fig. 1 Participant flow diagram. DASS = Depression Anxiety Stress Scale, HUQ = Health Update Questionnaire, NET = Neuro-Emotional Technique, SF-36v2 = Short Form 36 Version 2, TFT = Thyroid Function Test, Min = Minimum, Max = Maximum, IQR = Interquartile Range

Table 2 Demographic information

		Treatment (n = 44)	Placebo (n = 46)
Age	Median	46	43
	Minimum	20	20
	Maximum	72	75
	Mean	45.55	44.61
	Standard Deviation	11.21	11.32
Number of children	Mean	1.51	1.81
	Standard Deviation	1.30	1.20
Gender	Female	43	40
Ethnicity	Caucasian	40	38
	Asian	2	2
	Arab	1	0
	Aboriginal/Torres Strait Islander	0	1
	Unknown	1	5
Birthplace	Australia	26	29
Highest level of education	School Certificate	5	0
	HSC	3	10
	TAFE	13	8
	Undergraduate	13	15
	Postgraduate	8	11
	Unknown	2	2
Marital status	Married	20	27
	Separated	6	5
	Single	14	8
	Widowed	1	0
	Defacto	2	3
	Unknown	1	3
Employment	Full-Time	17	16
	Part-Time	11	13
	Retired	13	11
	Not Working	2	4
	Unknown	1	2

HSC higher school certificate, TAFE technical and further education

lower than normal heart rate compared to the normal range (NET = 37/44, Placebo 44/46).

In addition to the primary and secondary outcomes researchers also gathered data on the previous use of psychological services and concurrent use of medications and/or nutritional supplements. Thirty four percent (15/44) of the NET group and 37 % (17/46) of the placebo group reported that they had used support services (e.g. counselling service) in the past for emotional, psychological or lifestyle problems. At baseline, the vast majority of participants (NET 40/44, Placebo 43/46) reported currently using some form of thyroid medication for the

treatment of their condition. With respect to additional medication use, 21/44 of participants in the NET group and 20/46 of participants the placebo group reported using medications other than those prescribed for their thyroid condition. A substantial proportion of trial participants (NET 28/44, Placebo 27/46) reported taking nutritional products or supplements.

Analysis

The results from the linear mixed-effects modelling for the primary outcome may be seen in Table 4 and Fig. 3. Secondary outcomes that comprised of continuous data are presented in the remaining rows of Table 4. There was no significant interaction between time and treatment group for any of the outcome variables included in the study (final column of Table 4) indicating that there was no evidence of a difference between groups over time (Fig. 3 Primary outcome). There were no significant differences, at the 5 % significance level, between the NET and placebo groups at time seven weeks or six months (see the 3rd and 6th columns of Table 4) for any of the primary or secondary outcomes.

There were no significant differences between the NET and placebo groups for either RHR ($p = 0.20$) and RT ($p = 0.18$) readings over time.

The odds ratios and 95 % confidence intervals indicated no significant differences, at the 5 % significance level, between groups in the odds of demonstrating Tg-Ab concentrations outside of reference range at the seven weeks (OR: 0.65, 95 % CI: 0.24 to 1.73, $p = 0.38$) or the six month (OR: 1.24, 95 % CI: 0.45 to 3.38, $p = 0.68$) time points. Similar outcomes were observed with TPO-Ab concentrations (7 week OR: 0.94, 95 % CI: 0.32 to 2.74, $p = 0.90$; 6 month OR: 0.69, 95 % CI: 0.25 to 1.92, $p = 0.48$).

Sensitivity analysis was undertaken by using baseline outcome as a covariate in each of the continuous outcome models shown in Table 4. While the baseline value was consistently a highly significant factor ($p < 0.0001$), the interaction between time and group remained nonsignificant for all outcomes ($p > 0.3$). In other words, the only differences between groups, were those differences observed at baseline with no significant change over time.

Harms/adverse events

The harms/adverse events section has been written in accordance with the CONSORT document for the better reporting of harms in randomized trials [70]. No validated harms recording instruments were used.

Adverse events - NET group

Six (14 %) participants in the NET group reported adverse events that coincided with the application of intervention. One participant in the NET group reported feeling "sad" after the fifth treatment session. This same

Table 3 Mean baseline clinical characteristics

Outcome measure	Normal range	Treatment		Placebo	
		Median (Min, Max)	Mean (SD)	Median (Min, Max)	Mean (SD)
Thyroid function tests:					
TSH (mIU/L)	0.40–3.50	0.96 (0.00, 55.77)	2.98 (8.39)[a]	1.34 (0.01, 7.30)	1.85 (1.76)
FT4 (pmol/L)	9.0–19.0	15.00 (7.00, 26.00)	15.09 (3.22)	14.20 (3.80, 24.50)	14.51 (3.91)
FT3 (pmol/L)	2.6–6.0	4.06 (2.80, 7.45)	4.13 (0.80)	3.80 (3.00, 5.73)	3.95 (0.64)
DASS Scores:					
Depression	0–9	6.50 (0.00, 29.00)	9.43 (8.60)	6.00 (0.00, 41.00)	7.85 (8.52)
Anxiety	0–7	6.00 (0.00, 19.00)	6.79 (5.13)	4.00 (0.00, 30.00)	6.27 (7.73)
Stress	0–14	13.00 (3.00, 35.00)	13.71 (8.28)	11.00 (2.00, 38.00)	12.76 (8.53)
SF-36v2 Scores:	Normal Mean (SD)	Median (Min, Max)	Mean (SD)	Median (Min, Max)	Mean (SD)
Physical functioning	50 ± 3 (10)	52.82 (25.46, 57.03)	48.06 (8.36)	50.72 (29.68, 57.03)	48.66 (7.72)
Role physical	50 ± 3 (10)	49.51 (22.57, 56.85)	48.85 (8.60)	51.96 (17.67, 56.85)	46.32 (11.25)
Bodily pain	50 ± 3 (10)	46.06 (24.08, 62.12)	49.97 (9.87)	46.06 (24.08, 62.12)	46.53 (9.43)
General health	50 ± 3 (10)	45.31 (23.38, 57.70)	43.72 (11.26)	45.78 (23.78, 62.47)	45.16 (9.71)
Vitality	50 ± 3 (10)	39.60 (23.99, 58.33)	40.15 (8.88)	41.16 (20.87, 58.33)	41.68 (10.33)
Social functioning	50 ± 3 (10)	45.94 (13.22, 56.86)	42.09 (12.49)	45.94 (13.22, 56.85)	41.12 (12.82)
Role emotional	50 ± 3 (10)	48.10 (20.89, 55.88)	44.78 (10.71)	44.22 (20.89, 55.88)	43.58 (10.96)
Mental health	50 ± 3 (10)	44.38 (21.85, 61.27)	43.79 (11.04)	47.19 (16.22, 58.46)	43.03 (11.62)
Physical component summary	50 ± 3 (10)	50.46 (30.08, 61.73)	48.27 (7.76)	51.39 (16.70, 59.78)	48.45 (9.54)
Mental component summary	50 ± 3 (10)	42.59 (16.70, 60.18)	41.10 (11.49)	41.59 (16.40, 61.35)	40.79 (12.71)
	Normal Range	Median (Min, Max)	Mean (SD)	Median (Min, Max)	Mean (SD)
Resting temperature (°C)	35.5–37.03	35.8 (32.8, 37.0)	35.6 (0.9)	35.6 (33.4, 36.6)	35.6 (0.7)
Resting heart rate (bpm)	75–85	64 (30, 86)	65.7 (9.6)	64 (44, 86)	63.9 (11.3)

The SF-36v2 scores are based on the norm based scoring system (NBS) which is based on a mean score with a normal range between 47 and 53 NBS points. Resting temperature and resting heart rate data were analysed based on 'Day 1' dairy entries

[a]Strongly influenced by one person with very high TSH

DASS Depression, Anxiety, Stress Score, *NET* Neuro-Emotional Technique, *TSH* Serum thyroid stimulating hormone, *FT4* Free thyroxine, *FT3* Free triiodothyronine, *SF-36v2* Short Form-36 Version 2, *Min* minimum, *Max* Maximum, *SD* standard deviation

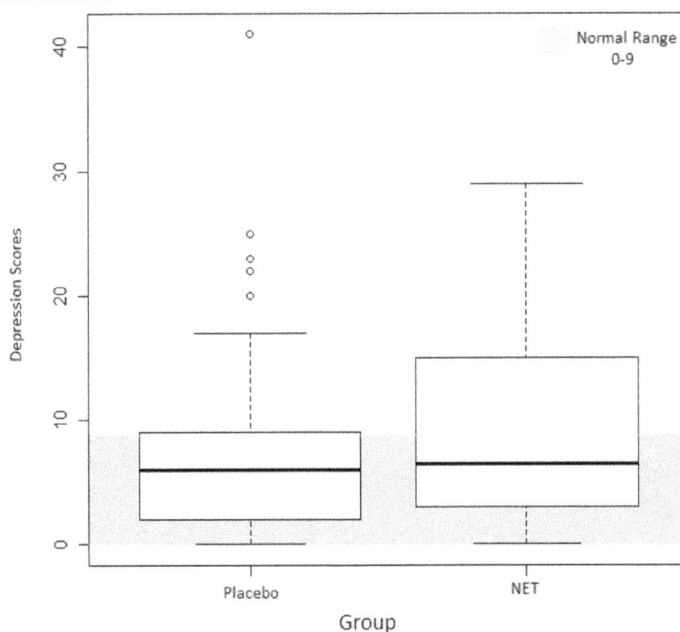

Fig. 2 Baseline depression scores

participant also described feeling "light-headed" after the sixth treatment session. One participant described feeling "drained" after the ninth treatment session. One participant described the sensation of her "head spinning" after the first treatment session. This same participant reported "pain in the lower neck" after the second session and reported a "light headed" feeling after treatments three, four, six and nine. On treatment number nine the participant reported "Always feeling a bit light headed". On visits seven and eight this same participant reported feeling "tired". One participant in the NET group developed a sore throat during the middle of the treatment phase which abated after two weeks. One participant reported feeling "a bit sad" after the ninth treatment session. One participant reported feeling "depressed" after the first and second treatment sessions. During the second treatment session, the participant felt uncomfortable while discussing a memory from her past that was prompted by the questioning associated with the intervention. The participant reported that a couple of hours after this treatment that she experienced a migraine headache that lasted for several hours. The participant was unhappy with the nature of treatment and withdrew herself from the trial. The vast majority of adverse events observed in the NET group occurred directly after the application of the intervention and were not reported at the time of subsequent interventions indicating that these events were of a limited duration. The participants who did experience

adverse events did not require any treatment aside from reassurance from the associated practitioner. No adverse events were reported in the NET group during the post-intervention phase of the clinical trial.

Adverse events - placebo group
Six (13 %) participants reported adverse events that coincided with the application of the placebo intervention. Five of the six described feeling "tired" directly after one or more of the placebo intervention sessions. One participant described feeling "sore" after the tapping applied by the treating practitioner to the right inferior angle of the scapula. No adverse events or harms were reported in the placebo group during or after the post-intervention phase of the clinical trial.

Blinding survey
Of the total number of participants that undertook the blinding survey ($n = 81$), 10/41 (24 %) of placebo participants correctly assumed that they were allocated to the placebo group. Two out of 40 (5 %) participants in the NET group correctly assumed their assignment to the NET group. There was a statistically significant difference between these two proportions (Fisher's exact test, $p = 0.025$). Based on these results, participants in the placebo group appeared more likely to correctly guess their group allocation compared to individuals in the NET group.

Table 4 Analysis of primary and secondary outcomes

Outcome	MCID (±)	Difference between groups 7 weeks (NET-Placebo)		Difference between groups 6 months (NET-Placebo)		Time x group interaction
		Mean difference (95 % CI)	P-value	Mean difference (95 % CI)	P-value	P-value
Depression	4	−0.58 (−4.62, 3.45)	0.78	−0.04 (−4.04, 3.96)	0.98	0.60
Anxiety	5	0.63 (−2.19, 3.46)	0.66	0.36 (−2.44, 3.16)	0.80	0.98
Stress	4	0.29 (−3.63, 4.21)	0.88	1.47 (−2.42, 5.35)	0.46	0.86
TSH	0.75	0.11 (−2.64, 2.88)	0.93	1.01 (−1.76, 3.77)	0.47	0.49
FT4	6.0	0.67 (−0.81, 2.15)	0.37	0.33 (−1.14, 1.80)	0.66	0.85
FT3	1.5	0.29 (−0.24, 0.83)	0.28	0.15 (−0.38, 0.68)	0.58	0.82
Physical functioning	3.5	−0.76 (−9.07, 7.56)	0.86	1.75 (−6.41, 9.91)	0.67	0.35
Role physical	3.2	4.25 (−7.31, 15.81)	0.47	4.35 (−6.93, 15.63)	0.45	0.99
Bodily pain	4.5	3.56 (−7.62, 14.73)	0.53	2.35 (−8.43, 13.13)	0.67	0.76
General health	5.7	2.11 (−8.20, 12.43)	0.69	3.35 (−6.78, 13.47)	0.52	0.28
Vitality	5.5	0.27 (−9.76, 10.30)	0.96	−0.10 (−9.84, 9.65)	0.98	0.76
Social functioning	5.0	9.05 (−4.55, 22.66)	0.19	5.58 (−7.54, 18.69)	0.40	0.65
Role emotional	3.8	2.12 (−8.72, 12.96)	0.70	1.13 (−9.36, 11.61)	0.83	0.86
Mental health	5.5	4.73 (−5.23, 14.72)	0.35	4.83 (−4.84, 14.49)	0.33	0.65
Mental component summary	3.1	4.11 (−1.58, 9.79)	0.16	0.22 (−5.25, 5.69)	0.94	0.36
Physical component summary	3.8	1.02 (−3.14, 5.18)	0.63	0.97 (−3.10, 5.03)	0.64	0.50

MCID minimal clinically important difference, *TSH* thyroid stimulating hormone (mIU/L), *FT4* free thyroxine (pmol/L), *FT3* Free triiodothyronine (pmol/L)

Discussion

This is the first randomized controlled trial investigating the short-medium term effects of NET treatment on individuals with primary hypothyroidism. Both treatment effects and harms data were captured in this study with the major findings presented below.

The NET and placebo groups were comparable with respect to clinical and demographic data at baseline. The vast majority of the study population were taking some form of thyroid medication, most commonly LT4, for their condition. The mean and median serum TSH, FT3, and FT4 concentrations were within the normal range. The

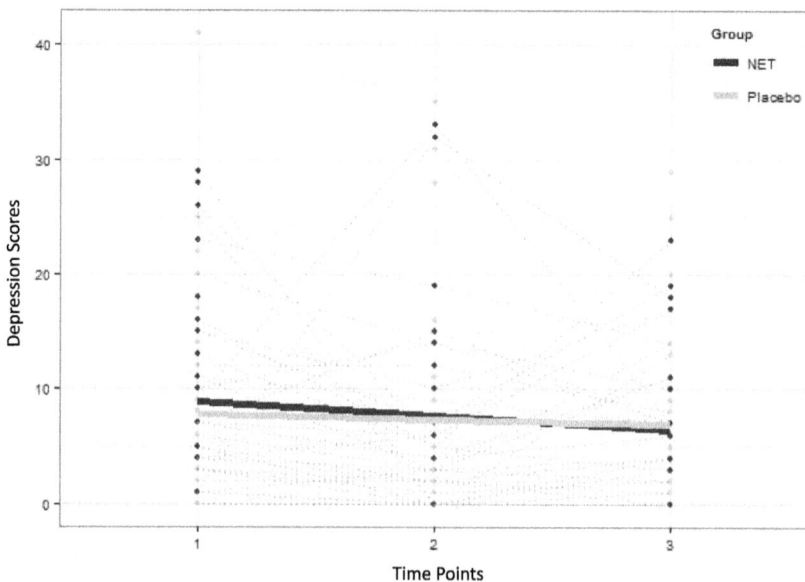

Fig. 3 Depression scores over time

majority of participants displayed abnormal TPO-Ab concentrations at baseline indicating the presence of thyroid autoimmunity. The mean and median depression scores were within normal range however, a substantial proportion of participants displayed abnormal depression scores at baseline. A similar scenario was observed with respect to the anxiety and stress scores at the time of the initial assessment. For the SF-36v2 data, mean self-reported general health, vitality, social functioning, and mental health scores were lower in the study population compared to normative data. These baseline neuropsychiatric findings were expected given the continued symptomatology reported large community based samples of patients with treated hypothyroidism [14, 16, 23].

The results of the analyses revealed that there were no significant differences, at the 5 % significance level, between the NET and placebo groups at time seven weeks or six months for any of the trial outcomes.

If NET has a stress-reducing effect, either; this has not been demonstrated in this particular study; or stress may not be a salient factor in onset and/or progression of this chronic disease. Further research, with much larger sample sizes, is required to ascertain the exact role of stress in the pathogenesis and progression of primary hypothyroidism.

With respect to harms, the way in which the NET treatment was applied, including the dosage, was well-tolerated by the study participants. There were some minor, short-lived adverse-events that followed the application of both the NET and placebo interventions.

Strengths of the study

This is the first RCT investigating the short-medium term treatment effects of NET in participants with primary hypothyroidism. Practitioners of varying backgrounds with similar clinical expertise in NET applied the intervention to the cohort. The approach to delivery, as well as the dosage of the intervention was based on a private practice model of care. The typical participant in the trial was a Caucasian female with a mean age of 45 years, with evidence of thyroid autoimmunity. This profile aligns strongly with epidemiological data regarding patients with primary hypothyroidism [3, 8, 97]. Due to the systemic influence of the thyroid hormones a wide selection of outcome measures were employed that would have captured any short-medium term physiological and psychological changes that coincided with the application of the intervention.

Limitations

Designing placebo interventions can be difficult in research when the underlying biological mechanism behind the therapy is unknown [98]. For this reason, designing a placebo in complementary and alternative medicine research is often dependent on unsubstantiated assumptions about the specificity of the intervention [99]. With this in mind, the placebo was designed via the collaboration of a group of NET certified practitioners, and members of the research team. The aim was to create a placebo intervention that would: closely mimic the NET intervention; would not provide any therapeutic benefit; would be considered credible by the participants; and would be of comparable duration to the NET procedure. The results from the analysis of the blinding survey results would suggest that the placebo intervention was more likely to be viewed as a 'sham' procedure compared to the NET treatment. As the practitioners were involved in the administration of both the NET and placebo interventions, it was not possible to blind these individuals to group allocation. However, to reduce the problem of non-blinding, practitioners were under strict instruction not to reveal group allocation to participants during the trial, and also to refrain from discussing any of the procedures in detail. Furthermore, as the treatment being provided by the practitioners in their private clinics was not recorded or monitored it was not possible to guarantee the fidelity of either of the treatment arms. Slight differences in the delivery of the NET and placebo intervention may account for the results observed in the blinding survey.

The participant's subjective report regarding reactions or adverse events associated with the intervention had the potential to be selectively-filtered by the treating practitioners. The majority of practitioners involved in the trial regularly use NET in their private clinics. These practitioners would presumably want to demonstrate the efficacy and safety of the intervention which may have introduced performance and/or reporting bias.

The study was designed to explore the influence of a biopsychosocial-based treatment approach on the clinical manifestations of primary hypothyroidism. The approach involved a diverse number of outcome measures, and multi-centre format in order to make use of all available resources. This scenario can be problematic in that it introduces the statistical problem of multiple comparisons in which the chances of obtaining a false positive result are increased [100]. While no corrections for multiple testing were used given the exploratory nature of the secondary outcomes this type of correction would not have changed the results obtained in this study.

A power analysis indicated that 51 participants per group would yield a more than 80 % chance of detecting a difference in depression scores of at least four points in NET group compared to the placebo group using a standard deviation of 6.97 based on normative data. The fact that the recruitment of participants fell short of the desired sample size means that there is reduced power to find a difference between groups. If we examine how many participants in each group achieved a four point decrease in depression scores at 7 weeks (11/22 for NET vs 7/18 for placebo) then a 95 % confidence interval for the number needed to treat before a positive treatment outcome occurred would be (–19 to 29). This wide interval indicates anything from no benefit to benefit for 1 in 29 participants and reflects the uncertainty in the data collected.

The sample that was obtained aligns well with profiles from large population studies regarding patients with primary hypothyroidism. There is however the potential that a specific type of participant responded to the recruitment advertisements. As the advertisements were calling for participation in research investigating a new, drug-free treatment for hypothyroidism, it is possible that individuals who were either: not taking medication; opposed to the concept of taking medication; poorly compliant with their current medication regimens; or dissatisfied with their current management regimens were more likely to respond. Furthermore, the advertisements made reference to the Department of Chiropractic at Macquarie University, as the host of this research. Proponents of chiropractic/complementary and alternative medicine, or individuals with positive past experiences with chiropractic treatment may therefore have been over represented in the sample population.

Both the DASS-42 and the SF-36v2 have recall periods of less than one month. For this reason, treatment effects with long latency periods may have been missed in between the seven-week and six-month assessments.

Dr Scott Walker [101], the creator of NET, originally designed the technique to be an adjunct to the usual manual therapy procedures he was using in his private practice. Walker deemed psychosomatic stress to be an important factor contributing to continued or cyclical symptomatology in his patients and designed NET to tackle this problem. The technique represented an additional tool that a practitioner could use if the standard manual procedures alone were not having a longstanding therapeutic effect in patients with musculoskeletal conditions [102]. Later on in the development of NET, Walker added nutritional elements and aspects of homeopathy to the NET procedure. In an attempt to make the investigation of NET more manageable, and the results from the study more comprehensible, the research team restricted the intervention to only the component of NET that deals with psychosocial stress. Based on reviews of homeopathy trials, the magnitude and plausibility of treatment effects of homeopathy for specific medical conditions remains poorly defined [103–105]. In a recent report from the National Health and Medical Research Council of Australia a working committee concluded that there were no health conditions for which there is reliable evidence that homeopathy is effective [106]. In the latest guidelines for the management of hypothyroidism, produced by the American Thyroid Association Taskforce, strong recommendations were made against the use of dietary supplements and nutraceuticals [12]. The main reasons for these recommendations were A)

the lack of evidence regarding the efficacy of these products and B) the potential risks associated with the use of these products for individuals with thyroid conditions. There is a dearth of high quality evidence regarding manual therapy for the treatment of hypothyroidism and a limited evidence-base for homeopathy and nutrition in this role. It is therefore difficult to ascertain what effect removing these components may have had on the overall efficacy of the NET procedure.

As stress is a potential environmental risk factor for the development of primary hypothyroidism, it is possible that NET treatment, a purported stress reduction technique, may function better in a preventative role. In cases of long standing autoimmune thyroid disease there is inflammation and subsequent destruction of the thyroid follicles. This results in the replacement of the thyroid parenchymal tissue with non-functional fibrous tissue [107]. In this scenario, the pathophysiological consequences of autoimmune thyroid disease have resulted in tissue that no longer has an endocrine function. While the disease process and the associated symptomatology continues, the damaged tissue is unlikely to respond, from an endocrine perspective, to any therapeutic intervention. To determine the preventative effect of NET treatment would require a large scale preventative trial which currently lacks evidential support and is beyond the scope of this discussion.

In obtaining ethics approval for this study researchers were required to outline the foreseeable risks associated with participation in the study. At the time of the trial design there were no published harms data regarding NET. As a result, an information and consent form was drafted that included likely potential adverse events such as muscle soreness, tiredness, and an uncomfortable recall of past events. These events were suggested as potential outcomes during consultation with experts in NET. While there were some minor adverse events that coincided with the intervention in both the NET and placebo groups, there is the possibility that participants were primed [108] to report certain events due to the content of this information and consent form.

Conclusions

In this study, NET intervention was not found to confer any clinical benefit to the participants in the short or medium term.

The data recorded on harms suggest that there are some minor, short-term, adverse events associated with the application of this procedure. These events however were predictable, relatively innocuous and did not require further intervention to remedy.

Appendix
Health update questionnaire

Name: _____ Date: _____

There are events and situations that occur in our lives that can influence our health and well-being. When running a clinical trial it is important for researchers to be aware of any events or situations that may influence the findings of the trial.

This questionnaire is designed to identify any factors that may influence the findings of the trial, and hence influence the final interpretation of results.

We ask that you fill out the questionnaire as accurately as possible. This information, when combined with the data obtained from initial and subsequent assessments, will help researchers accurately interpret the findings at the end of the trial.

Q1) Have you changed your medication or changed the way in which you are managing your condition (Hypothyroidism) in the last 6 months since beginning the trial? (Please circle one)

Yes   No
If so, what have you changed?

_____

_____

Q2) Have you tried any other forms of treatment for your condition in the last 6 months since beginning the trial? (Please circle one)

Yes   No
If so, what have you tried?

_____

_____

Q3) Have there been any major stressful situations or events in the last 6 months that may have influenced you general health and well-being? (Please circle one)

Yes   No
If so, what were these situations or events? (Optional)

_____

_____

Q4) Have you made any significant alterations to your life or your lifestyle in the last 6 months since beginning the trial? (Please circle one)

Yes   No
If so, what alterations have you made? (Optional)

_____

_____

Thank you for taking the time to fill out this questionnaire

Abbreviations
DASS-42: Depression anxiety stress scale-42 item; DQ: Demographic questionnaire; FT4: Free-Thyroxine; HPA: Hypothalamic-pituitary-adrenal; HUQ: Health update questionnaire; LT4: Levothyroxine; QOL: Quality of life; RCT: Randomized control trial; RHR: Resting Heart Rate; RT: Resting Temperature; SF-36v2: Short form 36 version 2; TFT: Thyroid function test; Tg-Ab: Thyroglobulin antibody; Tg: Thyroglobulin protein; TPO-Ab: Thyroid peroxidase antibody; TPO: Thyroid peroxidase enzyme; TSH: Thyroid stimulating hormone.

Competing interests
BTB is a chiropractor who works part-time in private practice. BTB has received training in NET and uses this technique in his private practice. HP was an employee of the ONE Research Foundation from 2002–2011. RB and PLG have no conflicts of interest to declare.

Authors' contributions
BTB wrote and compiled the manuscript. PLG, RB and HP were involved with the data collection and analysis and helped edit and review the final manuscript. BTB, RB and HP designed the trial. All authors read and approved the final manuscript.

Acknowledgements
The research project was funded (AUD $28,000) by the Australian Spinal Research Foundation (ASRF), as well as smaller ongoing contributions from the Macquarie University Postgraduate Research Fund (PGRF). The ASRF had no input into the design, conduct and publication of the study results. The authors would like to thank the individual practitioners who donated their time and expertise: Gerald Vargas, Bill Stathoulis, Nicholas Kovacs, Alison Griffiths, Luke Rossmanith, Peter O'Dwyer, Jackie Castell, Suzanne Labrie, Walter Kiris, and Alex McLennan. The authors would like to thank Peter Bablis for his advice and assistance in the design of the clinical trial.

Author details
[1]Department of Chiropractic, Macquarie University, Balaclava Road, North Ryde 2109NSW, Australia. [2]Department of Statistics, Macquarie University, Balaclava Road, North Ryde 2109NSW, Australia. [3]School of Health Professions - Murdoch University, 90 South Street, Murdoch 6150WA, Australia. [4]Private Practice, 84 Kingsway, Cronulla 2230NSW, Australia.

References
1. O'Leary PC, Feddema PH, Michelangeli VP, Leedman PJ, Chew GT, Knuiman M, et al. Investigations of thyroid hormones and antibodies based on a community health survey: the Busselton thyroid study. Clin Endocrinol (Oxf). 2006;64(1):97–104.
2. Vanderpump MP, Tunbridge WM, French JM, Appleton D, Bates D, Clark F, et al. The incidence of thyroid disorders in the community: a twenty year follow-up of the Wickham Survey. Clin Endocrinol. 1995;43(1):55–68.
3. Canaris GJ, Manowitz MR, Mayor G, Ridgway EC. The Colorado thyroid disease prevalence study. Arch Intern Med. 2000;160(4):526–34.
4. McLeod DSA, Cooper DS. The incidence and prevalence of thyroid autoimmunity. Endocrine. 2012;42(2):252–65.
5. McDermott MT. In the clinic. Hypothyroidism. Ann Intern Med. 2009;151(11):ITC61.
6. Monzani F, Del Guerra P, Carraccio N, Pruneti CA, Pucci E, Luisi M, et al. Subclinical hypothyroidism: neurobehavioural features and beneficial effect of L-thyroxine treatment. Clin Invest. 1993;71:367–71.
7. Roberts CGP, Ladenson PW. Hypothyroidism. Lancet. 2004;363(9411):793–831.
8. Hollowell JG, Staehling NW, Flanders WD, Hannon WH, Gunter EW, Spencer CA, et al. Serum TSH, T(4), and thyroid antibodies in the United States population (1988 to 1994): National Health and Nutrition Examination Survey (NHANES III). J Clin Endocrinol Metab. 2002;87(2):489–99.
9. O'Reilly DSJ. Thyroid hormone replacement: An iatrogenic problem. Int J Clin Pract. 2010;64:991–4.
10. Romijn JA, Lamberts JW, Smit SW. Intrinsic imperfections of endocrine replacement therapy. Eur J Endocrinol. 2003;149(2):91–7.

11. Fava GA, Sonino N, Morphy MA. Psychosomatic view of endocrine disorders. Psychother Psychosom. 1993;59(1):20–33.

12. Jonklaas J, Bianco AC, Bauer AJ, Burman KD, Cappola AR, Celi FS, et al. Guidelines for the treatment of hypothyroidism. Thyroid. 2014;24(12):1670–751. doi:10.1089/thy.2014.0028.

13. Saravanan P, Visser TJ, Dayan CM. Psychological well-being correlates with free thyroxine but not free 3,5,3'-triiodothyronine levels in patients on thyroid hormone replacement. J Clin Endocrinol Metab. 2006;91(9):3389–93.

14. Saravanan P, Chaut WF, Roberts N, Vedharas K, Greenwood R, Dayan CM. Psychological well-being in patients on adequate doses of L-thyroxine: results of a large, controlled community based questionnaire study. Clin Endocrinol. 2002;57:577–85.

15. Samuels MH, Schuff KG, Carlson NE, Carello P, Janowsky JS. Health status, psychological symptoms, mood, and cognition in L-thyroxine-treated hypothyroid subjects. Thyroid. 2007;17(3):249–58.

16. Wekking EM, Appelhof BC, Fliers E, Schene AH, Huyser J, Tijssen JG, et al. Cognitive functioning and well-being in euthyroid patients on thyroxine replacement therapy for primary hypothyroidism. Eur J Endocrinol. 2005;153(6):747–53.

17. Panicker VEJ, Bjøro T, Asvold BO, Dayan CM, Bjerkeset O. A paradoxical difference in relationship between anxiety, depression and thyroid function in subjects on and not on T4: findings from the HUNT study. Clin Endocrinol. 2009;71:574–80.

18. Ott J, Promberger R, Kober F, Neuhold N, Tea M, Huber JC, et al. Hashimoto's thyroiditis affects symptom load and quality of life unrelated to hypothyroidism: A prospective case–control study in women undergoing thyroidectomy for benign goiter. Thyroid. 2011;21(2):161–7.

19. Boelaert K, Newby PR, Simmonds MJ, Holder RL, Carr-Smith JD, Heward JM, et al. Prevalence and relative risk of other autoimmune diseases in subjects with autoimmune thyroid disease. Am J Med. 2010;123(2):183.e1–e9.

20. McDermott MT. Does combination T4 and T3 therapy make sense? Endocr Pract. 2012;18(5):750–7.

21. Peeters RP, van Toor H, Klootwijk W, de Rijke YB, Kuiper GG, Uitterlinden AG, et al. Polymorphisms in thyroid hormone pathway genes are associated with plasma TSH and iodothyronine levels in healthy subjects. J Clin Endocrinol Metab. 2003;88(6):2880–8.

22. Peeters RP, Attalki H, Toor H, de Rijke YB, Kuiper GG, Lamberts SW, et al. A new polymorphism in the type II deiodinase gene is associated with circulating thyroid hormone parameters. Am J Physiol Endocrinol Metab. 2005;289:E75–81.

23. Panicker V, Saravanan P, Vaidya B, Evans J, Hattersley AT, Frayling TM, et al. Common variation in the DIO2 gene predicts baseline psychological well-being and response to combination thyroxine plus triiodothyronine therapy in hypothyroid patients. J Clin Endocrinol Metab. 2009;94(5):1623–9.

24. Walsh JP, Ward LC, Burke V, Bhagat CI, Shiels L, Henley D, et al. Small changes in thyroxine dosage do not produce measurable changes in hypothyroid symptoms, well-being, or quality of life: Results of a double-blind, randomized clinical trial. J Clin Endocrinol Metab. 2006;91(7):2624–30.

25. Grozinsky-Glasberg S, Fraser A, Nahshoni E, Weizman A, Leibovici L. Thyroxine-Triiodothyronine combination therapy versus thyroxine monotherapy for clinical hypothyroidism: meta-analysis of randomized controlled trials. J Clin Endocrinol Metab. 2006;91:2592–9.

26. Wojcicka A, Bassett JHD, Williams GR. Mechanisms of action of thyroid hormones in the skeleton. Biochim Biophys Acta Gen Subj. 2013;1830(7):3979–86.

27. Joffe RT, Brimacombe M, Levitt AJ, Stagnaro-Green A. Treatment of clinical hypothyroidism with thyroxine and triiodothyronine: A literature review and metaanalysis. Psychosomatics. 2007;48(5):379–84.

28. Caturegli P, De Remigis A, Rose NR. Hashimoto thyroiditis: Clinical and diagnostic criteria. Autoimmun Rev. 2014;13(4–5):391–7.

29. Quaratino S. Models of autoimmune thyroiditis. Drug Discov Today. 2004;1(4):417–23.

30. Prummel MF, Strieder T, Wiersinga WM. The environment and autoimmune thyroid diseases. Eur J Endocrinol. 2004;150(5):605–18.

31. Tomer Y, Huber A. The etiology of autoimmune thyroid disease: A story of genes and environment. J Autoimmun. 2009;32:231–9.

32. Wasserman EE, Nelson K, Rose NR, Rhode C, Pillion JP, Seaberg E, et al. Infection and thyroid autoimmunity: A seroepidemiologic study of TPOaAb. Autoimmunity. 2009;42(5):439–46.

33. Oddie TH, Fisher DA, McConahey WM, Thompson CS. Iodine intake in the United States: a reassessment. J Clin Endocrinol Metab. 1970;30(5):659–65.

34. Hay ID. Thyroiditis: a clinical update. Mayo Clin Proc. 1985;60:836–43.

35. Krassas GE, Pontikides N, Tziomalos K, Tzotzas T, Zosin I, Vlad M, et al. Selenium status in patients with autoimmune and non-autoimmune thyroid diseases from four European countries. Expert Rev Endocrinol Metab. 2014;9(6):685–92.

36. Srivatsa B, Srivatsa S, Johnson KL, Samura O, Lee SL, Bianchi DW. Microchimerism of presumed fetal origin in thyroid specimens from women: a case–control study. Lancet. 2001;358(9298):2034–8.

37. Klintschar M, Schwaiger P, Mannweiler S, Regauer S, Kleiber M. Evidence of fetal microchimerism in Hashimoto's thyroiditis. J Clin Endocrinol Metab. 2001;86(6):2494–8.

38. Wang J, Zhang W, Liu H, Wang D, Wang W, Li Y, et al. Parvovirus B19 infection associated with Hashimoto's thyroiditis in adults. J Infect. 2010;60(5):360–70.

39. Antonelli A, Ferri C, Fallahi P, Ferrari SM, Ghinoi A, Rotondi M, et al. Thyroid disorders in chronic hepatitis C virus infection. Thyroid. 2006;16(6):563–72.

40. Winsa B, Karlsson A, Bergstrom R, Adami HO, Gamstedt A, Jansson R, et al. Stressful life events and Graves' disease. Lancet. 1991;338(8781):1475–9.

41. Gibson JG. Emotions and the thyroid gland: A critical appraisal. Psychosom Res. 1962;6:93–116.

42. Winsa B, Adami H, Bergström R, Gamstedt A, Dahlberg PA, Adamson U, et al. Stressful life events and Graves' disease. Lancet. 1991;338:1475–9.

43. Matos-Santos A, Lacerda Nobre E, Garcia E, Costa J, Nogueira PJ, Macedo A, et al. Relationship between the number and impact of stressful life events and the onset of Graves' Disease and toxic nodular goitre. Clin Endocrinol. 2001;55(1):15–9.

44. Boscarino JA. Posttraumatic stress disorder and physical illness: Results from clinical and epidemiologic studies. Ann N Y Acad Sci. 2004;1032:141–53.

45. Ferguson-Raypoht SM. The relation of emotional factors to recurrence of thyrotoxicosis. Can Med Assoc J. 1956;75:993–9.

46. Graves RJ. Newly observed affection of the thyroid gland in females. London Med Surg. 1835;7:516–7.

47. Glaser R, Kiecolt-Glaser JK. Stress-induced immune dysfunction: Implications for health. Nat Rev Immunol. 2005;5:243–51.

48. Juster R-P, McEwen BS, Lupien SJ. Allostatic load biomarkers of chronic stress and impact on health and cognition. Neurosci Biobehav Rev. 2010;35(1):2–16.

49. Segerstrom SC, Miller GE. Psychological stress and the human immune system: A meta-analytic study of 30 years of inquiry. Psychol Bull. 2004;130(4):601–30.

50. Elenkov IJ, Chrousos GP. Stress hormones, Th1/Th2 patterns, pro/anti-inflammatory cytokines and susceptibility to disease. Trends Endocrinol Metab. 1999;10(9):359–68.

51. Elenkov IJ. Glucocorticoids and the Th1/Th2 balance. Ann N Y Acad Sci. 2004;1024:138–46.

52. Chrousos GP. Stressors, stress, and neuroendocrine integration of the adaptive response. The 1997 Hans Seyle memorial lecture. Ann N Y Acad Sci. 1998;851:311–35.

53. Chrousos GP, Gold PW. The concepts of stress and stress system disorders: Overview of physical and behavioral homeostasis. JAMA. 1992;267(9):1244–52.

54. Wilder RL. Neuroendocrine-immune system interactions and autoimmunity. Ann Rev Immunol. 1995;13:307–38.

55. Ganesh BB, Bhattacharya P, Gopisetty A, Prabhakar BS. Role of cytokines in the pathogenesis and suppression of thyroid autoimmunity. J Interferon Cytokine Res. 2011;31(10):721–31.

56. Parish NM, Cooke A. Mechanisms of autoimmune thyroid disease. Drug Discov Today Dis Mech. 2004;1(3):337–44.

57. Trickett PK, Noll JG, Susman EJ, Shenk CE, Putnam FW. Attenuation of cortisol across development for victims of sexual abuse. Dev Psychopathol. 2010;22(1):165–75.

58. Danielson CK, Hankin BL, Badanes LS. Youth offspring of mothers with posttraumatic stress disorder have altered stress reactivity in response to a laboratory stressor. Psychoneuroendocrinology. 2015;53:170–8.

59. Bagnasco M, Bossert I, Pesce G. Stress and autoimmune thyroid diseases. Neuroimmunomodulation. 2007;13(5–6):309–17.

60. Strieder TGPM, Tijssen JG, Brosschot JF, Wiersinga WM. Stress is not associated with thyroid peroxidase autoantibodies in euthyroid women. Brain Behav Immun. 2005;19:203–6.

61. Strieder TG, Prummel MF, Tijssen JG, Endert E, Wiersinga WM. Risk factors for and prevalence of thyroid disorders in a cross-sectional study among healthy female relatives of patients with autoimmune thyroid disease. Clin Endocrinol. 2003;59(3):396–401.

62. Oretti RG, Harris B, Lazarus JH, Parkes AB, Crownshaw T. Is there an association between life events, postnatal depression and thyroid dysfunction in thyroid antibody positive women? Int J Soc Psych. 2003;49(1):70–6.

63. Bablis P, Pollard H. Hypothyroidism: A new model for conservative management in two cases. Chiropr J Aust. 2004;34:11–8.

64. Bablis P, Pollard H. A mind-body treatment for hypothyroid dysfunction: A report of two cases. Complement Ther Clin Pract. 2009;15:67–71.

65. Touzard JB, Busch-Pate T, Busch J. Thinking about a problem while getting adjusted? Dr Scott Walker may have the answer? The American Chiropractor. 2008.

66. Walker D, Walker S. Chiropractic technique summary: Neuro Emotional Technique (NET) 2010. http://www.chiroaccess.com/Articles/Chiropractic-Technique-Summary-Neuro-Emotional-Technique-NET.aspx?id=0000185. Last accessed 6th of May 2015.

67. Moher D, Hopewellb S, Schulzc FS, Montorid V, Gøtzschee PC, Devereauxf PJ, et al. CONSORT 2010 explanation and elaboration: updated guidelines for reporting parallel group randomized trials. BMJ. 2010;63:1–37.

68. Schulz KF, Altman DG, Moher D. Consort 2010 statement: updated guidelines for reporting parallel group randomized trials. Ann Intern Med. 2010;152(11):1–7.

69. Boutron I, Moher D, Altman DG, Schulz KF, Ravaud P. Extending the CONSORT statement to randomized trials of nonpharmacologic treatment: explanation and elaboration. Ann Intern Med. 2008;148:295–309.

70. Ioannidis JPA, Evans SJW, Gøtzsche PC, O'Neill RT, Altman DG, Schulz K, et al. Better reporting of harms in randomized trials: an extension of the CONSORT statement. Ann Intern Med. 2004;141:781–8.

71. The George Institute for Global Health. PEDro scale: The George Institute; 1999. http://www.pedro.org.au/english/downloads/pedro-scale/. Last accessed 6th May 2015.

72. Verhagen AP, de Vet HC, de Bie R, Kessels AG, Boers M, Bouter LM, et al. The Delphi list: a criteria list for quality assessment of randomized clinical trials for conducting systematic reviews developed by Delphi consensus. J Clin Epidemiol. 1998;51(12):1235–41.

73. Altman DG, Schulz KF, Moher D, Egger M, Davidoff F, Elbourne D, et al. The Revised CONSORT statement for reporting randomized trials: explanation and elaboration. Ann Intern Med. 2001;134(8):663–94.

74. Boutron I, Moher D, Altman DG, Schulz KF, Ravaud P. Methods and processes of the CONSORT group: example of an extension for trials assessing nonpharmacologic treatments. Ann Intern Med. 2008;148:60–6.

75. Horvath E, Kovacs K, Scheithauer BW. Pituitary hyperplasia. Pituitary. 1999;1(3–4):169–80.

76. Alkhani AM, Cusimano M, Kovacs K, Bilbao JM, Horvath E, Singer W. Cytology of pituitary thyrotroph hyperplasia in protracted primary hypothyroidism. Pituitary. 1999;1(3–4):291–5.

77. NET Inc. Seminar Information & Schedule. 2014. http://www.netmindbody.com/for-practitioners/seminar-information-and-schedule. Last accessed 6th of May 2015.

78. Karpouzis F, Pollard H, Bonello R. A randomized controlled trial of the Neuro Emotional Technique (NET) for childhood Attention Deficit Hyperactivity Disorder (ADHD): a protocol. Trials. 2009;10:6.

79. Karpouzis F. Clinical Investigation of Chiropractic Neuro Emotional Technique (NET) for Attention-Deficit/Hyperactivity Disorder (ADHD) in Children: [Master of Science (Honours)]. Sydney, Australia: Macquarie University; 2011.

80. Brown BT, Bonello R, Pollard H. The biopsychosocial model and hypothyroidism. BMC Chiropr Osteopat. 2005;13:5.

81. Brown BT, Bonello R, Pollard H. The use of traditional Chinese medical principles in chiropractic technique. Chiropr J Aust. 2008;38:18–26.

82. Bablis P, Pollard H, Bonello R. Neuro emotional technique for the treatment of trigger point sensitivity in chronic neck pain sufferers: a controlled clinical trial. Chiropr Osteopat. 2008;16:4.

83. Karpouzis F, Pollard H, Bonello R. Separation anxiety disorder in a 13-year-old boy managed by the Neuro Emotional Technique as a biopsychosocial intervention. J Chiropr Med. 2008;7(3):101–6.

84. Monti DA, Stoner ME, Zivin G, Schlesinger M. Short term correlates of the Neuro Emotional Technique for cancer-related traumatic stress symptoms: A pilot case series. J Cancer Surviv. 2007;1(2):161–6.

85. Brown BT, Bonello R, Pollard H, Graham P. The influence of a biopsychosocial-based treatment approach to primary overt hypothyroidism: A protocol for a pilot study. Trials. 2010;11(106). http://www.trialsjournal.com/content/11/1/106. last accessed accessed 6th of May 2105

86. Lovibond SH, Lovibond PF. Manual for the Depression Anxiety Stress Scales (DASS). 2nd ed. University of New South Wales, NSW 2052, Australia: Psychology Foundation Monograph; 2004.

87. Abbott. Architect System -TSH. Abbott Park, IL, USA: Abbott Ireland Diagnostic Division; 2005c.

88. Abbott. Architect System - Free T3. Abbott Park, IL, USA: Abbott Ireland Diagnostic Division; 2005a.

89. Abbott. Architect System -Free T4. Abbott Park, IL, USA: Abbott Ireland Diagnostic Division; 2005b.

90. Siemens. Immulite 2500 Anti-TG Ab. Los Angeles, CA, USA: Siemens Medical Solutions Diagnostics; 2005.

91. Siemens. Immulite 2500 Anti-TPO Ab. Los Angeles, CA, USA: Siemens Medical Solutions Diagnostics; 2005.

92. Ware JE, Kosinski M, Bjorner JB, Turner-Bowker DM, Gandek B, Maruish ME. User's manual for the SF-36v2 Health Survey. 2nd ed. Lincoln RI: Quality Metric Incorproated; 2007.

93. Brant R. Inference for means: comparing two independent samples 2015. http://www.stat.ubc.ca/~rollin/stats/ssize/n2.html. last accessed 6th of May 2015.

94. Random Sequence Generator. http://www.random.org/sform.html. Last accessed 6th of May 2015.

95. Hornik K. R: A Language and Environment for Statistical Computing. Vienna, Austria 2011.

96. Little D. Statistical Analysis with Missing Data. New York: Wiley; 1987.

97. Tunbridge WM, Evered DC, Hall R, Appleton D, Brewis M, Clark F, et al. The spectrum of thyroid disease in a community: The Whickham survey. Clin Endocrinol. 1977;7(6):481–93.

98. Schulz KF, Chalmers I, Hayes RJ, Altman DG. Empirical evidence of bias. Dimensions of methodological quality associated with estimates of treatment effects in controlled trials. JAMA. 1995;273:408–12.

99. Lewith G, Barlow F, Eyles C, Flower A, Hall S, Hopwood V, et al. The context and meaning of placebos for complementary medicine. Forsch Komplementmed. 2009;16:404–12.

100. Curran-Everett D. Multiple comparisons: philosophies and illustrations. Am J Physiol Regul Integr Comp Physiol. 2000;279(1):R1–8.

101. Walker S. The Amazing Story of NET [webpage]. 2000. https://www.netmindbody.com/about-us/the-amazing-story-of-net. Last accessed 6th of May 2015.

102. Walker S, NET Basic Seminar Manual 2005. Sydney, Australia.

103. Shang A, Huwiler-Müntener K, Nartey L, Jüni P, Dörig S, Sterne JA, et al. Are the clinical effects of homoeopathy placebo effects? Comparative study of placebo-controlled trials of homoeopathy and allopathy. Lancet. 2005;366(9487):726–32.

104. Cucherat M, Haugh MC, Gooch M, Boissel JP. Evidence of clinical efficacy of homeopathy. A meta-analysis of clinical trials. Eur J Clin Pharmacol. 2000;56(1):27–33.

105. Jonas WB, Kaptchuk TJ, Linde K. A critical overview of homeopathy. Ann Intern Med. 2003;138(5):393–9.

106. National Health and Medical Research Council. NHMRC Statement: Statement on Homeopathy. National Health and Medical Research Council. 2015. March 2015. Report No.: CAM02.

107. Burek CL, Talor MV. Environmental triggers of autoimmune thyroiditis. J Autoimmun. 2009;33(3–4):183–9.

108. Lang EV, Hatsiopoulou O, Koch T, Berbaum K, Lutgendorf S, Kettenmann E, et al. Can words hurt? Patient-provider interactions during invasive procedures. Pain. 2005;114(1–2):303–9.

17

Understanding clinical reasoning in osteopathy: a qualitative research approach

Sandra Grace[1*] (iD), Paul Orrock[1], Brett Vaughan[2], Raymond Blaich[1] and Rosanne Coutts[1]

Abstract

Background: Clinical reasoning has been described as a process that draws heavily on the knowledge, skills and attributes that are particular to each health profession. However, the clinical reasoning processes of practitioners of different disciplines demonstrate many similarities, including hypothesis generation and reflective practice. The aim of this study was to understand clinical reasoning in osteopathy from the perspective of osteopathic clinical educators and the extent to which it was similar or different from clinical reasoning in other health professions.

Methods: This study was informed by constructivist grounded theory. Participants were clinical educators in osteopathic teaching institutions in Australia, New Zealand and the UK. Focus groups and written critical reflections provided a rich data set. Data were analysed using constant comparison to develop inductive categories.

Results: According to participants, clinical reasoning in osteopathy is different from clinical reasoning in other health professions. Osteopaths use a two-phase approach: an initial biomedical screen for serious pathology, followed by use of osteopathic reasoning models that are based on the relationship between structure and function in the human body. Clinical reasoning in osteopathy was also described as occurring in a number of contexts (e.g. patient, practitioner and community) and drawing on a range of metaskills (e.g. hypothesis generation and reflexivity) that have been described in other health professions.

Conclusions: The use of diagnostic reasoning models that are based on the relationship between structure and function in the human body differentiated clinical reasoning in osteopathy. These models were not used to name a medical condition but rather to guide the selection of treatment approaches. If confirmed by further research that clinical reasoning in osteopathy is distinct from clinical reasoning in other health professions, then osteopaths may have a unique perspective to bring to multidisciplinary decision-making and potentially enhance the quality of patient care.

Where commonalities exist in the clinical reasoning processes of osteopathy and other health professions, shared learning opportunities may be available, including the exchange of scaffolded clinical reasoning exercises and assessment practices among health disciplines.

Background

Current health reforms have promoted team-based care, new scopes of practice, new health care roles and sharing of professional information [1, 2] which can cross professional boundaries and challenge our notions of professional identity. Professional boundaries are based on sets of competencies and unifying philosophies, and codified by formal education [3]. Professional identities,

created through monopolising a body of knowledge and skills [4], are challenged by practitioners who practise within advanced and extended scopes, as occurs when podiatrists perform minor surgical procedures, or when nurse practitioners prescribe medication. It has been suggested that knowledge in a particular area of discipline-specific expertise may be less important for future health practitioners than generic skills like teamwork, and sound and reasoned judgement [5].

Clinical reasoning broadly refers to the 'thinking and decision-making processes associated with clinical practice' [6]. Traditional models of clinical reasoning referred

* Correspondence: sandra.grace@scu.edu.au
[1]School of Health & Human Sciences, Southern Cross University, PO Box 157, Lismore NSW 2480, Australia
Full list of author information is available at the end of the article

to a cognitive practitioner-centred process whereby practitioners gather information about their patients, synthesise that information and develop treatment and management plans [7, 8]. Cognitive models tend to be very structured in their descriptions of how reasoning takes place. They also tend to be have little consideration for the patient's contribution to the reasoning process, despite practitioners' heavy reliance on context in the reasoning process [9].

How reasoning occurs for practitioners of varying experience (i.e. novice or experienced) has been a strong focus in the literature on clinical reasoning. Analytical or hypothetico-deductive reasoning was initially associated solely with the reasoning processes of novice practitioners. Expertise, on the other hand, was associated with intuitive reasoning or pattern recognition. Hallmarks of expertise included being able to identify and synthesise important clinical information, particularly for complaints that are ill-defined or complex [10], using metacognitive skills [11, 12], having life and clinical experience [13], and having insight into one's own reasoning processes [14]. It was previously thought that experienced practitioners, when presented with cases that did not fit into recognisable patterns, reverted to a hypothetico-deductive approach. However, it appears that these two approaches to problem solving are fluid and overlapping, practitioners dynamically moving between both, depending on the situation [15]. Peterson [16] demonstrated that radiology students who performed well on a radiology film-reading examination exhibited similar reasoning characteristics to those practitioners with many years' experience. Moreover, it appears that no two practitioners will follow the same reasoning process even if the presenting complaint is exactly the same and the same diagnosis is reached [17]. The dual processing theory of clinical reasoning [18] has been proposed to describe practitioners' use of both non-analytical processes (intuition or pattern recognition) and analytical ones (hypthetico-deductive) in clinical reasoning. This theory recognises the high level of interaction between the two processes.

Another approach to clinical reasoning in the health professions that has been described by Hamm [19] was based on the cognitive continuum theory proposed by Hammond [20]. In fact, it has been argued that that dual processing model should be replaced by cognitive continuum theory as the predominant theory to explain clinical reasoning [21]. Cognitive continuum theory is underpinned by the two concepts of cognition and task properties. Within cognition is a continuum from analysis (slow, deliberate task/data processing, high level of confidence in outcome) to intuition (fast task/data processing, low level of confidence in outcome). The central part of this continuum is referred to as quasirationality: a combination of analysis and intuition. Most clinical

reasoning is thought to lie within quasirationality [21]. Task properties can be described as well- and ill-structured: well-structured tasks require time to process and resolve, whereas ill-structured tasks require a quick resolution with little time devoted to contrasting different outcomes. Changing a task is likely to influence the point along the cognition continuum which describes a clinician's reasoning. It is the specific features of a task and mode of processing that Custers [21] suggests is an underdeveloped area in the clinical reasoning literature.

Sociocultural or interpretive models of clinical reasoning prioritise the centrality of the patient in clinical reasoning and emphasise the collaborative and interactive nature of the process [22, 23]. Edwards et al. [12] found that physiotherapists moved between reasoning about the patients' physical complaints (hypothetico-deductive or pattern recognition) and engaging with the patient or their carer (narrative reasoning) to understand the impact of the complaint. Higgs and Jones [24] described a number of contexts of clinical reasoning that included all aspects of the health encounter including patients, practitioners' interpersonal skills and personal values, teams, the workplace, and the local and global health systems where interactions take place (see Table 1). In this interpretation, collaborative reasoning could include interactions between patients and practitioners, and/or practitioners and other practitioners to co-create decisions about health care.

Clinical reasoning in specific health professions

Clinical reasoning has been described as a process that draws heavily on the professional learning, craft knowledge and intuition [25] that are particular to each health profession [26, 27]. Fleming and Mattingly [28] argued that the hypothetical deductive reasoning that emerged from the medical problem-solving tradition was too narrow to encompass 'the myriad ways in which health professionals devise solutions for clients' needs.' In an earlier work Fleming [29] compared medical and occupational therapy clinical reasoning and found both similarities that arose from using hypothetical reasoning and differences that arose from the 'particular focus, goals, and tasks of the two professions and the nature of the practice in those arenas.'

Metaskills can be broadly defined as higher-order skills that enable effective use of pre-existing skills (see Table 1). The use of metaskills has been identified as part of the clinical reasoning process in many health professions [30] Metaskills include: knowledge/hypothesis generation when differential diagnoses are formulated from information collected from or about patients [31, 32]; reflexivity that requires a combination of reflection on one's own clinical practice and identification of future learning needs; the ability to derive knowledge

Table 1 Key contexts and metaskills of clinical reasoning (adapted from Higgs and Jones [24])

Contexts	Practitioner	• Practice knowledge • Practice experience • Values and beliefs • Own professional practice
	Patient	• Values and beliefs • Health and illness experiences • Knowledge and experience of the health discipline • Knowledge and experience of other health disciplines and the health care system
	Community	• Patient's family and friends • The health discipline • Local and global health systems • Workplace
Metaskills		• Reflexivity • Metacognition • Emotional intelligence • Analytic skills and pattern recognition • Knowledge generation • Practice-model authenticity • Ability to derive knowledge and practice wisdom from reasoning and practice • Use of critical, creative conversation to make decisions

and practice wisdom from reasoning and practice; the use of critical, creative conversation to make decisions; and the ability to locate reasoning as behaviours and strategies within chosen practice models, each with an inherent philosophy of practice [24]. This last metaskill is also referred to as 'practice model authenticity' and suggests that clinical reasoning is likely to differ according to the underpinning philosophy and principles of a particular health profession.

Clinical reasoning in manual therapies

Manual therapies includes corrective exercise, chiropractic, osteopathy, physiotherapy, massage therapy, and muscle training [33]. The World Confederation for Physical Therapy [34] describes physical therapy as providing 'services that develop, maintain and restore people's maximum movement and functional ability. They can help people at any stage of life, when movement and function are threatened by ageing, injury, diseases, disorders, conditions or environmental factors ... Physical therapists help people maximise their quality of life, looking at physical, psychological, emotional and social wellbeing. They work in the health spheres of promotion, prevention, treatment/intervention, habilitation and rehabilitation.' Such a description could encompass the practices of many manual therapy professions.

A number of studies of the clinical reasoning practices in specific manual therapy professions are reported in

the literature. For example, Ajjawi [35] found that hypothetico-deductive reasoning was used as the predominant strategy in physiotherapy. Components of clinical reasoning that were originally described by Elstein in medicine [8], namely cue acquisition, hypothesis generation, cue interpretation and hypothesis evaluation, were still evident in physiotherapy although contemporary clinical reasoning took in case management as well as diagnosis [35]. Manual therapists have also been reported as embracing the biopsychosocial model, becoming more holistic in their approach, and having more focus on active management and patient participation [36].

Jones and Rivett [37] set out to develop the clinical reasoning skills of manual therapists using a series of cases with commentary. These authors argued that 'the original professional training of the manual therapists, whether it be in physiotherapy, chiropractic, osteopathy, medicine or another profession, is not important because the clinical reasoning process is universal' [37].

Clinical reasoning in osteopathy

Sociocultural and interpretive approaches to clinical reasoning may be particularly well suited to professions like osteopathy that are based on different philosophical foundations from medicine and that have traditionally emphasised holism, patient-centredness, and a wellness model of care [38]. The personal values of the practitioner and their professional belief system will influence their clinical reasoning [24]. The practice of osteopathy is reportedly founded on a set of principles [39], although it is unclear how these principles influence the clinical reasoning employed by osteopaths. A number of osteopathic reasoning models based on the relationship between structure and function in the human body have been developed to facilitate interpretation of subjective information collected from patients and objective data from diagnostic testing [40]. These structure-function relationships include biomechanical, psychosocial, neurological, nutritional, respiratory-circulatory and energy-expenditure models (see Table 2). The structure-function relationships are used to prioritise specific osteopathic treatment approaches and the order in which they are applied. However, despite the suggested inclusion of structure-function relationship models in osteopathic curricula and their use in practice, there is little in the literature that explores their application in osteopathic clinical reasoning. In fact, clinical reasoning in osteopathy has only recently been described in the literature. According to Thomson et al. [41], clinical reasoning for experienced practitioners lies along a continuum of practice from technical rationality (a practitioner-centred, physical, biomedical and biomechanical approach) to professional artistry (a patient-centred, biopsychosocial approach) - a continuum that encompasses hypothetico-

Table 2 Osteopathic diagnostic models

Biomedical	Consideration of signs and symptoms in the context of defined diseases and need for referral for further medical assessment and management (red flags).
Biomechanical	Assessment of the health of the musculoskeletal system, including how the structure (posture) and function are integrated.
Respiratory/ circulatory	Examination of the respiratory mechanism, ensuring that breathing function is optimal. Assessment of all tissues of the body for full blood supply and drainage, and of the structural and functional relationship between the two systems.
Neurological	Assessment of function in the central, peripheral and autonomic nervous systems, and the relationship of those systems to all tissues of the body.
Nutritional	Foundational dietary analysis for signs of deficiency or suboptimal nutritional status.
Behavioural	Consideration of the psychosocial factors influencing health, including relational, occupational and financial, and the need for multidisciplinary care.
Energy expenditure	Assessment of optimal energy utilisation, and consideration of issues that may affect the healing process (e.g. relatively minor mechanical or immune dysfunctions).

deductive reasoning, pattern recognition and narrative reasoning (collaborative dialogue between the patient and practitioner to co-produce treatments). In the current climate of health care reform, it is timely that the osteopathic profession explores its professional identity and the clinical reasoning that underpins it [42].

The purpose of this study was to explore osteopathic clinical educators' understanding of clinical reasoning in the broader context of clinical reasoning in the health professions, in order to ascertain commonalities and differences. Clinical educators were selected for this study because of their pivotal role in developing and assessing clinical reasoning skills in students. Osteopathic educators regularly engage with the design, conduct and marking of clinical assessments that purport to assess clinical reasoning in osteopathy. They are well positioned to reflect on their understanding of clinical reasoning and ways in which those understandings were shaped by their experiences as educators and practitioners. They are likely to have developed an understanding of the processes of clinical reasoning and of strategies to scaffold development of clinical reasoning in osteopathy students. The present study draws on the perspectives of clinical educators from osteopathic programs in Australia, New Zealand and the UK. Findings of this study will contribute to our understanding of clinical reasoning in osteopathy and will inform our understanding of the contribution of osteopathic clinical reasoning to patient health care and to curriculum development.

Methods

This research drew on elements of constructivist grounded theory. We assumed that clinical reasoning is created by practitioners as they interact with and interpret objects in the world [43]. In the present study 'objects' include patients' signs and symptoms, current literature, practitioners' previous experiences and colleagues' opinions. According to Charmaz [44], researcher and participant construct a shared reality through an iterative process of data collection and analysis. Researchers' perspectives formed part of the analysis in the present study. The research team comprised four osteopaths and one exercise physiologist, the latter also facilitated the focus groups. The strategy of using a facilitator from another discipline was to bring a perspective from another health discipline to the data analysis.

A purposive sample of participants from three Australian universities and two international osteopathic programs (one university in New Zealand and one college in the United Kingdom) were invited to contribute because of strong working relationships between the institutions. Four institutions accepted the invitation: four participants from Southern Cross University (SCU) (Australia), two participants from each of Victoria University (VU) (Australia), and Unitec (New Zealand), and one participant from the British School of Osteopathy (BSO) (United Kingdom), providing an appropriate cross-section of the profession for a preliminary investigation. This cross-section of participants is also relevant because of the capacity for osteopaths to move between these three countries to practise. Table 3 provides demographic data of the study participants. The study was approved by the SCU Human Research Ethics Committee (Approval number ECN-12-232). Data collection and analysis took place during 2013 and 2014.

Osteopathic educators were invited to participate in two data collection activities in which participants individually and collectively reflected on their understanding of clinical reasoning in osteopathy.

Focus groups

Three focus groups, each of 90 minutes duration, were conducted in a meeting room at SCU, at times convenient for all participants. A total of nine participants representing each participating institution (four from SCU, two from VU, two from Unitec and one from BSO) attended in person or by Skype. In Focus Group 1 four members from SCU met face to face with two representatives from VU. In Focus Group 2 all six attendees met with two representatives from Unitec, New Zealand via Skype. In Focus Group 3 the four members of SCU met with a representative of the BSO.

The facilitator used a semi-structured interview guide to explore two key questions:

Table 3 Participant demographics

	Gender	Age (years)	Institution	Years in practice	Years of clinical supervision
1[a]	M	51-60	SCU	25	22
2[a]	M	41-50	SCU	20	16
3[a]	F	51-60	SCU	32	30
4	F	51-60	SCU	25	22
5	F	41-50	VU	13	8
6[a]	M	41-50	VU	13	10
7	F	41-50	Unitec	21	20
8	M	41-50	Unitec	16	14
9	M	41-50	BSO	20	18
10[a]	F	51-60	SCU	12	5

[a]Members of the research team
Note: 10 was the facilitator; an exercise physiologist, not a registered osteopath

- What is clinical reasoning in osteopathy?
- Is clinical reasoning in osteopathy different from clinical reasoning in other health disciplines?

The interview guide was adapted after each round of data collection and analysis so that leads from previous focus groups could be pursued as they arose, and so that progressive data collection could generate and refine emerging theory.

Critical reflections

This study also drew on Brookfield's [45] theory of critical self-reflection. Critical self-reflection encourages a deep evaluation of reasons, both obvious and not-so-obvious, for thinking and acting. The focus groups allowed ideas and concepts about clinical reasoning in osteopathy to be discussed, challenged, refined and developed within the group. After the focus groups, participants were asked to further reflect on their understandings of clinical reasoning in osteopathy and to write their own definition of clinical reasoning. When all written reflections had been submitted, they were collated by one member of the research team and forwarded to the other members for reading and reflection.

Data analysis

Focus groups were audio recorded with participants' consent and each one analysesd before the following stage of data collection. This process was continued until redundancy of information was reached. Transcriptions and written definitions were thematically analysed using the following procedure: Each member of the research team independently scrutinized the transcripts by repeatedly reading and re-reading to generate conceptual categories. Next, the whole research team met to compare conceptual codes and to develop inductive categories.

Finally categories were compared and contrasted and searched for contradictions until agreement was reached. Theoretical sampling relied on the use of four education institutions in three continents, and a facilitator who provided a perspective from outside osteopathy.

Results

Five key themes emerged from the data:

Clinical reasoning does not lead to a single diagnosis

According to participants, the primary purpose of clinical reasoning in osteopathy was to develop a working diagnosis or rationale for treatment; practitioners were less concerned about naming a medical condition. As one participant said: *The aim isn't to come up with a diagnosis but with a treatment plan (Participant S).* Another commented:

> *In osteopathy you rarely come to a single label that conclusively says what this case is about … it's imprecise. There's no one answer like there is in a medical exam where the answer is infective endocarditis, for example. That single diagnosis is not there in osteopathy. (Participant P)*

In order to find ways of treating patients, practitioners synthesised findings from clinical histories, physical examinations and their own previous knowledge and experience. Clinical reasoning was used as a guide to the next phase of the consultation. Working diagnoses or hypotheses about patients' conditions involved likely aetiologies for presenting signs and symptoms, and precipitating and maintaining factors. An example of an osteopathic working diagnosis might be: *peripheral inflammatory nociception of radiocarpal joints, caused by rheumatoid arthritis and maintained by occupational stress and sedentary lifestyle* (Participant R). Participants acknowledged the importance of palpatory findings in their working diagnoses: *I always find something, something in the tissues - the quadratus lumborum might be tight so I'll work on it for a while (Participant M).* The working diagnosis for this patient was not a single, named medical condition.

Clinical reasoning occurs in many contexts

According to participants, clinical reasoning occurs in many contexts including those of the patient and the practitioner. Adopting a patient-centred approach clearly influenced the clinical reasoning process:

> *Typically [clinical reasoning] is collaborative – practitioner and patient, practitioner and patients' families, practitioner and other practitioners (Practitioner U).*

Participants spoke of the importance of cultivating a patient-centred approach in their students. Students needed to understand that their own values and beliefs, past experience and evidence-based knowledge had to be mitigated by those of their patients.

[We] encourage students to take a view of the patient that encompasses a whole range of attitudinal and affective components - not just facts-based or knowledge-based information on outcomes of clinical testing. While somebody may be experiencing significant lower back pain with high VAS [visual analogue pain scale] and limited ROM [range of motion] scores, it is the context that exists for the person in terms of their expectations of mobility, in terms of being able to get to the shops, look after two small children etc. - those things colour the value of that evidence in helping us establish what is important as an outcome for the patient. (Participant L)

The process of clinical reasoning was described as interactive and dynamic. Consistent with a patient-centred approach, the reasoning process engaged the patient through a continual and evolving sequence of data gathering (including history taking and physical examination) and feedback from patients, their families and other health practitioners. One participant emphasised the terms 'working diagnosis' and 'hypothesis' and discouraged using 'diagnosis' to highlight the fluid nature of the clinical reasoning process.

The practitioners' context was described as being strongly influenced by the challenges of practising a discipline that has a long tradition of anecdotal clinical efficacy but little scientific evidence specifically supporting osteopathic approaches. Where scientific evidence existed, it was used in the clinical reasoning process:

You look at the evidence, you look at the quality of that evidence, the context within which it sits and the relationship to the decision you are making. (Participant L)

Although osteopaths drew on evidence from other health disciplines (e.g. physiotherapy and chiropractic) that was relevant to their own practices, little research has been conducted on distinctly osteopathic approaches and treatments for a range of conditions. Participants' comments included:

We rely heavily on tacit knowledge and traditional knowledge. (Participant K)

You are left with very little evidence that guides you, and you have to reason from principles, past

experience, case series and the patient context. This would then also include so-called collaborative reasoning where the patient's previous experience, expectations and needs are brought into the equation. (Participant P)

Clinical reasoning also drew on environmental influences beyond the patient's and the practitioner's immediate context. One participant pointed out that the knowledge that was used in clinical reasoning could be drawn from many sources:

I think you draw on all knowledge when you are in clinic. It's not just about 'clinical knowledge'. I might have read a book or a patient might want to talk about something that comes from another realm, not a clinical realm, and these things influence your reasoning. (Participant R)

Clinical reasoning occurs in two different stages

Participants described two stages of clinical reasoning: the first involved an analysis of data to identify red flags for serious underlying pathology. Its purpose was specifically related to patient safety, namely, to identify patients requiring referral for medical or other health care. If patients were deemed suitable for osteopathic treatment, then osteopaths would attempt to clinically reason from a specifically osteopathic perspective.

I think the first thing is the orthopaedic and neurological level to rule out any nasties, anything that looks like an organic disease, and then take a look at what's happening in the physical body using all the osteopathic diagnostic techniques that give you information relative to the case. (Participant K)

I think there are two levels. The first is safety and I think in practice patient safety is reasonably assessed - cardinal signs, red flags. I think teachers and well-trained examiners know when to tick the patient safety box when they are assessing clinical reasoning. But that's only a chunk of the reasoning. It's not difficult. It's much more 'textbook' to learn. The second level is osteopathic reasoning. The osteopathic focus. (Participant P)

This osteopathic perspective referred to specific osteopathic diagnostic procedures, including diagnosis of soft tissue changes and diagnosis of restricted motion.

Clinical reasoning calls on a number of metaskills

Participants acknowledged that clinical reasoning in osteopathy required a number of metaskills on the part of the practitioner, including knowledge generation when practitioners analysed and synthesised data to form working diagnoses:

I see clinical reasoning as the process of gathering all relevant information including previous reports, imaging reports, test results, findings from physical examination etc., regarding a given patient, and processing it appropriately for the benefit of the patient. (Participant R)

Reflexivity - when practitioners reflected on their own abilities and limitations and how their personal insights influenced their clinical reasoning - was widely acknowledged by participants as an essential component of the clinical reasoning process:

Practitioners need to be able to reflect on action, but also importantly to reflect in action, that is, to analyse, synthesise, evaluate, and problem-solve many times as part of the normal business of practice. (Participant S)

Clinical reasoning in osteopathy is different from clinical reasoning in other health disciplines

Most participants stated that clinical reasoning in osteopathy was different from clinical reasoning in other health professions. It was acknowledged that the dual processes of hyptothetico-deductive reasoning and pattern recognition were at play in clinical reasoning in osteopathy as they appear to be in other health disciplines. However, according to participants, the difference was that clinical reasoning in osteopathy was guided by models that are grounded in osteopathic philosophy. These models were well known to the participants: not only had they been taught these models during their own pre-professional education, but also they were now involved in cultivating their use in the clinical reasoning processes of their students. These models are summarised in Table 2. Participants concurred with Participant U's comment below. Many had similar experiences with students from other disciplines:

We've taken physiotherapists into the masters' course. Our tutors pick up that they have a very different way of thinking and it's the clinical reasoning [in osteopathy] part that they struggle with the most. (Participant U)

One participant described her perception of a discipline-specific approach to clinical reasoning this way:

[The difference] has to be something to do with the osteopathic lens - the osteopathic way of looking at the world ... (Participant S)

Opinions were divided about the relationship between the clinical reasoning process and the osteopathic principles (the inter-relationship of body structure and function, the body's inherent self-regulation, the importance of the somatic tissues in overall health). On the one hand, they were envisaged as *forming an overarching framework (Participant S)* that rendered an osteopathic approach to clinical reasoning different from that of other health practitioners. Another participant disagreed: *The principles are vexatious really and we make little reference to them. (Participant U)*

Discussion

The purpose of this study was to understand clinical reasoning in osteopathy from the perspective of clinical educators and to determine the extent to which clinical reasoning in osteopathy was the same as, or different from, clinical reasoning in other health professions. Where commonalities exist, shared learning opportunities may be available, and osteopathic educators can confidently draw on scaffolded clinical reasoning exercises and assessment practices from other disciplines. Should further research confirm that clinical reasoning in osteopathy is distinct from other health professions, then clinical reasoning in osteopathy can contribute a different perspective to multi-disciplinary decision-making and potentially enhance the quality of patient care.

Similarities between clinical reasoning in osteopathy and other health professions

According to participants, the goal of clinical reasoning in osteopathy was not to reach a definitive medical diagnosis, but to identify and prioritise osteopathic treatment approaches. Clinical practice has been described as an encounter of considerable ambiguity [46] and perhaps even more so for osteopaths for whom a high proportion of their patients have chronic complex conditions for which medical diagnoses have not been found [47, 48]. Study participants used their clinical reasoning to direct their treatments based on osteopathic diagnosis, often in the absence of a named medical diagnosis. Research-informed practice calls on practitioners to consider all available evidence when formulating diagnoses and treatment plans [49]. This was achieved through a multi-stage reasoning process that usually began with a biomedical approach to identify red flags for serious underlying pathology, and culminated in specific osteopathic diagnostic techniques that included complex palpatory examination of all tissues of the body. This dependence on palpatory finding in the reasoning process has been established to varying degrees in other manual therapies, supported by clinical guidelines which argued for the use of these more subjective findings to guide appropriate management, even in the absence of definitive diagnosis of musculoskeletal conditions [50, 51]. However, this dependence on subjective palpatory findings is controversial. In fact, Jones and Rivett [37] argued against solely tissue-based reasoning in favour of management based on activity/participation for effective treatment while continuing to evaluate clinical impressions.

Much of the clinical reasoning literature supports health practitioners' use of multiple reasoning strategies (e.g. hypothetico-deductive and pattern recognition; diagnostic or procedural, interactive, and conditional or predictive reasoning; narrative reasoning; ethical reasoning; collaborative reasoning) [31, 32]. Participants in this study did not describe reasoning strategies beyond two diagnostic models: one grounded in biomedical science knowledge, and the other in osteopathy-specific knowledge. This may be a reflection of an approach in osteopathic curriculum to emphasise primary care responsibilities (i.e. initial screening for red flag conditions). However, although not explicitly described, the interactive process whereby data is gathered, including patient's response to treatment, is consistent with the collaborative reasoning model of occupational therapists described by Fleming and Mattingly [28].

Study participants described contexts that are similar to those described in other professions [24]. For example, participants were well aware of the patient's context (i.e. the acknowledgement and value of patient's personal health and illness experiences) and the practitioner's context (i.e. the influence that their own backgrounds, beliefs and biases could exert of their reasoning). Collaborations among practitioners are also likely to be confined to those with other osteopaths rather than with other health professions. This may ensue from and/or be the reason for the way that osteopathy is practised: most osteopaths in Australia work in sole practices or group practices with other osteopaths [52]. Although there is some evidence that osteopaths do engage in referral networks with other health professionals [48, 53], collaborative reasoning with other health professionals was not reported in our study. For osteopathy to fully contribute to multidisciplinary health care, sociocultural approaches to patient care, including collaborations concerning patient diagnoses and treatment, may need to be implemented in future osteopathic curricula. It is also worthy of note that the contexts of wider social responsibility and the global community described by Higgs and Jones [24] were not evident in the description of osteopathic clinical reasoning that emerged in this study.

Metaskills like hypothesis generation and reflexivity that were identified by study participants are also well described in other professions. For example, Jensen et al. [10], comparing occupational therapy and physical therapy, identified reflection and moral agency as critical aspect of clinical reasoning in both disciplines. Reflective self-awareness was also described in physiotherapy by Jones

et al. [32]. In fact, it has been argued that the ability to monitor and regulate cognitive processes appropriately is characteristic of expert performance in any profession [54].

Differences between clinical reasoning in osteopathy and other health professions

Clinical reasoning is grounded in the learning, craft knowledge and intuition of that profession [25]. Thompson et al. [55] described clinical reasoning in osteopathy as a spectrum of approaches from technical rationality to professional artistry, and this continuum incorporates the three aspects of reasoning identified by Paterson [25]. Being both practitioners and clinical educators, the participants in the present study described clinical reasoning from both perspectives. For example, one participant commented:

We assume there is a difference to find ... As practitioners we know there is a difference. We have got evidence from our students going in as physios (physiotherapists) in the Masters. They have little skills in clinical reasoning from an osteopathic perspective. (Participant M)

Participant M was able to bring perspectives from her own practice experience as well as her experience as a clinical educator to the discussion. In this case, her exposure to the clinical reasoning process of a student from a different discipline reinforced her own practice experience.

Participants were divided over how well osteopathic principles were applied in practice (*The principles are vexatious really and we make little reference to them. Participant U*). However, they all supported the idea of two phases of clinical reasoning in osteopathy, that is, using a biomedical approach to exclude red flag conditions, followed by reasoning through the lens of osteopathic structure-function models as part of the 'craft knowledge' of osteopathy. They argued that interpreting patient data through these structure-function relationships enabled practitioners to explore connections between seemingly unrelated things, for example, a headache with a dysfunctional breathing pattern or with restricted movement in one knee. How strongly other osteopaths support this two phase approach could be debated and will inevitability vary from practitioner to practitioner. There was general agreement among participants that the 'osteopathic lens' that was applied during the reasoning process, distinguished clinical reasoning in osteopathy from clinical reasoning in other professions. Whether a difference in fact exists, requires further exploration.

Implications

A focus on aspects of clinical practice that overlap across health professions may facilitate multidisciplinary health care. Global workforce reforms are driving many professions to re-evaluate their traditional boundaries and scopes of practice to make way for cross-boundary health care, such as advanced nursing practice and prescribing rights for podiatrists. Collaborations among practitioners from different disciplines may need to overcome preciously guarded professional boundaries if the patients' best interests are to be served. In fact, one of the trends in clinical reasoning identified by Higgs and Jones [24] was interdisciplinary reasoning that 'transcends the boundaries of professional groups (with their diverse backgrounds) and includes patients as part of multidisciplinary teams'. Future studies could look for similarities in clinical reasoning across related professions (e.g. physiotherapy, chiropractic and osteopathy) and across those professions with whom osteopaths share referral networks to identify how each profession can collaborate for optimal patient care. This process may also confirm or disprove the existence of an osteopathy-specific reasoning process. Should a clinical reasoning process that is unique to osteopathy be identified, osteopaths would need to be play a greater role in multidisciplinary decision making to bring their unique perspectives to patients' health care.

There are also important educational implications that derive from this study. Commonalities in clinical reasoning could be taught across disciplines and support the promotion of generalist training in some areas. Scaffolded learning activities to develop clinical reasoning and assessment rubrics could be shared across disciplines and marked by clinical educators of other health disciplines.

Limitations

The findings of this study are context-dependent and not intended to be generalised to other people or settings. Participants were both clinical educators and practitioners and their understandings of osteopathic clinical reasoning provided a rich data set. The rigour of the research was ensured by long engagement with the texts and triangulation with other literature in the field. There would be value in conducting a study similar to the present one with osteopaths who have no experience in an educational institution, in order to gather more practice-based opinions and reduce the possible influence of institutional and theoretical objectives in graduate outcomes that may be present in educators' opinions.

Conclusion

Study participants posited that clinical reasoning in osteopathy differed from clinical reasoning in other professions in its two-phase approach: using a biomedical approach to rule out red flag conditions initially, and then using an 'osteopathic lens' through which to interpret data and to inform treatment. This 'osteopathic lens' referred to diagnostic reasoning models that are based on the relationship between structure and function in the human body and guide the selection of treatment approaches. Such discipline-specific approaches to clinical reasoning can contribute to our understanding of professional identity, and to our understanding of the contributions that individual professions bring to multidisciplinary health care.

According to participants, clinical reasoning in osteopathy is used to guide treatment rather than to identify a named medical condition. Contexts (e.g. the patient's illness experiences, the practitioner's experience and biases), and metaskills (e.g. hypothesis generation, reflective self-awareness) were similar to those identified in the clinical reasoning processes of other health professions. Further emphasis may need to be given to collaborative clinical reasoning in osteopathy education and practice to ensure the best outcomes for patients.

Competing interests

The authors declare that they have no competing interests.

Authors' contributions

SG made a substantial contribution to conception and design of the study, acquisition of data, data analysis and interpretation of data, the initial draft of the manuscript and critical revision; PO made a substantial contribution to the conception and design of the study, acquisition of data, data analysis and critical revision of the manuscript; BV made a substantial contribution to the data acquisition, analysis and interpretation, and critical revision of the manuscript; RB contributed to data acquisition, analysis and interpretation, and critical revision of the manuscript; RC contributed to data collection, analysis and interpretation, and critical revision of the manuscript. All authors read and approved the final manuscript.

Authors' information

Sandra Grace is the Director of Research at the School of Health and Human Sciences, Southern Cross University and Course Co-ordinator of the Master of Osteopathic Medicine program. She is also an Adjunct Associate Professor at the Education for Practice Institute, Charles Sturt University, and a Visiting Associate Professor at the College of Health and Biomedicine, Victoria University. She is a health services researcher with particular focus on innovative models of care and interprofessional practice and education. Paul Orrock is an osteopathic clinician and academic. He has lectured in osteopathic courses at three Australian universities, and is Senior Lecturer, and inaugural Head of the Osteopathic Program at Southern Cross University. Paul has a Masters degree by research where he investigated the relationship between pelvic dysfunction and gait, and is currently studying for his PhD looking at pragmatic clinical trial methodology. Paul also has had a private practice as an osteopath for over 24 years integrating the use of natural medicines and osteopathy into family health care. Brett Vaughan is a lecturer in the College of Health & Biomedicine, Victoria University, Melbourne, Australia and a Professional Fellow in the School of Health & Human Sciences at Southern Cross University, Lismore, New South Wales, Australia. His interests centre on competency and fitness-to-practice assessments, and clinical education in allied health. Raymond Blaich is an osteopathic practitioner and educator. He is a lecturer at the School of Health and Human Sciences, Southern Cross University, in Lismore, New South Wales, Australia. Raymond has completed a Master's degree by research from the University of Sydney and is currently pursuing a PhD investigating the anatomical sciences in osteopathic education in Australia. Rosanne Coutts has 36 years of experience as an educator and is currently the Director of Teaching and Learning for the School of Health and Human Sciences at Southern Cross University. She has made a strong contribution to the ongoing development and restructure of curricula and has provided leadership for innovative educational advances. She has high level skills in the construction of educational environments relevant to the training of healthcare professionals preparing to work within the Australian healthcare system.

Author details

[1]School of Health & Human Sciences, Southern Cross University, PO Box 157, Lismore NSW 2480, Australia. [2]College of Health & Biomedicine, Victoria University, 301 Flinders Lane, Melbourne, Australia.

References

1. Clouston T, Whitcombe S. The professionalisation of occupational therapy: a continuing challenge. Br J Occup Ther. 2008;71:314–20.
2. Health Workforce Australia. National Health Workforce Innovation and Reform Strategic Framework for Action 2011–2015. Adelaide: Health Workforce Australia; 2011.
3. Nancarrow S. Six principles to enhance workforce flexibility. Hum Resour Health. 2015;13:9.
4. Allsop J, Saks M. Introduction: The Regulation of the Health Professions. In: Allsop J, Saks M, editors. The Regulation of the Health Professions. London: Sage; 2002.
5. Whitcombe S. Problem-based learning students' perceptions of knowledge and professional identity: occupational therapists as 'knowers'. Br J Occup Ther. 2013;76:37–42.
6. Higgs J, Jones M. Clinical Reasoning in the Health Professions. 2nd ed. Oxford: Butterworth Heinemann; 1995.
7. Arocha J, Patel V, Patel Y. Hypothesis generation and the coordination of theory and evidence in novice diagnostic reasoning. Med Decis Making. 1993;13:198–211.
8. Elstein A, Shulman L, Sprafka S. Medical problem solving: An analysis of clinical reasoning. Cambridge, MA: Harvard University Press; 1978.
9. Loftus S. Language in clinical reasoning: Learning and using the language of collective clinical decision making. Sydney: University of Sydney; 2006.
10. Jensen G, Resnik L, Haddad A. Expertise and clinical reasoning. In: Higgs J, Jones M, Loftus S, Christensen N, editors. Clinical reasoning in the health professions. Oxford: Butterworth Heinemann; 2008. p. 123–35.
11. Jensen G, Gwyer J, Shepard K, Hack L. Expert practice in physical therapy. Phys Thera. 2000;80:28–43.
12. Edwards I, Jones M, Carr J, Braunack-Mayer A, Jensen G. Clinical reasoning strategies in physical therapy. Phys Thera. 2004;84:312–30.
13. Simmons B. Clinical reasoning: concept analysis. Journal of Advanced Nursing. J Adv Nurs. 2010;66:1151–8.
14. Groves M, O'Rourke P. The clinical reasoning characteristics of diagnostic experts. Med Teach. 2003;25:308–13.
15. Sibbald M, de Bruin A. Feasibility of self-reflection as a tool to balance clinical reasoning strategies. Adv Health Sci Educ. 2012;17:419–29.
16. Peterson C. Factors associated with success or failure in radiological interpretation: diagnostic thinking approaches. Med Educ. 1999;33:251–9.
17. Charlin B, Desaulniers M, Gagnon R, Blouin D, Van der Vleuten C. Comparison of an aggregate scoring method with a consensus scoring method in a measure of clinical reasoning capacity. Teach Learn Med. 2002;14:150–6.
18. Croskerry P. A universal model of diagnostic reasoning. Acad Med. 2009;84:1022–8.
19. Hamm R. Clinical intuition and clinical analysis expertise and the cognitive continuum. In: Downie J, Elstein A, editors. Professional Judgement: A Reader in Clinical Decision Making. Cambridge: Cambridge University Press; 1988. p. 78–109.
20. Hammond K. Human Judgement and Social Policy: Irreducible uncertainty, inevitable error. New York: Oxford University Press; 1996.
21. Custers E. Medical education and cognitive continuum theory: An alternative perspective on medical problem solving and clinical reasoning. Acad Med. 2013;88:1074–80.
22. Unsworth C. Clinical reasoning: How do pragmatic reasoining, worldview and client-centredness fit? Br J Occup Ther. 2004;67:10–9.
23. Ersser S, Atkins S. Clinical reasoning and patient-centred care. In: Higgs J, Jones M, Loftus S, Christensen N, editors. Clinical reasoning in the health professions. 3rd ed. Oxford: Butterworth Heinemann; 2008. p. 77–87.
24. Higgs J, Jones M. Clinical decision making and multiple problem spaces. In: Higgs J, Jones M, editors. Clinical Reasoning in the Health Professions. Oxford: Butterworth-Heinemann; 2008. p. 3–23.
25. Paterson M, Higgs J, Wilcox S. Developing expertise in judgement artistry in occupational therapy practice. Br J Occup Ther. 2006;69:115–23.
26. Rose M, Best D. Transforming practice through clinical education, professional supervision and mentoring. London: Churchill Livingstone; 2005.
27. Etzioni A. The semi-professions and their organization. New York: Free Press; 1969.
28. Fleming MH, Mattingly C. Action and narrative: Two dynamics of clinical reasoning. In: Higgs J, Jones M, Loftus S, Christensen N, editors. Clinical reasoning in the health professions. 3rd ed. Amsterdam: Butterworth Heinemann; 2008.
29. Fleming M. Clinical reasoning in medicine compared with clinical reasoning in occupational therapy. Am J Occup Ther. 1991;45:988–96.
30. Ajjawi R, Higgs J. Learning to Reason: A Journey of Professional Socialisation. Adv Health Sci Educ. 2008;13:133–50.
31. Schwartz A, Elstein A. Clinical reasoning in medicine. In: Higgs J, Jones M, Loftus S, Christensen N, editors. Clinical reasoning in the health professions. 3rd ed. Oxford: Butterworth Heineman; 2008. p. 223–34.
32. Jones M, Jensen G, Edwards I. Clinical reasoning in physiotherapy. In: Higgs J, Jones M, Loftus S, Christensen N, editors. Clinical reasoning in the health professions. Oxford: Butterworth Heinemann; 2008. p. 246–56.
33. Farrell J, Jensen G. Manual therapy: A critical assessment of the role in the profession of physical therapy. Phys Thera. 1992;72.
34. World Confederation for Physical Therapy. What is physical therapy? http://www.wcpt.org/what-is-physical-therapy. Accessed 31 Aug 2015.
35. Ajjawi R. Learning to communicate clinical reasoning in physiotherapy practice. Sydney: The University of Sydney; 2006.
36. Twomey L. Foreword. In: Jones M, Rivett D, editors. Clinical Reasoning for Manual Therapists. Philadelphia, PA: Butterworth Heinemann; 2004. ix-x.
37. Jones M, Rivett D. Clinical reasoning for manual therapists. Edinburgh: Butterworth Heinemann; 2004.
38. Burns S, Burns J. Andrew Taylor Still, MD: founder of osteopathy. J Altern Complement Med. 1997;3:213–4.
39. Kuchera W, Kuchera M. Osteopathic principles in practice. Columbus: Greyden Press; 1994.
40. World Health Organization. Benchmarks for training in osteopathy. http://www.who.int/medicines/areas/traditional/BenchmarksforTraininginOsteopathy.pdf. Accessed 18 Oct 2010.
41. Thomson O, Petty N, Moore A. A qualitative grounded theory study of the conceptions of clinical practice in osteopathy – A continuum from technical rationality to professional artistry. Man Ther. 2014;19:37–43.
42. Thomson O, Petty N, Moore A. Clinical reasoning in osteopathy - More than just principles? Int J Osteopath Med. 2011;14:71–6.
43. Crotty M. The Foundations of Social Research. Meaning and perspective in the research process. St Leonards, Australia: Allen & Unwin; 1998.
44. Charmaz K. Constructing Grounded Theory: A Practical Guide through Qualitative Analysis London: Sage; 2006.
45. Brookfield S. Developing critical thinkers. Challenging adults to explore alternative ways of thinking and acting. San Francisco, CA: Jossey-Bass; 1989.
46. Dogra N, Giordano J, France N. Cultural diversity teaching and issues of uncertainty: the findings of a qualitative study. BMC Med Educ. 2007;7:8.
47. Orrock P. Profile of members of the Australian Osteopathic Association: Part 1 - The practitioners. Int J Osteopath Med. 2009;12:14–24.
48. Burke S, Myers R, Zhang A. A profile of osteopathic practice in Australia 2010–2011: A cross-sectional survey. BMC Musculoskelet Disord. 2013; 14:227–37.
49. Downing A, Hunter D. Validating clinical reasoning: A question of perspective, but whose perspective? Man Ther. 2003;8:117–9.
50. Group AAMPG. Evidence-based Management of Acute Musculoskeletal Pain. A Guide for Clinicians. Bowden Hills, Queensland: Australian Academic Press Pty Ltd; 2004.
51. Koes B, van Tulder M, Lin C-W, McAuley J. An updated overview of clinical guidelines for the managemetn of non-specific low back pain in primary care. Eur Spine J. 2010;19:2075–94.
52. Orrock P. Osteopathic Census 2004. Final Report to the Australian Osteopathic Association. In. Lismore: Southern Cross University; 2005.
53. Orrock PJ, Lasham K, Ward C. Allied health practitioners' role in the chronic disease management program: The experience of osteopathic practitioners. Int J Osteopath Med. 2014;18:97–101.
54. Alexander PA, Judy JE. The interaction of domain-specific and strategic knowledge in academic performance. Rev Educ Res. 1988;58:375–404.
55. Thomson O, Petty N, Moore A. Clinical reasoning and therapeutic approaches of experienced osteopaths. Int J Osteopath Med. 2013;16:e15–6.

18

Perceptions of the quality of the therapeutic alliance in chiropractic care in The Netherlands: a cross-sectional survey

Nicoline M. Lambers[*] and Jennifer E. Bolton

Abstract

Background: Research in various medical fields demonstrates a consistent and positive association between clinical outcomes and the quality of the therapeutic alliance between the patient and clinician. The aim of this study was to explore how well chiropractors and their patients in The Netherlands perceive the quality of their working relationship.

Methods: A nationwide survey of chiropractors and their patients was conducted in The Netherlands, using a validated Dutch translation of the Working Alliance Inventory (WAV-12). Data were collected over a 5-week period in September-October 2014. Both patients and chiropractors were requested to reflect on 12 statements about to how well they perceived their collaboration in reaching consensus on treatment goals and treatment strategies, and how well they perceived the existence of an affective bond in their working relationship. A 5-point Likert scale was used to answer each question. Higher ratings reflected a more positive perception of the therapeutic alliance. Furthermore, levels of agreement between patients' and chiropractors' perceptions of the quality of their therapeutic alliance were determined.

Results: In total, 207 working relationships between patients and their chiropractor were analysed. The quality of the therapeutic alliance was perceived as being very positive for both patients ($n = 183$, mean 49.14 ± 7.12) and chiropractors ($n = 202$, mean 50.48 ± 4.97). There was no difference in patients' perceptions whether treated by a male or female chiropractor, nor in relation to the chiropractor's years of experience. Nevertheless, poor agreement was found between perceptions of patients and chiropractors in the same relationship (ICC = 0.13).

Conclusions: Both patients and chiropractors perceived the quality of the therapeutic alliance as being very positive. Despite these positive results, patient and chiropractor pairs perceived the level of collaboration in order to reach agreement on treatment goals and strategies and the quality of their affective bond very differently. Clinically, these results suggest that chiropractors should, during the course of treatment, continue to collaborate with their patient and frequently verify whether their patient continues to agree with the treatment goals and treatment plan applied to further develop, improve and maintain a positive therapeutic alliance.

Keywords: Therapeutic alliance, Working alliance, Working relationship, Chiropractic, Doctor-patient relationship

Background

With regard to improving the quality of care, a paradigm shift is currently advocated in medicine from disease-centred care towards patient-centred care. One of the fundamental requirements for practising patient-centred care is developing a therapeutic working relationship with the patient [1]. In the literature, this therapeutic working relationship is interchangeably referred to as therapeutic alliance, working alliance or helping alliance [1–4].

There is consensus about the three essential elements of the alliance based on Bordin's concept of the Working Alliance [5]. The first two elements relate to the collaboration between the patient and clinician in reaching agreement on the treatment goals (goal dimension) and treatment strategies, or tasks, applied to achieve the goals (task dimension). The third element is the presence of an affective bond between the patient and clinician. An

---

* Correspondence: nlambers@aecc.ac.uk
Anglo-European College of Chiropractic, 13-15 Parkwood Road, Bournemouth BH5 2DF, UK

affective, emotional connection such as, for example, mutual trust and acceptance will favour collaboration and reaching consensus on treatment goals and treatment strategies [2–4, 6, 7].

The concept of the therapeutic alliance has become increasingly significant due to its positive and consistent association with treatment outcomes. This association was first identified in psychotherapy research [2–4] and more recently in research in the fields of general medicine [8–12] and physical therapy and rehabilitation [13–15]. To improve the quality of the therapeutic alliance, it is imperative for a clinician to understand which factors influence and enhance the quality of the therapeutic alliance.

A literature search (Additional file 1 and Fig. 1) was performed to identify the core components of the therapeutic alliance that determine its quality in relation to clinical outcomes in primary care settings. These were found to be: (1) empathy, (2) trust, (3) collaboration, (4) agreement on treatment goals and treatment strategies, and (5) patient-centred communication. Most research related to the association between empathy and trust with treatment outcomes, indicating the apparent relevance of the development of an affective bond as part of the alliance.

Empathy is a fundamental and crucial factor in the therapeutic alliance, and it is highly valued in relation to quality of care by both patients and clinicians [9, 16–19]. A recent systematic review found that an empathic behaviour on the clinician's side diminishes anxiety and distress in patients and improves patient satisfaction, patient adherence and patient enablement in medical settings [9].

Trust also influences the affective bond and is defined as 'the belief that the doctor is working in the patient's best interest'. It is found to be associated with increased patient satisfaction, adherence to treatment and continuity of care [12, 20–22]. Surprisingly to some, clinicians'

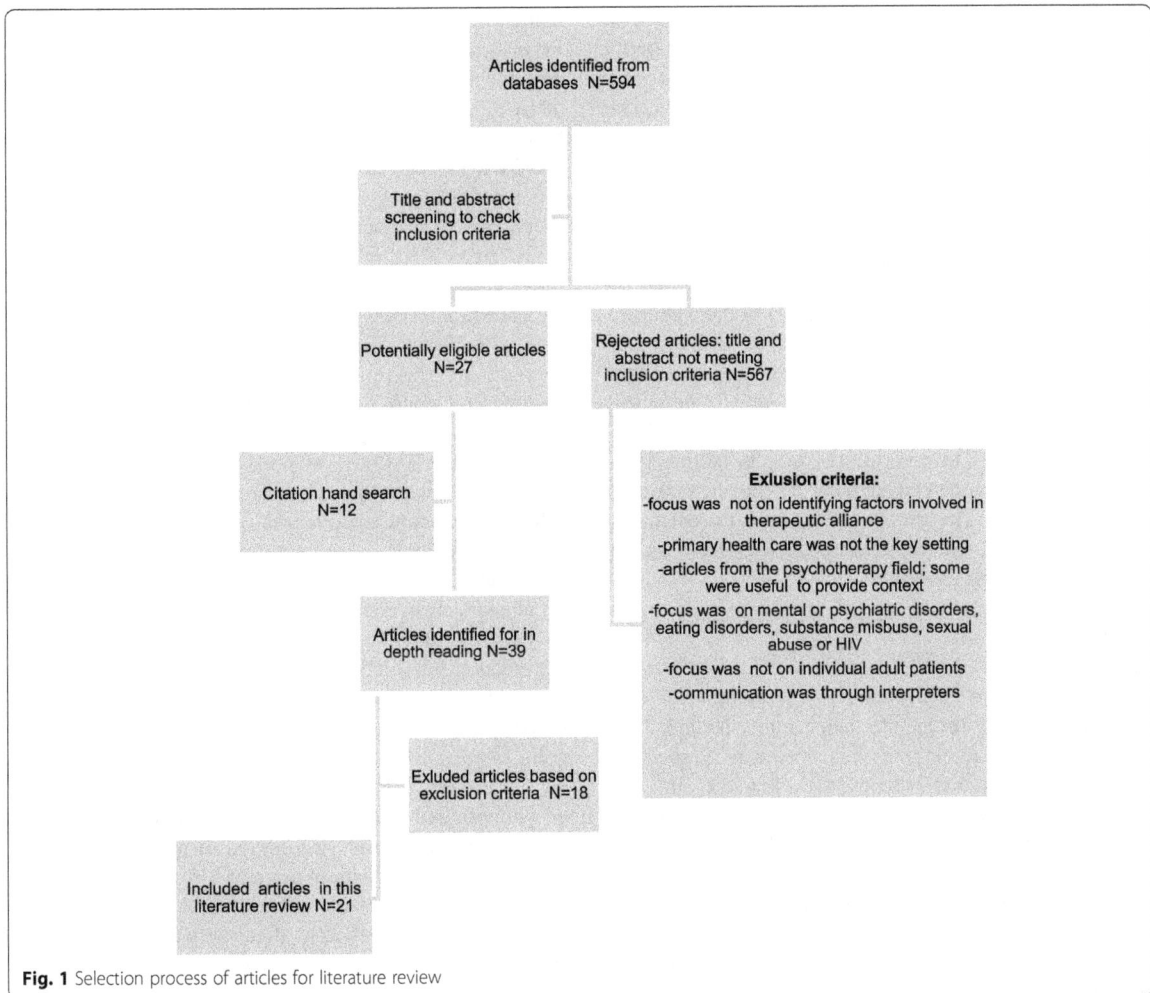

Fig. 1 Selection process of articles for literature review

behaviours that foster trust as perceived by patients are, above all, being comforting and caring, indicating that the affective characteristics of the clinician apparently provide the patient with more trust than do the technical competencies of the clinician [22].

Collaboration, or partnership, is considered another fundamental component of the therapeutic alliance [8, 23, 24] and is consistently associated with improved patient adherence and satisfaction with care [8, 25].

Although little research has been performed on the agreement on treatment goals and strategies component of the therapeutic alliance in primary care settings, it is also considered to be a fundamental part of the alliance [10, 11]. Positive outcomes are not very likely if there is no agreement on treatment goals and strategies between the patient and the clinician. Particularly in the case of chronic conditions, where self-management and self-efficacy are required from patients, consensus on treatment goals and strategies between the patient and the clinician have been found to improve treatment outcomes [26].

Finally, patient-centred communication is considered an essential and crucial component in the therapeutic alliance [11, 23, 27, 28], especially since it mediates the other core components of the alliance. Communication styles that help clinicians engage more with patients, and which facilitate patient participation, are associated with stronger therapeutic alliances [11].

Both understanding the concept of the therapeutic alliance and implementing the core components in clinical practice are essential in order to improve the quality of the working relationship. However, with respect to improving quality, it is important to know how patients and clinicians perceive the quality of the therapeutic alliance. Few studies have investigated this aspect, in particular in chiropractic care. The purpose of this study is, therefore, to describe the quality of the therapeutic alliance as perceived both by patients and by chiropractors in The Netherlands, and to determine whether patients and their chiropractors have similar perceptions of their encounter.

Methods
Participants
Participants were chiropractors working in The Netherlands and three of their adult patients. All members of the Netherlands Chiropractors' Association (NCA) who worked in private practice in The Netherlands ($n = 252$) were invited to participate in this study by email. Patients that were eligible to partake in this study were the participating chiropractor's first consecutive three patients after receiving the questionnaires who: (1) consulted their chiropractor for their third visit irrespective of their symptoms, (2) were over 18 years old, (3) were able to read and understand Dutch and (4)

had not consulted the same chiropractor in the last 3 years, except for the first and second consultation. In the case of an eligible patient refusing to participate, the chiropractor was requested to recruit the next eligible patient fulfilling the inclusion criteria.

Questionnaires
The questionnaires used to collect data for this survey were the client and therapist versions of the "Werkalliantievragenlijst (WAV-12) [29]. This WAV-12 is a translated (English to Dutch), shortened and revised version of the Working Alliance Inventory (WAI) [7, 30, 31]. This WAI is a self-report instrument based on Bordin's concept of the Working Alliance [5] to assess the quality of the working relationship as perceived by the client and the therapist. It is one of the most frequently used alliance measures, both in psychotherapy and other medical fields [15, 29, 32–34].

The WAV-12 client version has demonstrated good internal consistency reliability ($\alpha = 0.82\text{-}0.85$) and good construct validity (Goodness-of-Fit index 0.90) ([29]. Permission to use the WAV-12 for this study was received from Professor Horvath, the developer of the original WAI [30]. For this study, both the client and therapist versions of the questionnaire were slightly modified for use in a chiropractic setting by replacing the word client by patient, therapist by chiropractor, therapy by chiropractic and session by treatment.

Data collection
All chiropractors that agreed to enrol were sent an envelope with three chiropractor versions and three patient versions of the questionnaire in. For each patient-chiropractor encounter, the patient and the chiropractor each completed one questionnaire, resulting in "paired questionnaires". Both versions of the questionnaire consisted of twelve questions in the form of statements, reflecting patients' experiences with respect to collaboration in reaching agreement on treatment goals (goal dimension), agreement on treatment strategies (task dimension) and on the existence of an affective bond (bond dimension) in the working relationship, with four statements for each area. Patients and chiropractors were asked to rate how often they felt each statement to be true in their working relationship on a 5-point Likert scale ranging from (1) seldom or never, (2) sometimes, (3) fairly often, (4) very often, to (5) always. In addition, all patients and chiropractors were asked for their gender. Chiropractors were also asked to note their number of years of working experience as a chiropractor.

All participants were requested to complete their questionnaires immediately after the patient's third consultation. Research has shown that statistically reliable associations exist between the working alliance and clinical outcomes after the third consultation. Furthermore, the quality of the alliance early in the treatment was found to be a better predictor of outcomes than measured at later phases in the treatment [3, 30, 31]. In addition, as pointed out by Ferreira at al. (2013), assessing the alliance early in the treatment plan limits the influence of the clinical effect of the intervention [13]. Directly upon completion, all participants were instructed to put their questionnaire in an unmarked envelope, and personally seal it in order to safeguard anonymity and prevent anybody but the researcher from reading the answers. Data were collected over a five-week period in September-October 2014.

Data analysis
Variables retrieved from the questionnaires were the patients' and chiropractors' ratings (1–5) for each of the twelve questions, their gender and the chiropractors' years of working experience as a chiropractor. Data were analysed using SPSS (Version 20). To describe the overall quality of the working relationship, and the quality of the three separate elements (goal dimension, task dimension, bond dimension), as perceived by patients and chiropractors, descriptive statistics were used. Higher ratings indicated more positive perceptions of the alliance. The Intraclass Correlation Coefficient (ICC) was used to determine the level of agreement between patients' and chiropractors' perspectives of the alliance. The unpaired t-test was used to determine whether there was a difference in patients' perspective dependent on chiropractors' gender, and dependent on gender matching between the patient and their chiropractor. Finally, a one-way ANOVA test was used to determine the effect of the chiropractor's years of working experience on patients' perceptions.

Results
Participants
A total of 89 chiropractors (35.3 % of the invited NCA members) agreed to participate in this study. Of the 76 chiropractors (52.6 % female) that returned questionnaires, 60 (78.9 %) returned questionnaires on three working relationships, 12 (15.8 %) on two working relationships, and 4 (5.3 %) on one working relationship. One questionnaire was incomplete and excluded. Two reminders to participate were sent to all invited chiropractors and a further two emails were sent to remind chiropractors of returning their questionnaires. In total, data on 207 patient-chiropractor working relationships were included.

Demographic characteristics
Demographic characteristics of the participants are shown in Table 1.

Table 1 Demographic characteristics of the participants

Variable	Characteristic	N	%
Gender (Chiropractors)	Male	36	47.4
	Female	40	52.6
	Missing data	0	0
	Total	76	100
Gender (Patients)	Male	84	40.6
	Female	118	57.0
	Missing data	5	2.4
	Total	207	100
Gender matching in chiropractor-patient pairs	Matched	133	64.3
	Unmatched	69	33.3
	Missing data	5	2.4
	Total	207	100
Years of working experience (Chiropractors)	0–5 years	23	30.3
	6–14 years	28	36.8
	15+ years	25	32.9
	Total	76	100

WAV-12 scores and frequencies, overall and per dimension
As seen in Table 2, both patients ($n = 183$; mean 4.09 ± 0.59) and chiropractors ($n = 202$; mean 4.21 ± 0.41) rated their alliance very positive.

Compared to patients' perceptions, chiropractors perceived the quality of the working relationship slightly more positive, both on the quality of the therapeutic alliance overall, as well as on agreement on treatment goals and strategies and the presence of an affective bond separately. Both groups experienced the affective aspect within the alliance slightly more positive than the collaborative aspects. Agreement on goals, although still rated very positive, was perceived the least strong of the three dimensions. Fewer patients ($n = 183$, 88.4 %) than chiropractors ($n = 202$, 97.6 %) completed all twelve questions. Particularly questions exploring views on the quality of the affective bond (9.2 %) and agreement on treatment goals (4.8 %) were left unanswered by patients.

Figure 2 presents frequencies of scores on individual questions of the WAV-12, grouped per dimension, both for patients and chiropractors. Although perceptions were rated very positive, patients' ratings were more varied compared to the more skewed ratings of chiropractors.

Agreement between patients' and chiropractors' scores
Results in Table 3 showed that there was poor agreement (ICC < 0.40) [35] between patients' and chiropractors' perspectives on the same working relationships.

Influence of gender
Results in Tables 4 and 5 showed that there were no statistically significant differences in patients' perceptions

Table 2 Means of total scores and mean scores of patients and chiropractors on the WAV-12 overall and per dimension

Patient scores	N	Mean of total scores[a]	SD	Mean scores[b]	SD
Overall WAV-12	183	49.14	7.12	4.09	±0.59
Goal dimension	197	15.92	2.61	3.98	±0.65
Task dimension	201	16.39	2.46	4.10	±0.62
Bond dimension	188	16.89	2.80	4.22	±0.70
Chiropractor scores					
Overall WAV-12	202	50.48	4.97	4.21	±0.41
Goal dimension	206	16.18	2.21	4.04	±0.55
Task dimension	205	16.59	2.04	4.15	±0.51
Bond dimension	205	17.71	1.64	4.43	±0.41

[a]Overall WAV scores max 60; dimensional scores max 20
[b]Measured on a 1–5 point Likert scale, 5 representing an optimal alliance

of their working relationships between being treated by a male or female chiropractor.

Influence of working experience

The number of years of experience working as a chiropractor ranged from less than 1 to 31 years and was categorised into three similarly sized groups: 0–5 years (30.3 %), 6–14 years (36.8 %) and 15 years or more (32.9 %). The results in Fig. 3 showed that the differences in patients' perceptions on their working relationship were minimal between these three experience categories and were not statistically significant (Table 6).

Discussion

This study is the first to explore the quality of the therapeutic alliance between patients and chiropractors in The Netherlands as perceived by both patients and chiropractors. The measurement instrument used in this study assessed how both patients and chiropractors experienced collaboration in reaching agreement on treatment goals and treatment strategies to achieve their goals and how they perceived their affective bond. The results showed that, immediately after the third consultation, both patients and chiropractors perceived the quality of their working relationship overall to be very positive. Results on the quality of the three separate elements of the alliance showed that both patients and chiropractors slightly more often experienced the presence of the affective bond than collaboration in reaching consensus on treatment goals and treatment strategies. However, poor agreement was shown to exist between perceptions of patients and chiropractors of the quality of their alliance, both overall, and on the three elements of the alliance separately. Neither the chiropractors' gender nor their years of experience, nor gender matching between chiropractor-patient pairs was shown to influence perceptions of patients on the quality of the alliance significantly.

Whereas the results of this study are encouraging in that patients felt that their interaction with their chiropractor was very good, they do not permit chiropractors to sit back and relax. The therapeutic alliance is a dynamic and developing process of collaboration between the patient and clinician and its strength often fluctuates during the course of care [2, 29]. Understanding how clinician and patient factors, such as their present mood, preoccupation with personal issues and severity of symptoms, as well as situational factors, such as excessive workload, lack of time, waiting time, and delays in improvement, may cause fluctuations in the strength of the therapeutic alliance over time is imperative for chiropractors. To maintain a positive alliance between the patient and the chiropractor, both parties have to demonstrate a commitment to collaborate during the course of the treatment for however long that takes [2, 29]. Important to note in this respect is that although previous research has confirmed a positive and consistent association between therapeutic alliance and clinical outcomes, the term 'association' does not indicate that there is a causal relationship between the two [36]. However, a recent study in the field of physical therapy and rehabilitation found a clear dose–response effect between the therapeutic alliance and clinical outcomes. Outcomes were better when interventions were combined with enhanced therapeutic alliance applications, compared to a limited application of factors that have been shown to enhance the therapeutic alliance [14].

The small differences between patients' views and chiropractors' views might disguise the fact that there was poor agreement between these perceptions. The results showed that chiropractors and patients had very different perceptions of the same working relationship. A lack of agreement between patient views and therapist views is consistent with the literature in psychotherapy. It was suggested that patient perceptions are more predictive for clinical outcomes compared to therapist perceptions, on the basis that patient perceptions were

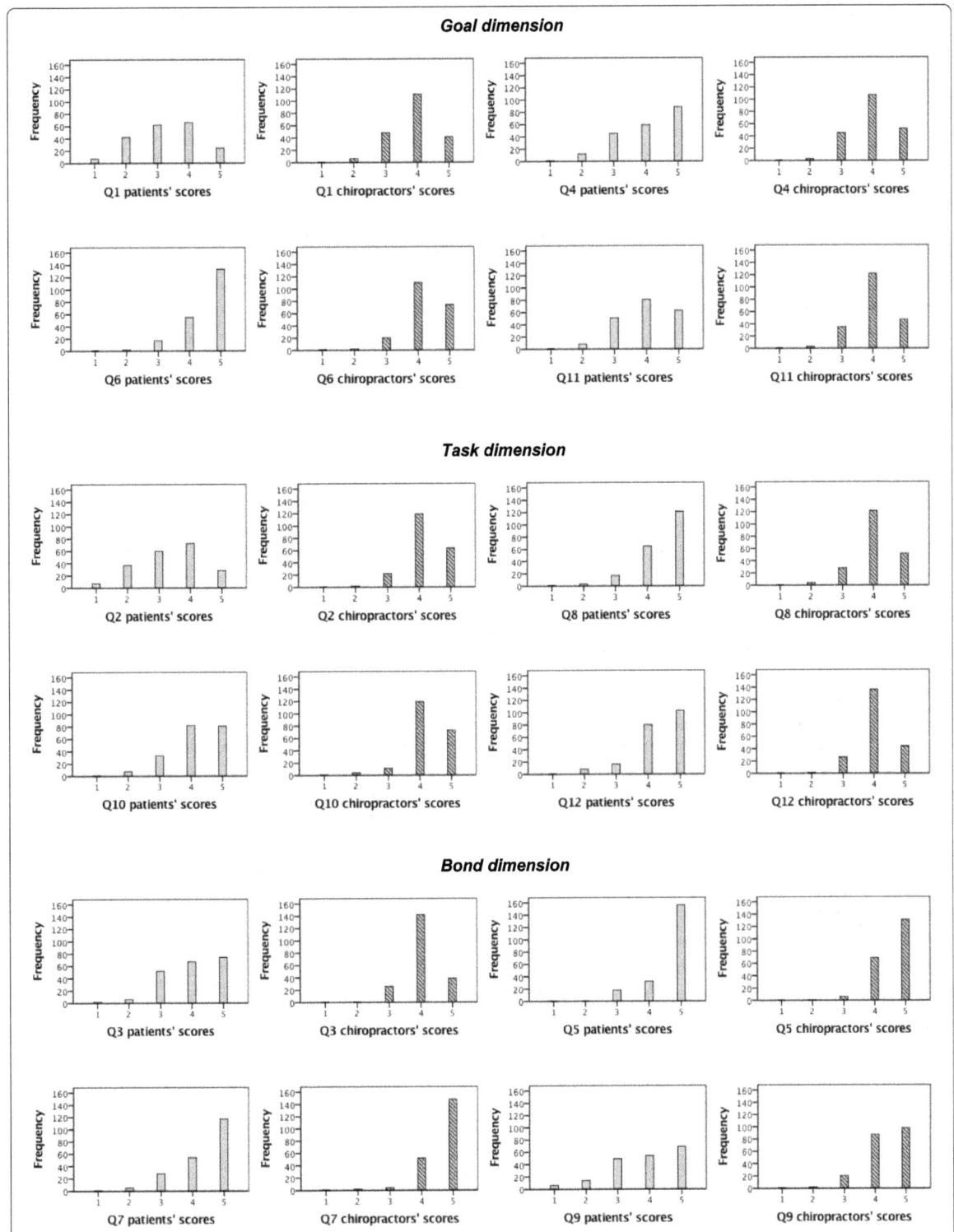

Fig. 2 Frequencies of patients' and chiropractors' scores on individual questions of the WAV-12, grouped per dimension

Table 3 Agreement between patients' and chiropractors' perceptions on their working alliance

Patients' and chiropractors' perceptions	N	ICC[a]
Overall WAV-12	180	0.13
Goal dimension	196	0.07
Task dimension	199	0.14
Bond dimension	186	0.10

[a]ICC < 0.40 indicates poor agreement

shown to remain more stable over time compared to therapists' perceptions [4, 6, 29]. However, no studies were conducted to test this hypothesis.

One could argue that the poor agreement between patients' and chiropractors' views is the most important finding of this study for clinical practice. Chiropractors should be aware of this possible dissonance and should verify their views with the patient, especially concerning views on setting treatment goals and treatment strategies. Dissonance in agreement on treatment goals and treatment strategies can jeopardise patient management, especially in the case of chronic disease, where self-management and self-efficacy from patients are essential [26].

Somewhat surprisingly, the results in the present study did not demonstrate any difference between the varying years of experience as a chiropractor on patients' perceptions of the quality of any of the elements of the therapeutic alliance. In a study in psychotherapy, which used the same version of the WAV-12 as the present study [29], interactions with respect to agreement on treatment strategies with therapists with over 20 years of experience were perceived significantly less positive compared to interactions with less experienced therapists (10–19 years). Besides a possible difference in education, it was postulated by the authors that a more experienced therapist may more frequently work on 'an automatic pilot', and spent less time and energy on discussing treatment strategies as to how to achieve the treatment goals with their patients. Working on the 'automatic pilot' may also be true for more experienced chiropractors. At the same time, as a result of patients

being informed better and having their own ideas about health, experienced chiropractors may have consciously or unconsciously adapted their patient management to accommodate for more collaboration, thereby improving the therapeutic alliance.

Studies on empathy and communication in relation to the therapeutic alliance [24, 37] found that female physicians displayed more empathy and active collaboration than male physicians, both of which behaviours are considered to improve the strength of the alliance. Although there might be differences in displaying empathy and active collaboration between male and female chiropractors, this study showed that patients' perceptions of the quality of the alliance did not differ for male and female chiropractors. This lack of difference might partly be explained by the fact that chiropractic care is considered as alternative medicine in The Netherlands and is still fairly unknown to many patients. Chiropractors will have to make an effort to explain and promote their care and might, therefore, be more motivated to engage and collaborate with the patient, independent of their gender. Educational differences between medicine and chiropractic might play a role as well. Historically, chiropractic has always advocated a holistic approach, in which patients are attended to in their whole identity as opposed to the former disease-centred approach in medicine. Chiropractors might, therefore, be more experienced in practising patient-centred care, which involves empathic and collaborative behaviour. Their training may thus diminish any gender differences in displaying empathy that was seen amongst male and female physicians. Furthermore, many chiropractors in The Netherlands decided to become a chiropractor because of their personal experience with chiropractic as a patient. It has been suggested that to improve empathic behaviour a clinician should be a patient himself [18]. Having started as a patient may be an advantage for many chiropractors, both female and male, in displaying empathy.

Some of these reasons could also explain the unexpected lack of difference in patients' perceptions of the therapeutic alliance between gender-matched and unmatched

Table 4 Patients' perceptions of the therapeutic alliance when treated by male and female chiropractors

Patients' perceptions	Gender chiropractor	N	Mean[a]	SD	t(df)	p
Overall WAV-12	Male	86	4.09	±0.60	t(181) = −0.18	0.86
	Female	97	4.10	±0.59		
Goal dimension	Male	93	3.98	±0.66	t(195) = −0.11	0.92
	Female	104	3.99	±0.65		
Task dimension	Male	96	4.11	±0.59	t(199) = 0.19	0.85
	Female	105	4.09	±0.64		
Bond dimension	Male	90	4.17	±0.74	t(186) = −1.07	0.29
	Female	98	4.28	±0.66		

[a]Measured on a 1–5 Likert scale, 5 representing an optimal alliance

Table 5 Patient's perceptions of the therapeutic alliance when treated by same sex and different sex chiropractors

Patients' perceptions	Gender match	N	Mean[a]	SD	t(df)	p
Overall WAV-12	No match	78	4.11	±0.54	t(179) = 0.46	0.64
	Match	103	4.07	±0.63		
Goal dimension	No match	85	4.03	±0.62	t(193) = 1.03	0.30
	Match	110	3.93	±0.67		
Task dimension	No match	87	4.10	±0.60	t(196) = 0.14	0.89
	Match	111	4.09	±0.63		
Bond dimension	No match	81	4.20	±0.66	t(183) = −0.24	0.81
	Match	104	4.23	±0.73		

[a]Measured on a 1–5 point Likert scale, 5 representing an optimal alliance

chiropractor-patient pairs. Other explanations for this lack of difference might be that patients who have a clear preference for a female or male chiropractor can often be booked with the chiropractor of their choice since many chiropractic clinics have both female and male chiropractors working in the clinic. Consulting a chiropractor of the gender of their preference may give patients a more positive stance in the working relationship. Recommendation by an acquaintance or family member might also positively influence the patient's stance in the working relationship at the start of the treatment, irrespective of factors such as gender or age of the chiropractor. Although this could be pure coincidence, the freedom of the patient to choose a chiropractor of the gender of preference may explain why almost two-thirds of the analysed working

relationships in this study involved gender-matched chiropractor-patient pairs.

There are several limitations to this study, which potentially compromise the external validity of this study. Firstly, participation in this study was on a voluntary basis. Chiropractors who advocate patient-centred care and have good communication skills could be overrepresented in this study. Secondly, questionnaires were sent to the participating chiropractors in advance, which allowed them to read the questions in advance, and as a result, allowed them to give their best performance to the patient with respect to the alliance. Thirdly, perceptions were observed at one moment in time and were, therefore, influenced by the mood of the participant at that particular moment. In addition, patients

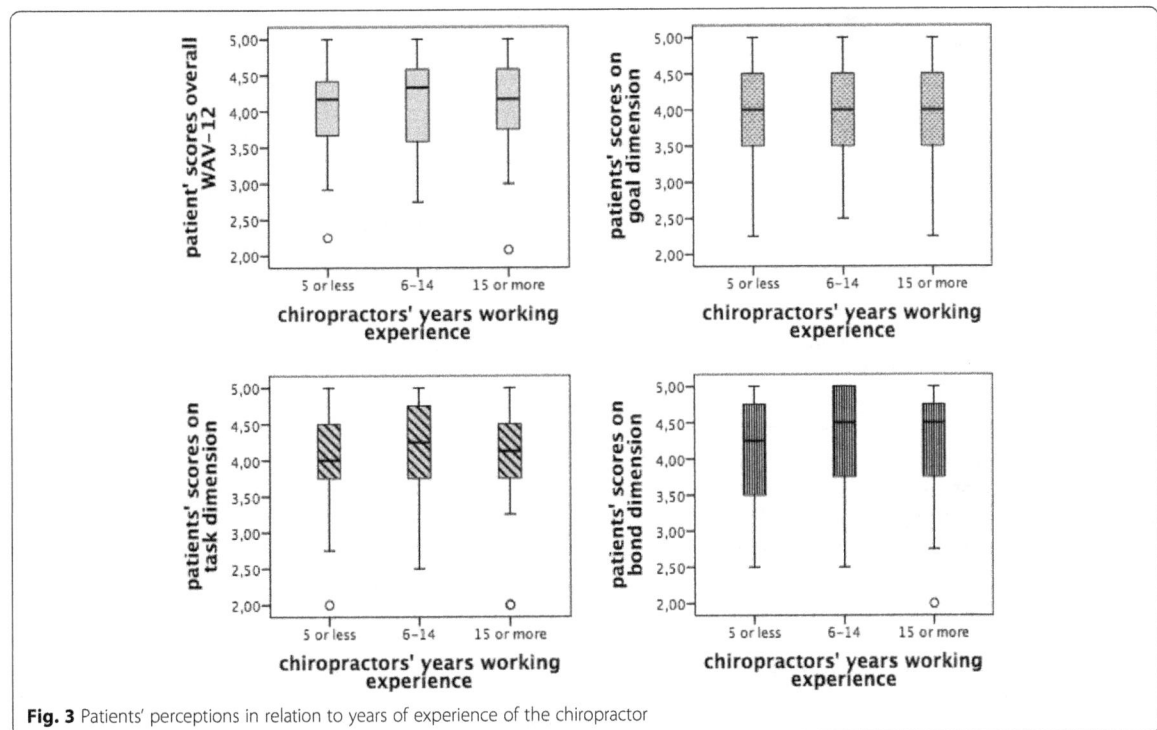

Fig. 3 Patients' perceptions in relation to years of experience of the chiropractor

Table 6 Patients' perceptions in relation to working experience of chiropractor

Patients' perceptions	Years experience	N	Mean[a]	SD	F(df)	p
Overall WAV-12	0–5	59	4.04	±0.59	F(2) = 0.60	0.55
	6–14	65	4.15	±0.64		
	15+	59	4.09	±0.55		
Goal dimension	0–5	62	3.93	±0.66	F(2) = 0.38	0.68
	6–14	72	4.03	±0.69		
	15+	63	3.95	±0.65		
Task dimension	0–5	63	4.03	±0.61	F(2) = 0.58	0.56
	6–14	74	4.15	±0.66		
	15+	64	4.07	±0.55		
Bond dimension	0–5	60	4.15	±0.71	F(2) = 0.55	0.58
	6–14	67	4.28	±0.75		
	15+	61	4.25	±0.62		

[a]Measured on a 1–5 point Likert scale, 5 representing an optimal alliance

who did not trust their chiropractor not to open the envelope and read their perceptions may have reported more positive perceptions. Furthermore, since all questions were scored in the same direction, participants may have failed to pay close attention to the questions and may have answered all items in the same way. The use of a questionnaire, which was developed in the field of psychotherapy, might be a further limitation. In the absence of a better alternative, the Working Alliance Inventory (WAI) has been proven valid and usable in physiotherapy settings [32]. Nevertheless, participants in the present study found some questions confusing or ambiguous. Noteworthy in this respect is that more than 10 % of patients did not complete all questions as requested. Particularly issues related to the quality of the affective bond between the patient and chiropractor were left unanswered. Although no feedback was requested from the participants, several patients reported questions exploring the quality of the affective bond to be irrelevant or inappropriate. And even though it could be argued that these questions were not relevant, some questions are considered less applicable in a chiropractic setting. Similar responses were found in a physiotherapy setting, and the authors suggested to develop a more conceptually sound measure of the therapeutic alliance for use in physiotherapy [32]. Furthermore, several chiropractors commented on the choice of response scale. The current options (seldom to always) were found inappropriate and not applicable to rating perceptions, and suggestions were made using options as to how much the participant agreed with each statement (strongly disagree to strongly agree). This modification was applied in a study on perceptions of the quality of the therapeutic alliance in a primary care setting, along with some modifications in the phrasing of the statements, and proved useful [10]. As in any observational

study, confounders could not be fully controlled for in this study. Specific patient or chiropractor characteristics could have influenced the results. Some patients might have had severe symptoms, unintentionally influencing their perceptions more negatively. Female and male chiropractors might have treated patients with different levels of symptoms, different levels of cognitive ability, and of different ages, which could all have influenced perceptions on gender and experience. These differences, however, reflect daily practice and were, therefore, considered acceptable.

One important recommendation for further research is to develop a uniform instrument to assess the quality of the therapeutic alliance, with an appropriate response scale that could be used in primary care settings. This uniform instrument should be translated and validated for use in different countries. The second recommendation for research is to further investigate the level of agreement on treatment goals and treatment strategies to achieve these goals between patients and chiropractors. In the present study, only perceptions of collaboration in reaching agreement were studied. It would be useful for clinical practice to conduct a study examining to what extent patients and chiropractors agree on treatment goals and treatment strategies, as was conducted for patients with diabetes and their physicians and showed poor levels of agreement [26].

Conclusion

The results of this study showed that both patients and chiropractors perceived their working alliances very positive. Contrary to what was expected, no significant differences were shown to exist in patients' perceptions in relation to the chiropractors' gender or years of working experience.

The most important finding with respect to clinical practice was that poor agreement was found between the perceptions of patients and chiropractors on the same working relationship. This dissonance in perceptions must be given serious consideration by chiropractors. In order to develop, improve and maintain a positive therapeutic alliance, chiropractors should, during the course of treatments, continue to collaborate with the patient and frequently verify their perception with the views of the patient, especially with respect to determining treatment goals and treatment strategies to achieve these goals.

Ethics approval and consent to participate

Ethics approval was applied for and granted by the Anglo-European College of Chiropractic (AECC) Research Ethics Subcommittee. All questionnaires were completed anonymously and consent to participate was implied by completion of the questionnaire in which an explanation of the study was given.

Consent for publication

Not applicable.

Availability of data and materials

The dataset supporting the conclusions of this article is included in an additional file.

Additional file

Additional file 1: Literature search and search strategy. (DOCX 96 kb)

Abbreviations

WAI: working alliance inventory; WAV: Werkalliantie Vragenlijst (Validated translation into Dutch from WAI).

Competing interests

The authors declare that they have no competing interests.

Authors' contributions

NL carried out the research and drafted the manuscript. JB acted as supervisor. Both authors read and approved the final manuscript.

Authors' information

This study was undertaken by NL (at that time in private chiropractic practice in The Netherlands) as part of a post-graduate MSc degree (Bournemouth University, United Kingdom). The study was supervised by JB, Vice Principal Post-Graduate Studies at the Anglo-European College of Chiropractic.

Funding

Not applicable.

References

1. Mead N, Bower P. Patient-centred consultations and outcomes in primary care: a review of the literature. Patient Educ Counsel. 2002;48:51–61.
2. Horvath AO, Del Re AC, Flückiger C, Symonds D. Alliance in individual psychotherapy. Psychotherapy (Chic). 2011;48:9–16.
3. Horvath AO, Symonds BD. Relation between working alliance and outcome in psychotherapy: A meta-analysis. J Couns Psychol. 1991;38:139–49.
4. Martin DJ, Garske JP, Davis MK. Relation of the therapeutic alliance with outcome and other variables: A meta-analytic review. J Consult Clin Psychol. 2000;68:438–50.
5. Bordin ES. The generalizability of the psychoanalytic concept of the working alliance. Psychotherapy Theory Res Practice. 1979;16:252–60.
6. Ardito RB, Rabellino D. Therapeutic alliance and outcome of psychotherapy: historical excursus, measurements, and prospects for research. Frontiers Psychol. 2011;2:270.
7. Hatcher RL, Gillaspy JA. Development and validation of a revised short version of the Working Alliance Inventory. Psychother Res. 2006;16:12–25.
8. Arbuthnott A, Sharpe D. The effect of physician-patient collaboration on patient adherence in non-psychiatric medicine. Patient Educ Couns. 2009;77:60–7.
9. Derksen F, Bensing J, Lagro-Janssen A. Effectiveness of empathy in general practice: a systematic review. Bri J General Practice J Royal College General Practitioners. 2013;63:e76–84.
10. Fuertes JN, Mislowack A, Bennett J, Paul L, Gilbert TC, Fontan G, Boylan LS. The physician-patient working alliance. Patient Educ Couns. 2007;66:29–36.
11. Pinto RZ, Ferreira ML, Oliveira VC, Franco MR, Adams R, Maher CG, Ferreira PH. Patient-centred communication is associated with positive therapeutic alliance: a systematic review. J Physiotherapy. 2012;58:77–87.
12. Rolfe A, Cash-Gibson L, Car J, Sheikh A, McKinstry B. Interventions for improving patients' trust in doctors and groups of doctors. Cochrane Database Syst Rev. 2014;3:CD004134.
13. Ferreira PH, Ferreira ML, Maher CG, Refshauge KM, Latimer J, Adams RD. The therapeutic alliance between clinicians and patients predicts outcome in chronic low back pain. Phys Ther. 2013;93:470–8.
14. Fuentes J, Armijo-Olivo S, Funabashi M, Miciak M, Dick B, Warren S, Rashiq S, Magee DJ, Gross DP. Enhanced Therapeutic Alliance Modulates Pain Intensity and Muscle Pain Sensitivity in Patients With Chronic Low Back Pain: An Experimental Controlled Study. Phys Ther. 2014;94:477–89.
15. Hall AM, Ferreira PH, Maher CG, Latimer J, Ferreira ML. The influence of the therapist-patient relationship on treatment outcome in physical rehabilitation: a systematic review. Phys Ther. 2010;90:1099–110.
16. Hojat M, Louis DZ, Markham FW, Wender R, Rabinowitz C, Gonnella JS. Physicians' empathy and clinical outcomes for diabetic patients. Acad Med J Assoc Am Med Colleges. 2011;86:359–64.
17. Jani BD, Blane DN, Mercer SW. The role of empathy in therapy and the physician-patient relationship. Forschende Komplementarmedizin. 2012;19:252–7.
18. Neumann M, Bensing J, Mercer S, Ernstmann N, Ommen O, Pfaff H. Analyzing the "nature" and "specific effectiveness" of clinical empathy: a theoretical overview and contribution towards a theory-based research agenda. Patient Educ Couns. 2009;74:339–46.
19. Norfolk T, Birdi K, Walsh D. The role of empathy in establishing rapport in the consultation: a new model. Med Educ. 2007;41:690–7.
20. Hall MA, Zheng B, Dugan E, Camacho F, Kidd KE, Mishra A, Balkrishnan R. Measuring patients' trust in their primary care providers. Med Care Res Rev. 2002;59:293–318.
21. Tarrant C, Stokes T, Baker R. Factors associated with patients' trust in their general practitioner: a cross-sectional survey. Bri J General Practice J Royal College General Practitioners. 2003;53:798–800.
22. Thom DH. Physician behaviors that predict patient trust. J Fam Pract. 2001;50:323–8.
23. Roter DL, Hall JA. Choices: biomedical ethics and women's health. Why physician gender matters in shaping the physician-patient relationship. J Women's Health. 1998;7:1093–7.
24. Roter DL, Hall JA, Aoki Y. Physician gender effects in medical communication: A meta-analytic review. J Am Med Assoc. 2002;288:756–64.
25. Jahng KH, Martin LR, Golin CE, DiMatteo MR. Preferences for medical collaboration: Patient-physician congruence and patient outcomes. Patient Educ Couns. 2005;57:308–14.
26. Heisler M, Vijan S, Ubel PA, Bernstein SJ, Hofer TP, Anderson RM. When Do Patients and Their Physicians Agree on Diabetes Treatment Goals and Strategies, and What Difference Does It Make? J Gen Intern Med. 2003;18:893–902.
27. Dahm MR. Tales of Time, Terms, and Patient Information-Seeking Behavior - An Exploratory Qualitative Study. Health Commun. 2012;27:682–9.
28. Levinson W, Gorawara-Bhat R, Lamb J. A study of patient clues and physician responses in primary care and surgical settings. J Am Med Assoc. 2000;284:1021–7.

29. Stinckens N, Ulburghs A, Claes L. De werkalliantie als sleutelelement in het therapiegebeuren. Meting met behulp van de WAV-12, de Nederlandstalige verkorte versie van de Working Alliance Inventory. Tijdschrift Klinische Psychologie. 2009;39:44–60.

30. Horvath AO, Greenberg LS. Development and validation of the Working Alliance Inventory. J Couns Psychol. 1989;36:223–33.

31. Tracey TJ, Kokotovic AM. Factor structure of the Working Alliance Inventory. Psychol Assess J Consult Clin Psychol. 1989;1:207–10.

32. Besley J, Kayes NM, McPherson KM. Assessing the measurement properties of two commonly used measures of therapeutic relationship in physiotherapy. N Z J Physiother. 2011;39:75–80.

33. Elvins R, Green J. The conceptualization and measurement of therapeutic alliance: an empirical review. Clin Psychol Rev. 2008;28:1167–87.

34. Miller SEKM. An Examination of Therapeutic Alliance in Chinese Medicine. Aust J Acupuncture Chinese Med. 2011;6:17–22.

35. Cicchetti DV. Guidelines, criteria, and rules of thumb for evaluating normed and standardized assessment instruments in psychology. Psychol Assess. 1994;6:284–90.

36. Lucas RM, McMichael AJ. Association or causation: evaluating links between "environment and disease". Bull World Health Organ. 2005;83:792–5.

37. Hojat M, Gonnella JS, Nasca TJ, Mangione S, Vergare M, Magee M. Physician empathy: definition, components, measurement, and relationship to gender and specialty. Am J Psychiatr. 2002;159:1563–9.

19

Nonfunctioning pituitary macroadenoma: a case report from the patient perspective

Craig A. Bauman[1,2*], James D. Milligan[1,2], Tammy Labreche[3] and John J. Riva[1,4]

Abstract

Background: Nonfunctioning pituitary macroadenoma (NFPA) is a tumour of the endocrine system that is virtually always benign and can be difficult to detect. This case report is presented from the patient's perspective to highlight experiences that led to the eventual diagnosis of this condition.

Case presentation: A 48 year-old male experienced prolonged and unexplained reduced athletic performance worsening over five years. The patient reported decreased libido, which initiated a testosterone blood test. This confirmed reduced testosterone levels and resulted in an endocrinology referral. A subsequent dynamic contrast MRI of the pituitary region revealed a mass. The most frequent symptoms of NFPA are visual field defects, headaches and features of hypopituitarism (includes fatigue, dizziness, dry skin, irregular periods in women and sexual dysfunction in men).

Conclusion: Clinicians should consider this differential diagnosis in middle-aged athletes with diminished athletic performance from an unknown cause, test visual fields and inquire if symptoms of headaches or hypopituitarism are present.

Keywords: Pituitary, Adenoma, Macroadenoma, Nonfunctioning, Middle-aged, Athletic, Performance

Background

Chiropractors are commonly utilized by middle-aged athletes to determine sources of reduced athletic performance [1]. Such clinicians are also often consulted for headache treatment [2]. For this reason chiropractors need to be aware of the potential diagnosis of nonfunctioning pituitary macroadenoma.

The pituitary is an endocrine (hormone-producing) gland that is located immediately below the base of the brain (Figs. 1 and 2) [3]. It approximates the size of a pea and is regulated by the hypothalamus [3]. It produces hormones that impact numerous parts of the body and stimulates all the other endocrine glands to produce their own hormones [3]. As a result of its complex tasks, it is frequently referred to as the 'master gland' [3].

Nonfunctioning pituitary macroadenoma (NFPA) is a nearly always benign tumour of the endocrine system [3, 4]. NFPA is the most common adenoma in the pituitary gland, accounting for 25–33 % of these tumours [5, 6]. At the time of diagnosis, most NFPAs are macroadenomas (greater than 1 cm in diameter) [5, 6]. The prevalence of NFPA has been estimated at 22 cases per 100 000 in cross-sectional studies [4]. They frequently present in those greater than 50 years of age [5], and the progression can vary widely, with some growing slowly and others becoming rapidly invasive [5].

The gold standard method of management of NFPA is surgical resection of the tumour via endoscopy using a transsphenoidal approach through the nasal cavity [4]. Prognosis for treated patients is generally very good [4]. Although NFPA is benign in nature, patients often need individualized management, lifelong diagnostic imaging and endocrinological monitoring [7]. This paper describes a specific case presentation around diminished athletic performance to highlight typical features related to NFPA from the patient perspective.

Case Presentation

History

I am a Canadian Doctor of Chiropractic and chiropractic clinician who is sharing their experience with NFPA.

* Correspondence: bauman@mcmaster.ca
[1]Department of Family Medicine, McMaster University, Hamilton, ON, Canada
[2]The Centre for Family Medicine Family Health Team, 25 Joseph Street, Kitchener, ON, CanadaN2G 4X6
Full list of author information is available at the end of the article

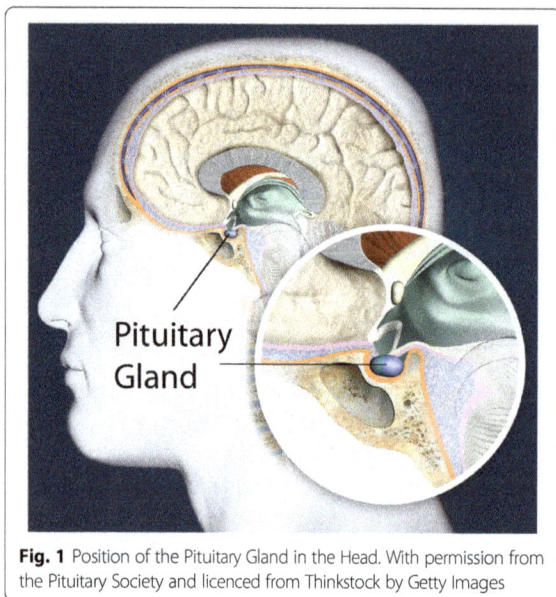

Fig. 1 Position of the Pituitary Gland in the Head. With permission from the Pituitary Society and licenced from Thinkstock by Getty Images

Fortunately, through fate or luck, circumstances led to successful management. My story starts as an age 43 male, five years prior to diagnosis. After an afternoon nap, I arose from bed quickly and had a brief intense pain sensed in the centre of my head. For 1 month afterwards, I had a mild sharp pain in the centre of my head for the first 200 m of a recreational run. I attended my family physician for this complaint and had a neurological examination, which was normal, and I was advised to come back if the pain returned. In hindsight, I felt this head pain was related to the NFPA; however this was not the typical type of headache presentation. Over the next 5 years I noticed a slow progressive reduction in strength that corresponded to a 30 % decrease in my weight training ability. Also, I noticed a weight gain of 5–10 lb that was mostly abdominal which I initially thought was attributed to "getting older". When I ran a competitive 5-km race which resulted in me being 2 min and 12 s slower than the previous year despite increased training, this prompted me to return to my family physician.

Bloodwork was ordered. A mild anemia (normochromic normocytic) was detected, with hemoglobin of 117 g/L (normal 135–175 g/L), hematocrit of 0.36 L/L (normal 0.40–0.50 L/L), and red blood cell count of 3.83 x E12/L (normal 4.50–6.00 x E12/L). Investigations to determine the etiology of the anemia included a chest x-ray, colonoscopy, gastroscopy and abdominal ultrasound, all of which were normal. During this time I reported to my family physician I was losing hair on my legs, my libido was very low along with having acquired cold sensitivity, hot flashes, anxiety and some noticeable hair growth on the

scalp where I had been losing hair. By chance, during the period of when various diagnostic tests were occurring, I attended a family medicine continuing education conference where an endocrinologist spoke of the connection between low testosterone and a pituitary tumour. I later discussed this possibility with my family physician and a testosterone blood test was ordered.

Physical examination
The results of the testosterone tests showed testosterone was nearly absent at 0.5 nmol/L (normal 8.4–28.8 nmol/L) and bioavailable testosterone was 0.1 nmol/L (normal is 3.6–11.2 nmol/L). I was referred to an endocrinologist. A dynamic contrast MRI of the pituitary region (specifically the sella turcica) was ordered. A large 2.5 cm diameter mass was discovered in my pituitary region. A subsequent referral was made to a pituitary neurosurgical team and a series of tests and consults were booked (further bloodwork, neuro-opthalmology and endocrinology appointments). My bloodwork identified reduced pituitary hormone levels, which suggested the tumour was nonfunctioning. The luteinizing hormone (LH) at 0.8 IU/L (normal male 1.7–8.6 IU/L) and follicle stimulating hormone (FSH) at 1.1 IU/L (normal male 1.5–12.4 IU/L) were also reduced. Diminished levels of these hormones were causing my testosterone to be low, which compromised hematopoiesis (i.e. the production of all types of blood cells) and resulted in the anemia [8]. Prolactin was elevated to 51 ug/L (normal male 4–15 ug/L) due to the tumour stalk effect (i.e. mass effect from the tumour on the pituitary infundibulum) [7, 9]. Thyroid function was also compromised by the NFPA. My Free T4 was 11 pmol/L (normal 12–22 pmol/L) and Free T3 was 2.8 pmol/L (normal 3.1–6.8 pmol/L). I was prescribed testosterone gel and levothyroxine medication for replacement.

While frequently affected in NFPA, the neuro-ophthamologist concluded my visual fields were normal. A consult with an otolaryngologist (ENT) surgeon was required to evaluate the size of my nasal cavity in preparation for the surgical endoscopy procedure. In surgery, the endoscope is passed through the nasal cavity to make an opening in the sphenoid sinus, to access the pituitary region allowing the neurosurgeon to remove the tumour. This is called the transsphenoidal approach and its advantages are being less invasive and no visible scaring following neurosurgery [9].

Imaging
The neurosurgeon and the neuroradiologist reviewed my imaging (the previous dynamic contrast MRI and a recent CT) and had a high degree of suspicion of a NFPA. Only after surgery and pathological sectioning of the tumour can a confirmatory diagnosis be made.

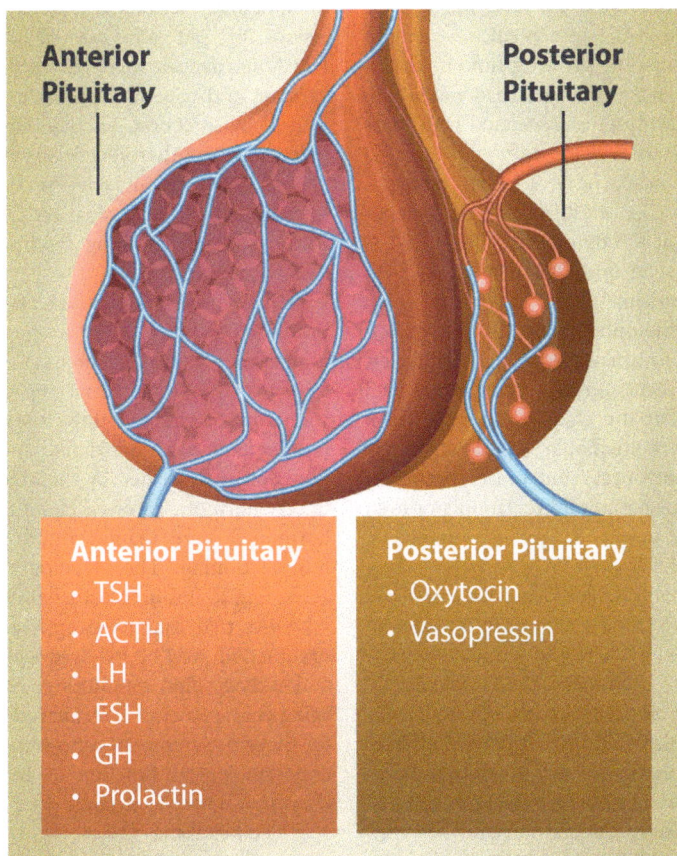

Fig. 2 Hormones of the Anterior and Posterior Pituitary Gland. TSH is thyroid stimulating hormone, ACTH is adrenocorticotropic hormone, LH is luteinizing hormone, FSH is follicle-stimulating hormone and GH is growth hormone. With permission from the Pituitary Society and licenced from Thinkstock by Getty Images

Intervention

Prior to surgery, I received meningococcal B immunizations as ENT surgery has an eleven-fold and neurosurgery has a seven-fold, increased risk of meningitis in the first 10 days following surgery [10]. With a MRI just before surgery, adhesive stickers known as fiducial markers were attached to my head. This assists the neuro-navigation of the neurosurgeon to help orient themselves relative to the tumour position in my head during the surgery. In the operating room, my head was placed in a form-fitting cradle for stabilization. Later, when under anesthetic, a series of pins were screwed into my skull to further stabilize it, as the surgeon has to be very precise during the procedure. The entire surgical procedure typically takes up to 5 h.

Conclusions

The surgery was completed without incident and I was returned to the recovery room after approximately 4 h. I had a subsequent follow up with my care team one month after surgery, where the pathological sectioning confirmed

a NFPA. This was a tremendous relief as other, more sinister tumours were a possibility. Radiation therapy was considered but not deemed required. Future ongoing screening recommendations for recurrence includes annual MRI monitoring.

Discussion

Clinical presentation

Clinically, NFPA comprise about 80 % of all pituitary macroadenomas [5]. It is likely there are many in the population with undetected macroadenomas [11]. Imaging of the head is now commonly implemented as part of the workup of many unrelated medical cases [5] and as a result, pituitary lesions are often detected incidentally [5]. Nonfunctioning categorizes the tumour cells as not secreting hormones versus functioning adenomas. This can be advantageous; but also can make discovery difficult as there is absence of a readily identifiable syndrome of pituitary hormone hypersecretion often leading to growth of these tumours for many years before discovery [9]. Many cases presenting with NFPA have at least some pituitary insufficiency [7]. The majority of patients who have NFPA will seek medical attention because of a mass effect (i.e. the growing tumour applying pressure to tissues) from the macroadenoma [9]. The main complaints or symptoms associated with mass effect are visual field defects with or without decreased visual acuity, unspecified headache and effects of hypopituitarism (Table 1) [3]. As a result, many macroadenomas are often uncovered at the optometrist [9].

Visual field defects exist in 60–70 % of patients with NFPA at the time of suspicion of the diagnosis, which results from pressure on the optic chiasm by the tumour [7, 9]. Patients are usually unaware of the deficiency, which only becomes apparent during formal visual field testing [9]. Compression of the chiasm can result in a symmetrical bi-temporal hemianopia (i.e. loss of the outer field of vision in both eyes), but more commonly there is an asymmetrical bi-temporal hemianopia or even a unilateral temporal field defect [5, 7]. The chiropractic clinician could test visual fields if NFPA is suspected using the confrontation visual field test. Headache, often localized to the brow or periorbital region, is present in 40–60 % of all patients and is generated by increased intracranial pressure and/or stretching of the dura mater [7, 12]. The neurosurgeon stated that NFPA, along with some other pituitary tumours, are increasingly detected in middle-aged athletes with reduced athletic performance and signs of hypopituitarism. Inquiry as to the presence of these symptoms should be made in the patient history. As chiropractors are consulted by mature athletes, NFPA should remain in their differential diagnosis when such signs are present and a referral made to their physician with a note.

Differential diagnoses of NFPA includes craniopharyngiomas, germinomas, metastatic tumours and vascular aneurysms [13]. Differential diagnoses for NFPA visual field defects includes compressive lesions (eg, craniopharyngiomas), ischemic lesions (eg, pituitary apoplexy), inflammatory lesions (eg, multiple sclerosis), and toxic lesions (eg, pheniprazine) [12]. Differential diagnoses of NFPA headaches includes cluster headaches, migraine variants and trigeminal neuralgia [14]. Fatigue could be caused by infection, anemia, endocrinopathies (eg, diabetes and hypothyroidism), sleep disturbances (eg, sleep apnea), medication side-effects, adrenal insufficiency (usually other symptoms and signs) and malignancies (rare) [15]. Overtraining syndrome in athletes can also lead to fatigue [16].

Pituitary tumours can be classified by size or by function [5]. The best current diagnostic imaging method for evaluating pituitary adenomas is MRI [7]. Size, as determined by MRI, less than 1 cm in diameter is considered a microadenoma and those tumours greater than 1 cm in diameter are considered a macroadenoma [5, 11]. Function is described by the detectable increase of a pituitary hormone through blood tests [5]. Therefore, if no hormones were manufactured, the tumour is defined nonfunctioning. These tumours may also be classified according to immunohistochemistry [11].

NFPAs that touch the optic apparatus, without visual dysfunction, may be followed with close ophthalmological and radiographic monitoring, pending tumour and imaging characteristics [17]. Surgery should be contemplated for those patients with concerning tumour growth, loss of endocrinological function, a lesion close to the optic chiasm, a desire to become pregnant, or unremitting unspecified headaches [18].

Treatment

The majority of patients with a large NFPA should have pituitary surgery [5, 6, 9]. Surgical morbidity and cure rate have been found to be highly reliant on the skill of the pituitary surgeon [7, 9, 19]. The favoured surgery is a transsphenoidal approach, due to less associated morbidity and mortality [9]. The surgical management of

Table 1 Symptoms and Signs of Pituitary Hormone Deficiency. With permission from the Pituitary Society

Pituitary Hormone	Target Organs	Effect of Deficiency
ACTH	Adrenal glands: cortisol and DHEA	Fatigue, low sodium in blood, weight loss, skin pallor
TSH	Thyroid gland: thyroid hormone	Fatigue, weight gain, dry skin, sensitivity to cold, constipation
LH and FSH in Women	Ovaries: estrogen, progesterone; ovulation	Loss of periods, loss of sex drive, infertility
LH and FSH in Men	Testes: testosterone, sperm production	Loss of sex drive, erectile dysfunction, impotence, infertility
GH in Children & Adolescents	Bone, muscle, fat	Lack of growth (height); increased body fat, failure to achieve normal peak bone mass
GH in Adults	Whole body	Poor quality of life, increased body fat, decreased muscle and bone mass
PRL	Breast	Inability to breast feed
Oxytocin	Breast, Uterus	Complete deficiency could make breast feeding difficult
Antidiuretic hormone (vasopressin)	Kidney	Frequent urination (day & night), dilute urine, excessive thirst

macroadenomas (greater than 1 cm) is precipitated by the greater probability that these tumours will increase in size over time leading to resultant mass effects. The initial goals of post surgical therapy are to mitigate any future mass effect and to return normal endocrine function [9].

Because there is a known correlation between the severity of visual loss before surgery and persisting visual field defects after treatment, the wait time for surgery is typically expedited [7]. Besides the improvement of visual function, full cessation of headaches is likely to occur after surgery for NFPA [7]. During post surgical follow-up, careful assessment and replacement of pituitary deficiencies is implemented [7]. It is possible that future advancements in the field of neurosurgery, such as endoscopic techniques utilizing combination with neuronavigation, will further improve surgical outcomes and improve the long-term prognosis [7].

NFPA treatment can involve single or combinations of surgical intervention, radiotherapy or pharmacological treatment [5]. It is essential that all options for therapy are discussed and inclusion of surgical, endocrine and oncology providers is often provided in a multidisciplinary team setting [5]. For those adenomas less than 1 cm in diameter and restricted to the sella, a strategy of watchful waiting and serial MRI scans is often employed [5]. It is necessary to have ruled out any secondary hormonal deficiencies to optimize quality of life [5].

Assuming hormonal normality, then close monitoring may be all that is needed [5]. With no hormone irregularity present, follow up in this instance relies upon serial screening [5]. For those adenomas larger than 1 cm (the majority), after excluding hormone deficiencies, it is common to proceed to surgical management [5]. These macroadenomas more commonly exert pressure effects [5].

Pharmacological treatment of the NFPA tumour itself is typically unsuccessful [5, 9]. Medical management is frequently based around regular follow-up, monitoring of visual problems and secondary hormone deficiencies [5]. Periodically, tissue regrowth develops post surgically and, although a repeat surgical intervention can be pursued, adjunctive radiotherapy also remains a useful option [5]. Indeed, radiation therapy may be proposed if the patient is not suited for surgery or if complete tumour removal is not achievable [5, 20, 21]. Radiosurgery for NFPAs is quite effective, with usually around a 90 % success rate for tumour control [20, 21].

The greatest risk of transsphenoidal neurosurgery is a postoperative cerebrospinal fluid leak [4]. When this occurs, a clear fluid drips out of the nose quite steadily when leaning forward. Symptoms of a leak may also include a headache, however headache can also be expected after the neurosurgical procedure itself.

Post-surgery, rest and avoidance of straining activities (valsalva) is required with an anticipated return to work in approximately 2 months.

All patients that require hydrocortisone replacement should carry a steroid card (e.g. instructions in case of an emergency) and participate in education about sick day rules (sickness stress requires increased cortisol which can no longer be produced) [5]. These sick day rules will be advised by a physician and frequently involves doubling the usual hydrocortisone dose for 1 to 3 days [22]. An adrenal crisis (acute cortisol insufficiency) can ensue during times of illness which can be life threatening and must be managed promptly [23]. Symptoms include unusual tiredness and weakness, dizziness when standing up, nausea, vomiting, diarrhea, loss of appetite, stomach ache and joint aches and pains [22].

Prognosis and adverse events

In NFPA, no single conclusive predictive factor has been identified that is associated with recurrence [24]. NFPAs, with or without perceptible residual tumour, need stratification of treatment and radiological/endocrinological follow-up strategies [6]. The tumour growth-free survival rates at 5 years are 85 % with intrasellar remnant and 49 % with extrasellar remnant and at 10 years are 58 % with intrasellar remnant and 23 % with extrasellar remnant [6]. Fortunately, 54 % of residual tumours will not regrow again after surgery [6, 9]. Therefore, it is advised that MRI should be repeated annually in these patients [6]. Reoperation or radiotherapy should be contemplated only when the tumoural regrowth is confirmed, except where the adenomatous residue is voluminous and close to the optic nerves/chiasm [6]. Whether NFPAs are associated with an increased mortality or reduced lifespan is still unknown [8].

Adverse events from a transsphenoidal approach were linked with 1 % mortality and 5 % important complications (e.g. cerebrospinal fluid leakage, fistula, meningitis, persistent diabetes insipidus or new visual field defect) [4]. Olfaction may be impacted by this surgical technique [25, 26]. Of patients with visual field defects prior to surgery, 78 % had recovery in their visual field defects [4]. Conversely, gains in pituitary function occurred in less than a third of the patients [4]. Complete removal of the lesions, as evaluated by the operating surgeons, occurs in approximately 20 % of the cases [4].

Limitations

A key limitation of this paper may be the inherent/unintentional bias that the principal author may bring to the report since it's from the patient-perspective. This case report may have biased observations in how the principal author recounted the details.

Case conclusion

One month after surgery, I was able to stop taking hydrocortisone as my pituitary returned to producing sufficient hormone. I was off work a total of 6 weeks. Six months post surgery, I felt I was in excellent health, had returned to running and strength training and my body weight had returned to the level it was 5 years prior. The 6 month follow up dynamic contrast MRI showed no definite tumour residual. Ongoing yearly MRIs will occur to monitor for regrowth. I will continue on testosterone and levothyroxine medication indefinitely and levels monitored. Truly, I am delighted with the outcome and decided to share the learning experience through a case report for other clinicians as a patient may describe these slowly progressive symptoms during a consultation.

Take home points

- Nonfunctioning pituitary macroadenoma can be difficult to detect
- Vision changes, headaches and symptoms of hormone irregularity offer clues to the tumour's presence
- Unexplained reduced performance in middle-aged athletes may be an indicator
- Post-surgery, yearly imaging may be required to monitor for tumour recurrence
- Life-long hormone replacement therapy may be required

Consent

Written informed consent was obtained from the patient for publication of this case report. A copy of the written consent is available for review by the Editor-in-Chief of this journal.

Competing interests
The authors declare that they have no competing interests.

Authors' contributions
CB contributed to the literature review. CB, JM and JR contributed to the writing of the manuscript. All authors read and approved the final manuscript.

Authors' information
CB and JR are members of the McMaster Chiropractic Working Group, which receives in kind support from the Canadian Chiropractic Association.

Acknowledgements
The patient in this case review is the principal author. This paper is dedicated to Mr. Thomas Hunter, partner at Gowlings Law Firm Waterloo Region Office. John Riva is supported by a PhD training award from the NCMIC foundation. A special thank you to Dr. Neil Duggal and the entire pituitary neurosurgical team at London Health Sciences, London, Ontario, Canada.

Author details
[1]Department of Family Medicine, McMaster University, Hamilton, ON, Canada. [2]The Centre for Family Medicine Family Health Team, 25 Joseph Street, Kitchener, ON, CanadaN2G 4X6. [3]School of Optometry and Vision Science, University of Waterloo, Waterloo, ON, Canada. [4]Department of Clinical Epidemiology & Biostatistics, McMaster University, Hamilton, ON, Canada.

References
1. Miners AL. Chiropractic treatment and the enhancement of sport performance: a narrative literature review. J Can Chiropr Assoc. 2010;54(4):210–21.
2. D'Sylva J, Miller J, Gross A, Burnie SJ, Goldsmith CH, Graham N, Haines T, Brønfort G, Hoving JL. Manual therapy with or without physical medicine modalities for neck pain: a systematic review. Man Ther. 2010;15(5):415–33.
3. The pituitary society. Viewed April 27, 2015. http://www.pituitarysociety.org.
4. Murad MH, Fernández-Balsells MM, Barwise A, Gallegos-Orozco JF, Paul A, Lane MA, et al. Outcomes of surgical treatment for nonfunctioning pituitary adenomas: a systematic review and meta-analysis. Clin Endicrinol (Oxf). 2010;73:777–91.
5. Saunders S, Vora JP. Endocrine evaluation of pituitary tumours. Br J Neurosurg. 2008;22(4):602–8.
6. Chen Y, Wang CD, Su ZP, Chen YX, Cai L, Zhuge QC, Wu ZB. Natural history of postoperative nonfunctioning pituitary adenomas: a systematic review and meta-analysis. Neuroendocrinology. 2012;96:333–42.
7. Dekkers OM, Pereira AM, Romijn JA. Treatment and follow-up of clinically nonfunctioning pituitary macroadenomas. J Clin Endocrinol Metab. 2008;93(10):3717–26.
8. Ellegala DB, Alden TD, Couture DE, Vance ML, Maartens NF, Laws Jr ER. Anemia, testosterone, and pituitary adenoma in men. J Neurosurg. 2003;98(5):974–7.
9. Jaffe CA. Clinically non-functioning pituitary adenoma. Pituitary. 2006;9:317–21.
10. Howitz MF, Homøe P. The risk of acquiring bacterial meningitis following surgery in Denmark, 1996–2009: a nationwide retrospective cohort study with emphasis on ear, nose and throat (ENT) and neurosurgery. Epidemiol Infect. 2014;142:1300–9.
11. Ezzat S, Asa SL, Couldwell WT, Barr CE, Dodge WE, Vance ML, et al. The prevalence of pituitary adenomas: a systematic review. Cancer. 2004;101(3):613–9.
12. Lee AG, Lai KE, Jirawuthiworavong GV. Pituitary adenoma. Eyewiki. Viewed January 24, 2016. http://eyewiki.aao.org/Pituitary_Adenoma.
13. Mulinda JR: Pituitary macroadenomas differential diagnosis. Medscape. Viewed January 24, 2016. http://emedicine.medscape.com/article/123223-differential
14. Blanda M: Cluster Headache Differential Diagnoses. Medscape. Viewed January 24, 2016. http://emedicine.medscape.com/article/1142459-differential
15. Ponka D, Kirlew M. Top 10 differential diagnoses in family medicine: fatigue. Can Fam Physician. 2007;53(5):892.
16. Budgett R. Fatigue and underperformance in athletes: the overtraining syndrome. Br J Sports Med. 1998;32(2):107–10.
17. Ryu WH, Tam S, Rotenberg B, Labib MA, Lee D, Nicolle DA, et al. Conservative management of pituitary macroadenoma contacting the optic apparatus. Can J Neurol Sci. 2010;37:837–42.
18. Freda PU, Beckers AM, Katznelson L, Molitch ME, Montori VM, Post KD, et al. Pituitary Incidentaloma: An Endocrine Society Clinical Practice Guideline. J Clin Endocrinol Metab. 2011;96(4):894–904.
19. Leach P, Abou-Zeid AH, Kearney T, Davis J, Trainer PJ, Gnanalingham KK. Endoscopic transsphenoidal pituitary surgery: evidence of an operative learning curve. Neurosurgery. 2010;67(5):1205–12.
20. Ding D, Starke RM, Sheehan J. Treatment paradigms for pituitary adenomas: defining the roles of radiosurgery and radiation therapy. J Neurooncol. 2014;117:445–57.
21. Brada M, Jankowska P. Radiotherapy for Pituitary Adenomas. Endocrinol Metab Clin N Am. 2008;37:263–75.
22. National institutes of health clinical center. Managing adrenal insufficiency. Viewed April 26, 2015. http://www.cc.nih.gov/ccc/patient_education/pepubs/mngadrins.pdf.
23. Corenblum B, Mulinda JR, Romesh K: Hypopituitarism (panhypopituitarism). Medscape. Viewed October 30, 2015. http://emedicine.medscape.com/article/122287-overview.
24. Roelfsema F, Biermasz NR, Pereira AM. Clinical factors involved in the recurrence of pituitary adenomas after surgical remission: a structured review and meta-analysis. Pituitary. 2012;15:71–83.
25. Rotenberg BW, Saunders S, Duggal N. Olfactory outcomes after endoscopic transsphenoidal pituitary surgery. Laryngoscope. 2011;121(8):1611–3.
26. Tam S, Duggal N, Rotenberg BW. Olfactory outcomes following endoscopic pituitary surgery with or without septal flap reconstruction: a randomized controlled trial. Int Forum Allergy Rhinol. 2013;3(1):62–5.

20

Spinal manipulative therapy, Graston technique® and placebo for non-specific thoracic spine pain: a randomised controlled trial

Amy L. Crothers[1], Simon D. French[2,4], Jeff J. Hebert[3] and Bruce F. Walker[2*]

Abstract

Background: Few controlled trials have assessed the efficacy of spinal manipulative therapy (SMT) for thoracic spine pain. No high quality trials have been performed to test the efficacy and effectiveness of Graston Technique® (GT), an instrument-assisted soft tissue therapy. The objective of this trial was to determine the efficacy of SMT and GT compared to sham therapy for the treatment of non-specific thoracic spine pain.

Methods: People with non-specific thoracic pain were randomly allocated to one of three groups: SMT, GT, or a placebo (de-tuned ultrasound). Each participant received up to 10 supervised treatment sessions at Murdoch University chiropractic student clinic over a 4 week period. The participants and treatment providers were not blinded to the treatment allocation as it was clear which therapy they were receiving, however outcome assessors were blinded and we attempted to blind the participants allocated to the placebo group. Treatment outcomes were measured at baseline, 1 week, and at one, three, six and 12 months. Primary outcome measures included a modified Oswestry Disability Index, and the Visual Analogue Scale (VAS). Treatment effects were estimated with intention to treat analysis and linear mixed models.

Results: One hundred and forty three participants were randomly allocated to the three groups (SMT = 36, GT = 63 and Placebo = 44). Baseline data for the three groups did not show any meaningful differences. Results of the intention to treat analyses revealed no time by group interactions, indicating no statistically significant between-group differences in pain or disability at 1 week, 1 month, 3 months, 6 months, or 12 months. There were significant main effects of time ($p < 0.01$) indicating improvements in pain and disability from baseline among all participants regardless of intervention. No significant adverse events were reported.

Conclusion: This study indicates that there is no difference in outcome at any time point for pain or disability when comparing SMT, Graston Technique® or sham therapy for thoracic spine pain, however all groups improved with time. These results constitute the first from a fully powered randomised controlled trial comparing SMT, Graston technique® and a placebo.

Trial Registration: This trial was registered with the Australia and New Zealand Clinical Trials Registry on the 7th February, 2008. Trial number: ACTRN12608000070336

Keywords: Chiropractic, Spinal manipulation, Graston Technique®, Back pain, Thoracic spine

* Correspondence: bruce.walker@murdoch.edu.au
[2]School of Health Professions, Discipline of Chiropractic, Murdoch University, South Street, Murdoch, WA, Australia
Full list of author information is available at the end of the article

Background

Thoracic spinal pain is common with most occupational groups having 1-year prevalence around 30 % [1]. Commonly used treatment options for non-specific thoracic spine pain include manual therapies such as massage, mobilisation, and spinal manipulative therapy (SMT) [2], however there are no high quality studies evaluating these modalities. To date there are only two published randomised controlled trials whose primary aim was to assess the effectiveness of SMT on thoracic spinal pain [3, 4]. In the first study by Schiller [3] the author conducted a small study of 30 patients with 'mechanical thoracic spine pain' where SMT was compared to a sham comprising non-functional ultrasound. While patients in the SMT group reported lower pain intensity and greater lateral flexion range of motion immediately following the 2 to 3 week treatment period, there were no differences after 1 month. Concurrently, there were no between-group differences in McGill Pain and Oswestry Disability scores at any point of the trial.

In the second study by Lethola et al. [4], thoracic spinal manipulation and needle acupuncture led to similar outcomes as placebo electrotherapy in reducing pain in female patients with recent-onset mechanical thoracic spinal pain. This three arm study randomised 114 females aged 20–60 with thoracic spine pain (≤3-month duration) between the third and eighth thoracic vertebrae to receive a high-velocity thrust spinal manipulation, needle acupuncture, or placebo electrotherapy with intermittent suction. All interventions were provided by the same physiotherapist 4 times per week for 3 weeks. The study results showed small differences in pain reduction favouring manipulation 1-week post-intervention. However, these differences were not clinically important.

A third study was identified in a systematic review [5] of non-invasive interventions for musculoskeletal chest wall pain and thoracic pain, in this study [6] Stochkendahl et al. used a secondary outcome measure of severity of thoracic pain associated with their primary interest of acute chest wall pain. They studied 115 patients aged 18–75 years presenting to an emergency cardiology department in Denmark. Fifty-nine patients were randomised to receive a multimodal program of care provided by a chiropractor (up to 10 visits/4 weeks) including manipulation to the cervical and/or thoracic spine, combined with any or all of the following: joint mobilization, soft tissue therapy, stretching, stabilizing or strengthening exercises, heat or cold, and advice. There were 56 in the control group who received a single 15 min session of education provided by a chiropractor, which included reassurance and advice promoting self-management and individualized instruction on posture and home exercises to increase spinal movement or muscle stretch. While this study's primary outcome was acute chest pain, data on thoracic pain was obtained and there were no differences between the groups at 4, 12 and 52 weeks.

The results of the trials above are similar to those found in systematic reviews of manual therapy for neck pain [7] and low back pain [8, 9].

For the purposes of this study we chose to evaluate SMT, Graston technique® (GT) [10] and a placebo treatment. The reasons for these choices are that SMT is a commonly used treatment worldwide [11] and GT is a popular soft-tissue technique in the United States and becoming more popular in other developed countries [12, 13]. GT is an instrument-assisted soft-tissue therapy involving the use of hand-held stainless steel instruments. The promoters of the GT [10] claim that the instruments resonate in the clinician's hands allowing the clinician to isolate soft-tissue "adhesions and restrictions", and treat them precisely. While there are two preliminary studies that show a) an increased blood flow with the use of GT [12] and b) improvements in shoulder ranges of motion among baseball players with its application [13] we are not aware of any high level evidence to support claims or the effectiveness of GT for spinal pain.

Given the lack of scientific evidence for the use of this modality and its apparent popularity for spinal pain a high quality trial was deemed necessary to determine efficacy.

Accordingly, we conducted a study to determine the efficacy of SMT and GT compared to sham therapy for the treatment of non-specific thoracic pain.

Methods

The full protocol of this study has been published in free full text format elsewhere [14]. In summary, the study was a three-arm randomised, placebo-controlled trial, conducted between March 2008 and July 2009, comparing two treatment modalities to a sham intervention for people with acute or sub-acute thoracic spine pain. The therapy arms consisted of SMT and GT and the sham was non-functional ultrasound. Ethics approval was granted by Murdoch University Human Research and Ethics Committee (2007/274).

Study sample and participant enrolment

The study was conducted at the Murdoch University Chiropractic student clinic in Perth, Western Australia. Participants were recruited using advertisements posted around the Murdoch University Campus, on local community boards and in newspapers.

Potential participants were screened with a detailed history and physical examination by a research assistant who applied the inclusion and exclusion criteria. Eligible participants were invited to enter the trial and asked to read and sign a consent form.

Inclusion criteria

People were included if they met the following criteria:

1. Age 18 years or older with non-specific thoracic spine pain of any duration, which was defined as pain in the region from T1 to T12 (Fig. 1) and complied with the descriptive classification by Triano et al. [15] (Table 1).
2. A Visual Analogue Score (VAS) pain score of at least 2 out of 10 and an Oswestry Disability Index (ODI) score of greater than 15 % at baseline [16, 17].

Exclusion criteria

People were excluded if they met any of the following criteria:

1. Had a contraindication to manual therapy including osteoporosis, thoracic fracture, spinal infection, neoplastic disorders, spondyloarthropathy, and clinical examination suggestive of frank disc herniation or generalised infection such as influenza.
2. Had a contraindication to Graston technique including neoplastic disorders, kidney infection, anticoagulant medication, rheumatoid arthritis, uncontrolled hypertension, thoracic fracture, osteomyelitis or generalised infection.

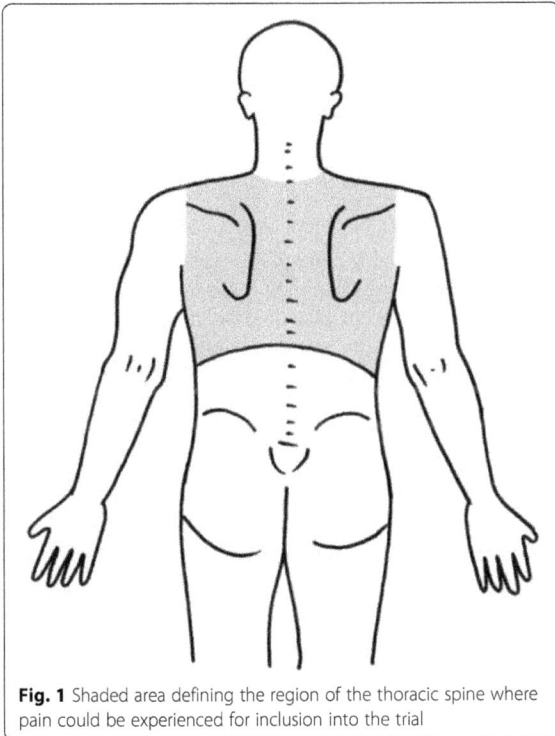

Fig. 1 Shaded area defining the region of the thoracic spine where pain could be experienced for inclusion into the trial

Table 1 Definition of non-specific thoracic spine pain [15]

- Midline back pain - for the purposes of this trial, the pain will be bound by the lateral margins of the thorax laterally and the trapezium superiorly
- Non dermatomal referred pain difficult to localise
- No signs of nerve root tension
- No major neurological deficit
- Pain with compression over the thoracic spine into spine extension
- Reduced range of motion

3. Had somatic conditions found on examination to refer pain to the thoracic spine from outside the defined area (including cervical zygapophyseal joints, muscles and discs).
4. Had an active history of visceral conditions referring pain to the thoracic spine including myocardial ischaemia, dissecting thoracic aortic aneurysm, peptic ulcer, acute cholecystitis, pancreatitis, renal colic, acute pyelonephritis
5. Had a current substance abuse problem.
6. Was not fluent and/or literate in the English language.
7. Was currently receiving care for thoracic pain from any other healthcare provider.
8. Could not commit to the full study protocol.
9. Was currently seeking compensation or had commenced litigation for thoracic spine pain.

Treatment allocation

Randomisation occurred directly after baseline measures were taken, after the participant had been screened for inclusion and informed consent provided. An online randomisation site, Research Randomiser [18], was used to generate treatment allocation. This online randomisation module is a web browser application that supports online randomisation of patients into healthcare trials. 150 random basis sequences without blocs were generated, and then placed in sequentially numbered, opaque, sealed envelopes and stored in a sealed box. As each participant entered the trial the next consecutive opaque, sealed envelope was given to the treating student and supervising clinician by the research assistant.

Interventions and treatment

Participants were randomised to one of three treatment arms as follows:

1. Chiropractic group: a series of high velocity low amplitude chiropractic manual adjustments (SMT) to the thoracic spine were administered by a registered chiropractor or a final year chiropractic student under the direct supervision of a registered chiropractor. The thrust direction was at the discretion of the treating chiropractor or student.

2. Graston Technique group: Graston Technique was administered by final year chiropractic students who were certified in module one of the Graston Technique, under the direct supervision of a registered chiropractor who attended each consultation and in addition placed their hands on the anatomical regions involved;

3. Placebo group: participants received a session of de-tuned ultrasound administered by a final year chiropractic student, under the direct supervision of a registered chiropractor who attended each consultation and also placed their hands on the anatomical regions involved.

The reason for the random placement of hand near the painful area by the chiropractors for participants in groups 2 and 3 was designed to mitigate any lack of confidence in a student intern interaction and to provide a hands-on component to the therapy and make it more equivalent to the group 1 experience.

All treating students and chiropractors were briefed on the administration of the study and trained to show the same enthusiasm for all three treatment modalities. To minimise potential for attention effects, we standardised the delivery of therapy such that all sessions lasted 10–15 min, irrespective of treatment group. The administration of the various modalities and monitoring of progress is described in detail elsewhere [14] however, we aimed to administer 10 treatments of each of the "therapies" over 3–4 weeks to each participant.

Change in inclusion criteria from the protocol

Initially, eligible participants were people with non-specific thoracic pain of less than 3 months duration. However, recruitment was slow so this was amended to also include participants with any duration of pain.

Outcome measures and baseline data

Treatment outcomes comprised self-reported pain intensity with a 100 mm Visual Analogue Scale (VAS) and pain-related disability measured with a version of the Oswestry Disability Index (ODI) modified for patients with thoracic spine pain. These instruments are discussed in detail in the study protocol [14]. Outcomes were administered at baseline, 1 week after treatment commenced, upon completion of the 4-week intervention period and at three, six and 12 months.

A variation to the published protocol occurred with the decision to not obtain some baseline measures of race/ethnicity, education, household income, marital status, current employment status and general health status using the Short-Form Health Survey (SF-36). This was partly due to anticipated participant fatigue and that these extra baseline questions would likely put them off participating in the trial.

Adverse effects

Participants were provided with a list of potential adverse effects in an information letter prior to giving consent. Participants recorded information about adverse events in a log book.

Blinding

The two outcome measures were self-administered instruments. Participants were given blank questionnaires in a package by a research assistant following their first treatment. Participants were instructed to complete the instruments at each assessment time point. After completion of the forms the participant posted them back to the Murdoch University Chiropractic Clinic. Research assistants remained blind to the outcome data for the entire study period. The participants and treatment providers were not blinded to the treatment allocation as it was clear that the groups were receiving different treatments. Participants in the placebo group were blinded to their placebo allocation until follow-up was complete at 12 months. Participants were surveyed for the adequacy of the placebo blinding at the end of the study.

Sample size calculations

To calculate the sample size, we used the means of 23.9, 18.9 and 13.9 and assumed a standard deviation of 12.1 of the ODI derived in a study by Hoiriis et al. [19] in a similar chiropractic teaching setting. The clinical effect size used for the ODI was 10 % [17], alpha was set at .05. Recruiting 30 participants per group was calculated to provide 80 % power to identify between-group differences this large or larger. Sample size calculations using the VAS from the previous study resulted in a smaller n value for each group, therefore the ODI was used. We used 30 as a minimum requirement for each group.

Data analysis

A researcher blinded to group allocation analysed the data. Statistical analyses were performed using IBM SPSS Statistics v21. The statistical analysis varied from the published protocol in the following way. Treatment effects were estimated using separate, random-intercept linear mixed models for each outcome variable. Time (1 week, 4 weeks, 3 months, 6 months, and 12 months) and treatment group (placebo, MT, Graston) were modelled as fixed effects. The hypothesis of interest was the time by group interaction which we further examined with pairwise comparisons of the estimated marginal means. We included the baseline outcome score as a covariate in each model. Consistent with the intention to treat principle, the linear mixed models estimated values for missing data based on available scores; therefore all participants randomised to a treatment group were included in the analyses of clinical outcomes. Alpha level was 0.05 for all analyses.

Results

The participant flow through the trial is presented in Fig. 2; 376 people responded to advertisements and after screening 144 patients were considered eligible for the study and were randomised to a study group. One participant was omitted from the study and their data not included in the analysis; this participant was excluded after being incorrectly randomised leaving 143 participants. It was discovered that the randomisation sequence for this one participant was interrupted and the participant was incorrectly allocated by a clinic supervisor holding an envelope up to a bright light in advance of allocation. Demographic and clinical information at baseline is described in Table 2. There were no important differences in prognostic

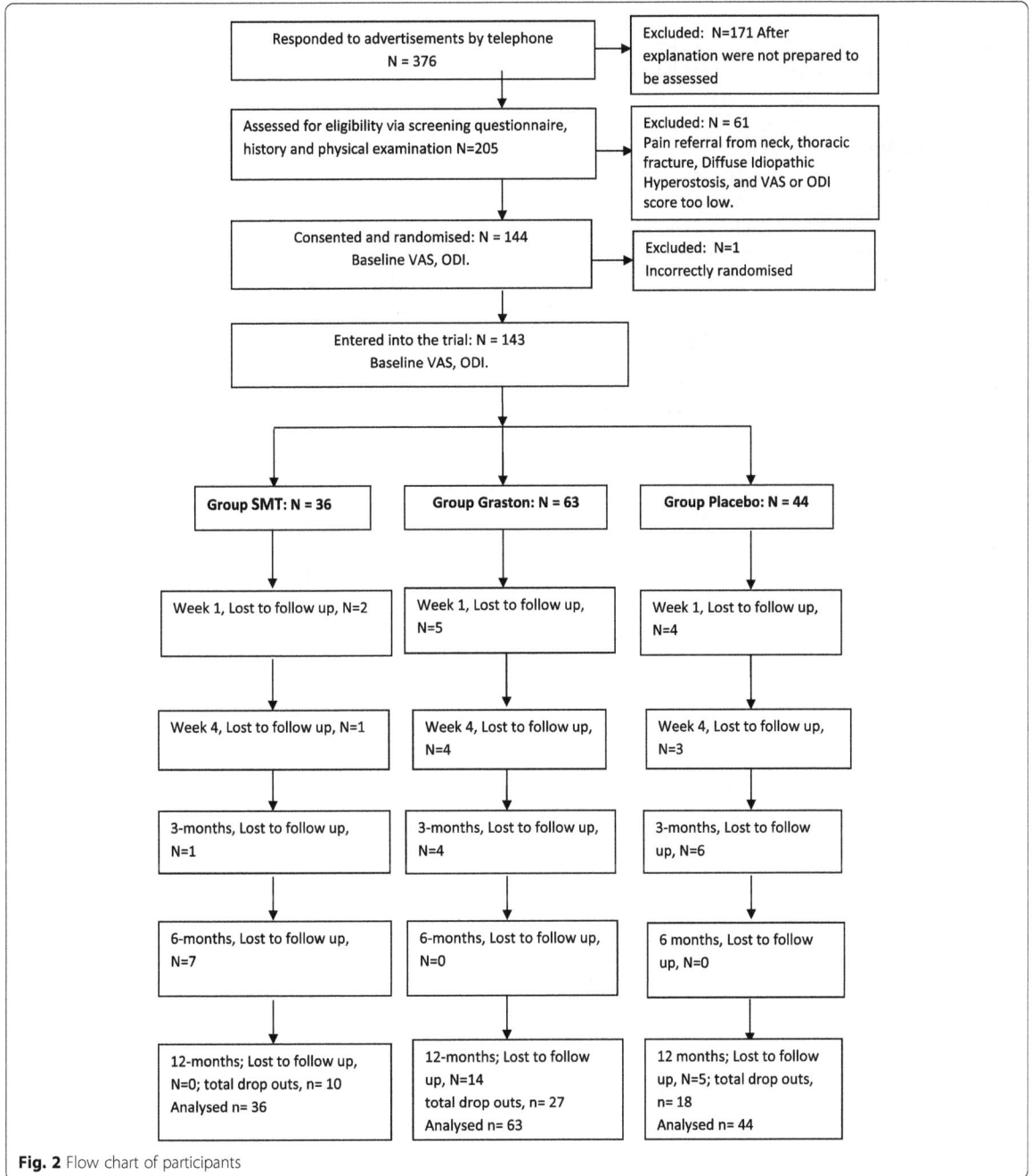

Fig. 2 Flow chart of participants

Table 2 Baseline data for the entire sample and the three treatment groups

Variable	All (N = 143)	SMT (N = 36)	Graston (N = 63)	Placebo (N = 44)
Age (years)	45.8 (13.7)	44.4 (13.0)	44.8 (14.3)	48.5 (13.0)
Sex (% Male)	53.2	55.6	50.2	54.6
Pain (0-10 VAS)	5.6 (2.0)	5.5 (2.0)	5.7 (2.1)	5.5 (2.0)
Disability (0-100 ODI)	28.5 (10.4)	27.2 (10.2)	29.6 (11.1)	28.1 (9.9)
Pain duration (years)	9.2 (12.0)	9.0 (16.0)	8.2 (11.0)	10.9 (9.4)

Values are mean (standard deviation) unless otherwise indicated

variables between the groups and it can be seen that our recruitment strategy resulted in an overwhelming number of participants with long standing pain.

Of the total enrolled participants, there was a similar loss to follow up from each treatment group. Based upon results in Fig. 2, at 12 months the numbers lost to follow-up between groups compared to baseline, was SMT (28 %), Graston (45 %) and Placebo (41 %). Drop outs were unable to be contacted to determine the reason for loss to follow up.

Table 3 shows the pain (VAS) and disability (ODI) scores for the three treatment groups from baseline through all time points of follow up.

Analysis demonstrates that there was no difference between the treatment groups for pain (Fig. 3) or disability (Fig. 4) at any time point.

Results of the intention to treat analyses revealed no time by group interactions, indicating no significant between-group differences in pain or disability at 1 week, 4 weeks, 3 months, 6 months, or 12 months (Table 3). There were significant main effects of time ($p < 0.01$) for both pain and disability indicating improvements in pain

and disability from baseline among all participants (Table 3).

No significant adverse events were notified in this trial, however one participant reported increased pain after the placebo therapy. The participant dropped out of the study at this point and was lost to follow up.

Blinding

Participants in the placebo group were asked at 12 months about the group to which they were allocated SMT, "other physical therapy" or just "other". Only 8 participants responded to the question, 5 of whom thought they were in the SMT group and 3 in the "Other PT group", none thought they were allocated to the "Other group" i.e. the placebo group.

Discussion

Our study indicates that there is no difference in outcome at any time point for pain or disability when comparing SMT, Graston technique or placebo therapy for long standing thoracic spine pain, however all groups improved with time. These results constitute the first

Table 3 Results of the intention-to-treat analysis comparing clinical outcomes between treatment groups

	Mean (SD) for each group			Adjusted mean difference between groups (95 % CI)		
	Graston	SMT	Placebo	Graston vs MT	Graston vs placebo	SMT vs placebo
Disability (0-100)*						
Baseline	29.6 (11.0)	27.2 (10.0)	28.1 (9.8)	-	-	-
1 week	22.6 (11.8)	22.3 (10.0)	23.7 (12.1)	-0.58 (-4.7,3.6)	-1.9 (-5.8,2.0)	-1.3 (-5.8,2.0)
1 month	18.1 (12.0)	19.8 (11.7)	21.5 (12.3)	-3.4 (-7.7, 0.9)	-4.5 (-8.6, -0.4)	-1.1 (-5.7, 3.6)
3 months	16.2 (13.1)	21.0 (14.3)	18.7 (15.0)	-4.6 (-9.5, 0.4)	-2.1 (-7.0, 2.8)	2.5 (-2.9, 7.9)
6 months	16.2 (13.1)	18.2 (14.2)	16.9 (14.1)	-1.9 (-6.9, 2.9)	-0.4 (-4.9, 4.2)	1.6 (-3.7, 6.9)
12 months	16.3 (13.5)	21.2 (16.0)	16.1 (16.3)	-4.8 (-10.5, 0.9)	-1.2 (-6.8, 4.4)	3.6 (-2.5, 9.7)
Pain intensity (0-10)†						
Baseline	5.7 (2.1)	5.5 (2.0)	5.5 (1.9)	-	-	-
1 week	4.7 (1.9)	5.1 (2.0)	4.7 (1.8)	-0.3 (-1.2, 0.5)	0.1 (-0.7, 0.8)	0.4 (-0.5, 1.2)
1 month	3.4 (1.9)	4.3 (2.0)	4.2 (2.4)	-1.0 (-1.9, -0.2)	-0.9 (-1.7, -0.1)	0.1 (-0.8, 1.0)
3 months	3.2 (2.6)	4.0 (2.2)	3.5 (2.3)	-0.8 (-1.8, 0.1)	-0.3 (-1.3, 0.6)	0.5 (-0.5, 1.5)
6 months	3.5 (2.5)	3.6 (2.2)	3.6 (2.5)	-0.4 (-1.4, 0.7)	-0.2 (-1.2, 0.8)	0.2 (-1.0, 1.3)
12 months	3.2 (2.3)	3.8 (2.4)	3.3 (2.5)	-0.8 (-1.9, 0.3)	-0.4 (-1.5, 0.7)	0.4 (-0.8, 1.6)

*Time by treatment group interaction $p = 0.24$
†Time by treatment group interaction $p = 0.58$

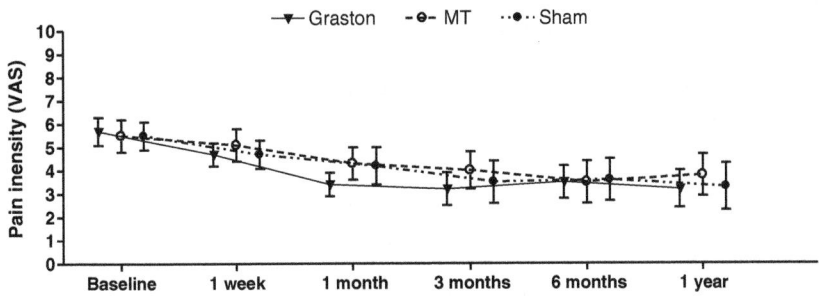

Fig. 3 Mean group visual analogue scale pain scores over time with 95 % confidence intervals

from an adequately powered randomised controlled trial comparing spinal manipulation, Graston technique and a placebo. It appears that our findings differ from the one other randomised trial [3] that reported SMT to be superior to sham for thoracic spine pain reduction, however that trial was inadequately powered and a Type II error was likely.

The results of our study are similar to those published for manipulation for low back pain [8] and for neck pain [7] where comparisons of manipulation to other modalities show only small treatment effects. The anatomy and biomechanics of the lumbar and cervical spines differ to that of the thoracic spine in that, among other things, the thoracic vertebrae are bound by ribs. However, our results suggest that these anatomical differences have not made any difference to clinical outcome after manual therapy is applied.

The strengths of this study lie in its randomised design and the inclusion of a sham or placebo arm for comparison of the active therapies involved. Another strength was the power of the study which was pre-determined and met by an initially adequate sample size.

Limitations to our study were the use of a modified Oswestry Disability Index (ODI) for the thoracic spine. We modified the original ODI [20] by replacing the words "low back pain" with "mid back pain" and doing

this to the commonly used version where sexual difficulties had been removed. Otherwise the ODI was left intact. However it should be noted that the ODI was constructed for low back pain disability and as such may not be valid for mid back pain disability. Nevertheless there were no validated instruments to specifically measure thoracic spine pain related disability. Further validity studies should be undertaken to test this instrument for use in measuring thoracic spine disability. Even though dropout rates were similar between groups the lack of information regarding reasons for drop outs is also a limitation. This lack of information was caused by logistics and funding constraints that prevented us employing the human resources necessary to follow participants up. In addition, while we recorded the number of drop outs per group we did not record if a participant was pain free after less than 10 consultations and as such we are unable to report the average number of treatments per group or their range. Because of the size of the drop out rate treatment effect estimates beyond 3 months should be interpreted with caution. One participant was omitted from the study because they were incorrectly randomised and their data not included in the analysis when it was discovered that a clinic supervisor held an envelope up to a bright light in advance of allocation. This occurred despite briefing all clinical supervisors about the

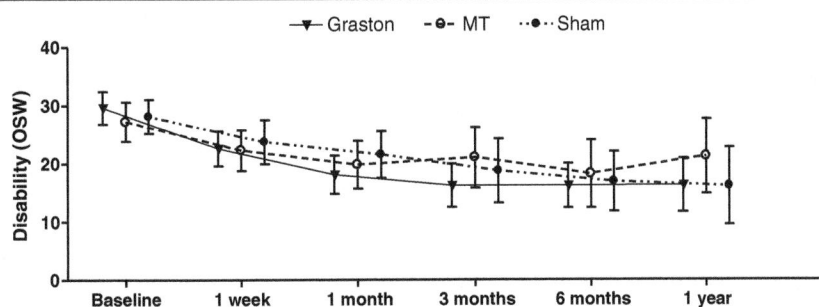

Fig. 4 Mean group Oswestry disability scores over time with 95 % confidence intervals

trial including randomisation. To prevent any further breach the randomisation sequence cards were wrapped in aluminium foil and placed back into their envelopes and the supervisor was counselled.

Another possible limitation is the use of final year chiropractic interns to deliver the SMT and Graston therapy whose therapy outcomes may differ from more experienced clinicians. We did not record whether the intern or the practitioner delivered the treatment but it was under the supervision of the practitioner and had to be performed to their satisfaction. This was in accord with the published protocol. In addition, there is some evidence that therapist-related factors of increased experience and specialty certification status do not result in an improvement in patients' disability associated with back pain [21]. All students had been certified in Stage I Graston therapy use by a certified Graston therapist. Regarding blinding of the placebo group we were unable to draw any conclusion on its success given the poor response to the question.

A final limitation occurred in the disproportionate numbers randomly allocated to the three groups, i.e. 36, 63 and 44. This imbalance resulted from the use of simple randomisation wherein each participant had an equal likelihood of being assigned to the groups. However, by chance an unequal number of individuals were assigned to each arm of the study and this may have adversely affected an optimum level of statistical power. Block randomization is a commonly used technique in clinical trial design to reduce bias and achieve balance in the allocation of participants to treatment arms, especially when the sample size is small [22]. In hindsight we should have used block randomisation as this would have resulted in equal group sizes.

The clinical implications and generalisability of this study are limited because while the results suggest that all of the methods tested provided benefit for chronic mid back pain this benefit included the placebo/sham arm. This apparent lack of effect may be due, at least in part, to the tendency to treat non-specific mid-back pain as a homogenous condition, rather than a heterogeneous collection of as yet undefined but differing conditions, some of which might respond and others that do not respond to a particular therapy. Research to identify diagnostic subsets within non-specific mid-back pain may be worthy and if successful, individual therapies such as manual therapy or Graston technique may be better directed.

Conclusion

This study indicates that there is no difference in outcome at any time point for pain or disability when comparing spinal manipulative therapy, Graston Technique®

or sham therapy for non-specific thoracic spine pain, however all groups improved with time. These results constitute the first from a fully powered randomised controlled trial comparing spinal manipulative therapy, Graston technique® and a placebo.

Competing interests
The authors declare that they have no competing interests.

Authors' contributions
AC contributed to the review, design, writing and performance of the research, SF contributed to the review, design and writing, JH contributed to the statistical design, coordination and writing, BW contributed to the review, design, writing and performance of the research. All authors read and approved the final manuscript.

Author details
[1]Private practice of chiropractic, Geraldton, WA 6530, Australia. [2]School of Health Professions, Discipline of Chiropractic, Murdoch University, South Street, Murdoch, WA, Australia. [3]School of Psychology and Exercise Science, Murdoch University, South Street, Murdoch, WA, Australia. [4]School of Rehabilitation Therapy, Faculty of Health Sciences, Queen's University, Ontario, Canada.

References
1. Briggs AM, Bragge P, Smith AJ, Govil D, Straker LM. Prevalence and associated factors for thoracic spine pain in the adult working population: a literature review. J Occup Health. 2009;51(3):177–92.
2. Hegmann K. Cervical and thoracic spine disorders. In: Hegman KT, editor. Occupational medicine practice guidelines Evaluation and management of common health problems and functional recovery in workers. 3rd ed. Elk Grove Village, Illinois, USA: American College of Occupational and Environmental Medicine (ACOEM); 2011. p. 1–332.
3. Schiller L. Effectiveness of spinal manipulative therapy in the treatment of mechanical thoracic spine pain: a pilot randomized clinical trial. J Manip Physiol Ther. 2001;24(6):394–401.
4. Lehtola V, Korhonen I, Airaksinen O. A randomised, placebo-controlled, clinical trial for the short-term effectiveness of manipulative therapy and acupuncture on pain caused by mechanical thoracic spine dysfunction. Int Musculoskelet Med. 2010;32:25–32.
5. Southerst D, Marchand AA, Cote P, Shearer HM, Wong JJ, Varatharajan S, Randhawa K, Sutton D, Yu H, Gross DP, et al. The effectiveness of noninvasive interventions for musculoskeletal thoracic spine and chest wall pain: a systematic review by the Ontario Protocol for Traffic Injury Management (OPTIMa) collaboration. J Manip Physiol Ther. 2015;38(7):521–31.
6. Stochkendahl MJ, Christensen HW, Vach W, Hoilund-Carlsen PF, Haghfelt T, Hartvigsen J. A randomized clinical trial of chiropractic treatment and self-management in patients with acute musculoskeletal chest pain: 1-year follow-up. J Manip Physiol Ther. 2012;35(4):254–62.
7. Gross A, Langevin P, Burnie SJ, Bedard-Brochu MS, Empey B, Dugas E, Faber-Dobrescu M, Andres C, Graham N, Goldsmith CH, et al. Manipulation and mobilisation for neck pain contrasted against an inactive control or another active treatment. Cochrane Database Syst Rev. 2015;9:Cd004249.
8. Rubinstein SM, van Middelkoop M, Assendelft WJ, de Boer MR, van Tulder MW. Spinal manipulative therapy for chronic low-back pain: an update of a Cochrane review. Spine. 2011;36(13):E825–846.
9. Walker BF, French SD, Grant W, Green S. A cochrane review of combined chiropractic interventions for low-back pain. Spine. 2011;36(3):230–42.
10. Graston Technique [http://www.grastontechnique.com/]. Accessed 18 Apr 2014.
11. Hurwitz EL. Epidemiology: spinal manipulation utilization. J Electromyogr Kinesiol. 2012;22(5):648–54.
12. Portillo-Soto A, Eberman LE, Demchak TJ, Peebles C. Comparison of blood flow changes with soft tissue mobilization and massage therapy. J Altern Complement Med. 2014;20(12):932–6.

13. Laudner K, Compton BD, McLoda TA, Walters CM. Acute effects of instrument assisted soft tissue mobilization for improving posterior shoulder range of motion in collegiate baseball players. Int J Sports Phys Ther. 2014;9(1):1–7.
14. Crothers A, Walker B, French SD. Spinal manipulative therapy versus Graston Technique in the treatment of non-specific thoracic spine pain: design of a randomised controlled trial. Chiropr Osteopat. 2008;16:12.
15. Triano JJ, Hondras MA, McGregor M. Differences in treatment history with manipulation for acute, subacute, chronic and recurrent spine pain. J Manip Physiol Ther. 1992;15(1):24–30.
16. Kelly AM. The minimum clinically significant difference in visual analogue scale pain score does not differ with severity of pain. Emerg Med J. 2001;18(3):205–7.
17. Ostelo RW, de Vet HC. Clinically important outcomes in low back pain. Best Pract Res Clin Rheumatol. 2005;19(4):593–607.
18. Research Randomizer [http://www.randomizer.org/]. Accessed 18 Apr 2014.
19. Hoiriis KT, Pfleger B, McDuffie FC, Cotsonis G, Elsangak O, Hinson R, Verzosa GT. A randomized clinical trial comparing chiropractic adjustments to muscle relaxants for subacute low back pain. J Manip Physiol Ther. 2004;27(6):388–98.
20. Fairbank JC, Couper J, Davies JB, O'Brien JP. The Oswestry low back pain disability questionnaire. Physiotherapy. 1980;66(8):271–3.
21. Whitman JM, Fritz JM, Childs JD. The influence of experience and specialty certifications on clinical outcomes for patients with low back pain treated within a standardized physical therapy management program. J Orthop Sports Phys Ther. 2004;34(11):662–72.
22. Efird J. Blocked randomization with randomly selected block sizes. Int J Environ Res Public Health. 2011;8(1):15–20.

21

Quality of reporting of randomised controlled trials in chiropractic using the CONSORT checklist

Fay Karpouzis[1*], Rod Bonello[2], Mario Pribicevic[3], Allan Kalamir[3] and Benjamin T. Brown[3]

Abstract

Background: Reviews indicate that the quality of reporting of randomised controlled trials (RCTs) in the medical literature is less than optimal, poor to moderate, and require improving. However, the reporting quality of chiropractic RCTs is unknown.

As a result, the aim of this study was to assess the reporting quality of chiropractic RCTs and identify factors associated with better reporting quality. We hypothesized that quality of reporting of RCTs was influenced by industry funding, positive findings, larger sample sizes, latter year of publication and publication in non-chiropractic journals.

Methods: RCTs published between 2005 and 2014 were sourced from clinical trial registers, PubMed and the Cochrane Reviews. RCTs were included if they involved high-velocity, low-amplitude (HVLA) spinal and/or extremity manipulation and were conducted by a chiropractor or within a chiropractic department. Data extraction, and reviews were conducted by all authors independently. Disagreements were resolved by consensus. Outcomes: a 39-point overall quality of reporting score checklist was developed based on the CONSORT 2010 and CONSORT for Non-Pharmacological Treatments statements. Four key methodological items, based on allocation concealment, blinding of participants and assessors, and use of intention-to-treat analysis (ITT) were also investigated.

Results: Thirty-five RCTs were included. The overall quality of reporting score ranged between 10 and 33 (median score 26.0; IQR = 8.00). Allocation concealment, blinding of participants and assessors and ITT analysis were reported in 31 (87 %), 16 (46 %), 25 (71 %) and 21 (60 %) of the 35 RCTs respectively. Items most underreported were from the CONSORT for Non-Pharmacological Treatments statement. Multivariate regression analysis, revealed that year of publication ($t_{32} = 5.17$, $p = 0.000$, 95 % CI: 0.76, 1.76), and sample size ($t_{32} = 3.01$, $p = 0.005$, 95 % CI: 1.36, 7.02), were the only two factors associated with reporting quality.

Conclusion: The overall quality of reporting RCTs in chiropractic ranged from poor to excellent, improving between 2005 and 2014. This study suggests that quality of reporting, was influenced by year of publication and sample size but not journal type, funding source or outcome positivity. Reporting of some key methodological items and uptake of items from the CONSORT Extension for Non-Pharmacological Treatments items was suboptimal. Future recommendations were made.

Keywords: Manipulation, Chiropractic manipulation, Spinal manipulative therapy, Spine, Musculoskeletal, Quality of reporting, Randomised controlled trials, The CONSORT statement

* Correspondence: faykchiro@optusnet.com.au
[1]PO Box 2108, Rose Bay Nth 2030, NSW, Australia
Full list of author information is available at the end of the article

Background

Randomised controlled trials (RCTs) are considered to be the "gold standard" of clinical research [1, 2], by which health care professionals make decisions about the efficacy and effectiveness of interventions [3–6]. However, poorly designed and reported studies continue to be published, leading to a compromised evidence base [7]. This can adversely influence meta-analysis findings and clinical practice recommendations [7–10]. As a result of the poor reporting of RCTs, the CONSORT (Consolidated Standards of Reporting Trials) statement was developed in 1996 [6], and updated in 2010 [11], with the aim of improving the quality of reporting of RCTs through standardization, comprehensiveness and transparency [6, 11].

Reporting research in manual therapies presents obstacles not experienced in medical pharmacological trials. Non-pharmacological trials, such as chiropractic RCTs, test complex therapeutic interventions, which tend to be multi-faceted [12]. As a result, they are more challenging to describe, standardise, reproduce and administer consistently to all participants involved in a clinical trial [12]. These variants, along with others, such as care provider's expertise may substantially impact estimates of treatment effect [12]. This makes it imperative for such studies to adhere to the CONSORT 2010 [13] and CONSORT for Non-Pharmacologic Treatments statements criteria [12].

Reviews indicate that the quality of reporting of RCTs in the medical literature is less than optimal [14–18]. As a result, many reviewers have drawn conclusions that the overall quality of reporting was poor to moderate [7, 9, 19–21], and require improving [22–26].

To our knowledge there has not been an assessment of the quality of reporting of RCTs in chiropractic. As a result, the aim of this study was to assess the reporting quality of RCTs in chiropractic and to identify factors associated with better reporting quality. The candidate factors that were chosen for this study, have previously been identified in the medical literature as influencing the reporting quality of RCTs [8, 9, 18].

The objectives of this study were to:

1. Assess the overall quality of reporting of RCTs in chiropractic using a customised tool, based on the CONSORT 2010 and CONSORT for Non-Pharmacologic Treatments statements.
2. To report on 4 key methodological items that minimise bias, based on allocation concealment, blinding of participants and assessors, and use of intention-to-treat analysis.
3. To determine factors associated with higher quality of reporting.

We hypothesized that quality of reporting was influenced by industry funding, positive findings, larger sample sizes, latter year of publication and publication in non-chiropractic journals.

Methods

This study has ethics approval from Murdoch University, Research Ethics and Integrity Office: Ethics #2014/119. The study protocol has been published previously, [27] however an outline is presented below.

Study selection

We searched ten clinical trial registers (refer to Fig. 1) and two electronic databases (PubMed and the Cochrane Database of Systematic Reviews), to identify publications of RCTs involving chiropractic studies, published between January 2005 to July 2014. The search terms used were: "Spine" OR "Lower Extremity" OR "Upper Extremity" AND "Musculoskeletal Manipulations" OR, "Manipulation, Chiropractic" OR "Spinal Manipulative Therapy" AND "Chiropractic". Full text articles of RCTs in the English language were included if they met inclusion criteria as outlined in Table 1. Article selection and data extraction was conducted by all authors independently, and disagreements were resolved by consensus.

We chose to limit this review to high-velocity, low-amplitude (HVLA) studies only, as manual manipulative procedures are the basis of training for all chiropractors. Furthermore, HVLA procedures are reported to be the most popular chiropractic adjusting techniques, used by 93 % of chiropractic practitioners in the US, with similar numbers internationally [28].

It should be recognised that, for the purpose of this study we have included RCTs where both chiropractors and non-chiropractors were involved in the delivery of the interventions, such as physiotherapists, physical therapists and osteopaths [29–32]. However, the HVLA interventions were all delivered by a chiropractor who was part of the study team. We also included studies where the HVLA intervention was the comparator rather than the primary intervention [32–36].

Pilot and feasibility studies were not included as the CONSORT checklist could not be applied to such studies without them being disadvantaged during scoring, in that they typically do not include all items from the CONSORT, such as a power analysis and ITT analysis. Similarly, studies not published as full papers were not included, as it is impossible to properly assess those papers against the CONSORT criteria.

Review strategy

The characteristics of included studies have been reported in Additional file 1. The characteristics of excluded studies have been reported in Additional file 2.

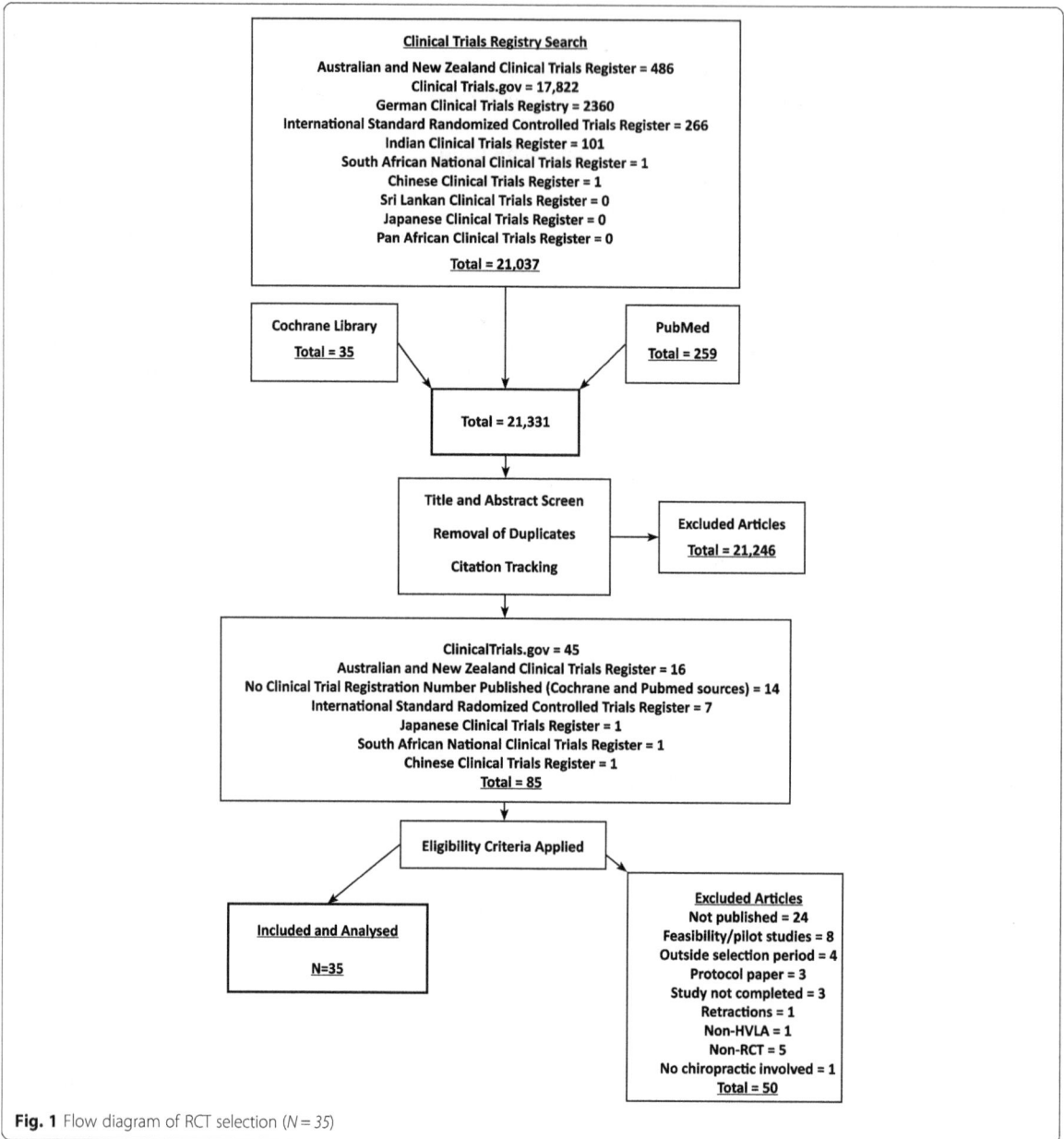

Fig. 1 Flow diagram of RCT selection (N = 35)

Rating the overall reporting quality

This study was modeled upon previously published medical studies assessing the quality of reporting RCTs [9, 14, 16, 18, 19, 37], which used the CONSORT checklists. Furthermore, the CONSORT was used, as it is considered to have both face and content validity and is a measure of methodological quality [38].

A 39-point customised CONSORT checklist was developed by three authors (FK, RB and BB) in order to ascertain the overall quality of reporting of chiropractic RCTs. The overall quality of reporting checklist was developed by integrating items from the CONSORT 2010 [13], and the CONSORT for Non-Pharmacological Treatments statements [12]. Twenty-two items were included from the CONSORT 2010 statement [13], i.e. items one through to 25, excluding items 21, 22 and 24. Items 21 (generalizability [external validity] of the trial findings) and 22 (interpretation of results), which are included in the discussion section, were excluded from the customised checklist because it is challenging to objectively evaluate them [7, 39]. Item 24 (access to trial protocol), was also excluded, as historically it was not a

Table 1 Inclusion and exclusion criteria

Inclusion Criteria

RCTs with parallel or cross-over study design

Adult study populations with musculoskeletal and non-musculoskeletal with conditions or no condition

Chiropractic high-velocity, low-amplitude (HVLA), musculoskeletal manipulation

Treatment must include chiropractic manipulation, either spinal or peripheral (or both) with/without adjunctive therapy (mobilization, soft tissue therapy, massage, traction, electro-therapies, ultrasound, exercise advice, ergonomic advice, hot/cold therapy, back education)

Comparators: HVLA, placebo, sham treatment or conventional/standard/usual care treatment, or no treatment

Exclusion Criteria

Reviews, systematic reviews and meta-analyses

Non-randomised trial designs (quasi-experimental, observational studies)

Pilot or feasibility studies

Studies with n-of-1

Studies evaluating diagnostic tests, prevention, prognosis, cost-effectiveness, pathophysiological or mechanophysiological mechanisms, validation of questionnaires

Trials not reported as full papers (abstracts), editorials, commentaries, letters, case reports or series, audits, guidelines, historical articles

Methodological/Protocol, epidemiological and qualitative studies

Studies reporting updates of previously published RCTs

requirement to publish protocols prior to publication of results. Items from the CONSORT 2010 checklist included in our assessment tool are outlined in Table 2. In addition, nine items from the CONSORT for Non-Pharmacological Treatments statement [12], were included i.e. Extensions 1, 3, 4a, 4b, 4c, 8, 13, 15 and 'New Item' and are outlined in Table 3.

The assessment of the adequacy of reporting, was based on the CONSORT 2010 guidelines and its extensions [12, 13, 40]. Items were defined as 'yes' if they were clearly and adequately reported and received a score of 1; or 'no' if they were unclear or not reported at all, and received a scored of 0. Items that were not applicable to a specific study were defined as 'not applicable' ('N/A') and were coded 9. The overall quality of reporting score of the trial was calculated as a percentage of the items rated as 'yes' (with a score ranging between 0 and 39 points).

Key methodological items, that safeguard against biases [9, 18, 39], have also been reported in the literature [16], such as: allocation concealment (Item 9), blinding (Item 11), and use of ITT analysis (Item 16). The separate assessment of the key methodological items was deemed necessary because, even within published articles with high overall reporting scores, these are often under reported [38] (Table 4). Blinding of participants was scored separately to blinding of assessors. The question of blinding of care-providers was excluded

for pragmatic purposes. It has been established that blinding manual therapy practitioners is virtually impossible [41, 42], with similar constraints to the blinding of surgeons in medical clinical trials [14].

All authors were involved in the scoring of the RCTs. Each RCT was scored by at least two authors, who were blinded to each other's results. Results were collated, and any discrepancies were resolved via consensus.

Definition of trial characteristics

A "positive finding" in a trial was defined as a trial in which the chiropractic intervention was deemed by authors to have statistically significant results and hence was considered superior to the comparator (i.e. placebo/sham, usual care, standard care, medical care, other health care modality, no care or other chiropractic intervention). If the trial produced results that stated that the chiropractic manipulative therapy and the comparator both produced positive outcomes in the study, then the RCT was rated as "no" to the question of "positive finding", as the chiropractic intervention was not deemed superior to comparator (Refer to Additional file 1).

Trials were considered to be industry-funded, if there was at least partial industry funding. Industry funding included chiropractic research organizations, chiropractic governing bodies or other industry organizations with potentially vested interests in the research. Chiropractic departments funding research within private chiropractic colleges were also deemed to be industry funding, whereas chiropractic and non-chiropractic departments within government educational institutions were considered to be non-industry. Trials that did not have any funding, were also classified as non-industry funding (Refer to Additional file 1).

Trials were considered as published in chiropractic journals, if the journal was dedicated predominantly to the advancement of chiropractic research, education and health care (Refer to Additional file 1).

Statistical analysis description

This study used descriptive statistics to characterise the overall quality of reporting of chiropractic RCTs, as well as the key methodological items. The percentage of trials that scored 'yes' to each CONSORT 2010 item were tabulated and are presented in Table 2. The percentage of trials that scored 'yes' to each item from the CONSORT for Non-Pharmacological Treatments, are presented in Table 3. The key methodological items are presented in Table 4.

Two continuous variables were dichotomised. The sample size variable was divided into a smaller group with $n = 1$–100 and a larger group where $n > 100$. The 'year of publication' variable was also divided into two time periods (2005–2007 and 2008–2014), which were

Table 2 Frequencies of CONSORT 2010 items from customized overall quality of reporting checklist (*N* = 35)

Item	Criterion	CONSORT Description	Total	%
1a	Title	Identification as a randomised trial in the title	26	74
1b	Abstract	Structured summary of trial design, methods, results, and conclusions	35	100
2a	Background	Scientific background and explanation of rationale	35	100
2b		Specific objectives or hypotheses	34	97
3a	Trial Design	Description of trial design (such as parallel, factorial)	18	51
4a	Participants	Eligibility criteria for participants	34	97
4b		settings and locations where the data were collected	17	49
5	Interventions	The interventions for each group with sufficient details to allow replication, including how they were administered	32	91
6a	Outcomes	Completely defined pre-specified primary and secondary outcome measures	32	91
7a	Sample size	How sample size was determined	25	71
8a	Sequence generation	Method used to generate the random allocation sequence	29	83
9	Allocation concealment	Mechanism used to implement the random allocation sequence (such as sequentially numbered containers), describing any steps taken to conceal the sequence until interventions were assigned	31	87
10	Implementation	Was implementation discussed. Who generated the random allocation sequence, who enrolled participants, and who assigned participants to interventions	26	74
11ai	Blinding	Whether or not participants, were blinded to group assignment	16	46
11aii		Whether those assessing the outcomes were blinded to group assignment	25	71
12a	Statistical methods	Statistical methods used to compare groups for outcome(s)	35	100
13a	Participant flow	For each group, the numbers of participants who were randomly assigned, received intended treatment, and were analysed for the primary outcome	29	83
13b		For each group, losses and exclusions after randomization, together with reasons	20	57
14a	Recruitment	Dates defining the periods of recruitment and follow-up	23	66
15	Baseline data	A table showing baseline demographic	32	91
16i	Numbers Analysed	Number of participants (denominator) in each group included in each analysis; state the results in absolute numbers when feasible (e.g., 10/20, not 50 %)	16	46
16ii		"Intention-to-treat" analysis	21	60
17ai	Outcomes and estimation	Primary outcome: a summary of results for each group and the estimated effect size and its precision (e.g., 95 % confidence interval)	26	74
17aii		Secondary outcome: a summary of results for each group and the estimated effect size and its precision (e.g., 95 % confidence interval)	25	71
17b		For binary outcomes, presentation of both absolute and relative effect sizes is recommended	4	11
18	Ancillary Analyses	Results of other analyses performed, including subgroup analyses and adjusted analyses, distinguishing pre-specified	7	20
19	Adverse events	All adverse events or side effects in each intervention group	22	63
20	Limitations	Trial limitations	31	89
23	Registration	Registration number	19	54
25	Funding	Sources of funding and other support	32	91

Legend: Total: Total number of trials reporting item; %: Percentage of trials reporting item

used in an additional analysis. These time periods were created to distinguish between chiropractic RCTs published before and after the publication of the CONSORT Extension for Non-Pharmacological Treatments statement.

All univariate regression analyses explored associations between the outcome, i.e. the overall quality of reporting score and the exploratory variables (i.e. industry funding, positive findings, sample size group, year of publication and journal type). To test these five exploratory variables, we constructed five univariate models, which included each of the exploratory variables. The exploratory variables that produced results that had a $p \leq 0.1$, in the univariate regression analysis, were included in the

Table 3 Frequencies of CONSORT for Non-Pharmacological Treatment statement items from customised overall quality of reporting checklist (N = 35)

Item	Criterion	CONSORT Description	Total	%
1ext	Abstract	Does abstract include-description of the experimental treatment, comparator, care providers, centers, and blinding status	11	31
3ext	Methods	When applicable, eligibility criteria for centers and those performing the interventions (at least one)	13	37
4aext	Interventions	Description of the different components of the interventions and, when applicable, descriptions of the procedure for tailoring the interventions to individual participants	29	83
4bext		Details of how the interventions were standardised (if training was administered)	11	31
4cext		Details of how adherence of care providers with the protocol was assessed or enhanced	1	3
8ext	Randomization	When applicable, how care providers were allocated to each trial group	11	31
13ext	Flow Diagram	The number of care providers or centers performing the intervention in each group and the number of patients treated by each care provider or in each center	3	9
New Item		Details of the experimental treatment and comparator as they were implemented	8	23
15ext	Baseline data	Description of care providers (case volume, qualification, expertise, etc.) and centers	8	23

Legend: Total: Total number of trials reporting item; %: Percentage of trials reporting item; ext: extension criteria from CONSORT for Non-Pharmacological Treatments

multivariate model [22, 39]. The intention for building this multivariate regression model, was in order to ascertain which of the exploratory variables were independently associated with higher overall quality of reporting scores for the 35 RCTs included in this study. The method used in the multivariate regression analysis was stepwise approach. In the final multivariate regression analysis, variables were considered statistically significant if $p < 0.05$.

An additional 'final' multivariable model was created. This model differed in that, the year of publication, which was originally used as a continuous variable, was substituted for the dichotomous variable (as described above). By dividing the year of publication variable into two time periods, pre and post introduction of the CONSORT Extension for Non-Pharmacological Treatments statement, we could analyse the data to investigate whether this new CONSORT statement, impacted the overall quality of reporting.

Variation Inflation Factors (VIFs) were used to test collinearity between exploratory variables. None of the VIFS were >10, indicating that there was no collinearity among the variables. All assumptions for normality and linearity were checked using the Mahalanobis' and

Cook's Distance statistics. Statistical analyses were conducted using SPSS © 22.0.0.0 (IBM Corporation 2013).

Results

Sources yielded a total of 21,331 trials. Of the 85 studies that met the first round of inclusion criteria, only 35 (41 %) involving 4435 participants, were published as full-text articles in English journals (Refer to Fig. 1 and Additional file 1). These 35 articles, were assessed for their overall quality of reporting. The RCTs involved adult populations ranging between 17 and 78 years of age. Twenty-five of the 35 (71 %) RCTs reported positive findings in favour of the chiropractic intervention. Seventeen of the 35 (49 %) RCTs were published in a chiropractic journal. Only 43 % (15/35) of the RCTs were industry funded. The sample sizes of the included RCTs ranged between 20 and 444 participants with a mean of 127 (SD ± 102).

Overall quality of reporting score

The overall quality of reporting score, ranged between 10 and 33 with median score of 26.0 (IQR = 8.00). Individual scores are outlined in the Additional file 1. With regard to reporting frequencies of individual CONSORT items, refer to Tables 2 and 3.

Table 4 Frequencies of key methodological items from the customised CONSORT checklist (N = 35)

Item No.	Criterion	CONSORT Description	Total	%
9	Allocation concealment	Mechanism used to implement the random allocation sequence (such as sequentially numbered containers), describing any steps taken to conceal the sequence until interventions were assigned	31	87
11ai	Blinding	Whether or not participants, were blinded to group assignment	16	46
11aii	Blinding	Whether those assessing the outcomes were blinded to group assignment	25	71
16ii	Numbers Analysed	"Intention-to-treat" analysis	21	60

Legend: Total: the total number of RCTs that reported this item; %: Percentage of trials reporting item

Items that were most poorly reported from the CONSORT 2010 checklist were as follows: item 4b (settings and locations where data were collected), with 17/35 (49 %) of trials reporting this; item 11(a)(i) (whether participants were blinded) with 16/35 (46 %) of trials reporting this; item 13b (the description of each groups losses, exclusions and reasons within the flow diagram), with 20/35 (57 %) reporting on this; item 16 (i) (numbers analysed....in absolute numbers e.g. 10/20, not 50 %) with 16/35 (46 %) of trials reporting this; item 19, (the reporting of adverse events), with 22/35 (63 %) of trials reporting this; and item 23, (the reporting of clinical trial registration) with only 19/35 (54 %) of trials reporting this (Refer to Table 2).

The items that were most underreported, were from the CONSORT Extension for Non-Pharmacological Treatments checklist, with only one of the nine items achieving a high score. Item 4(a) extension requires the reporting of the description of the different components of the interventions and whether they were tailored to individuals, with 29/35 (83 %) of RCTs reporting this item. All other items from the CONSORT for Non-Pharmacological Treatments checklist were very poorly reported with an overall quality of reporting score ranging between 1/35 (3 %) for item 4c extension, (which details how adherence of care providers with the protocol was assessed or enhanced) through to 13/35 (37 %) for item 3 extension, (which describes the eligibility of centers or care providers of the interventions) (Refer to Table 3).

The scoring of the key methodological items also revealed some areas of weakness. Poor reporting of item 11(a)(i) (the blinding of participants) which was reported in 16/35 (46 %) of RCTs, and item 16(ii) (the ITT analysis) which was reported in 21/35 (60 %) of RCTs. The other two items were reported more frequently (Refer to Table 4).

Results of statistical analyses

The univariate regression analysis revealed that year of publication ($t_{33} = 4.99$, $p = 0.000$), journal type ($t_{33} = 3.28$, $p = 0.002$), and sample size group ($t_{33} = 2.75$, $p = 0.010$), were all individually and significantly associated with overall quality of reporting (Refer to Table 5 and Figs. 2, 3, and 4 respectively).

The multivariate regression analysis subsequently revealed that year of publication ($t_{32} = 5.17$, $p = 0.000$), and sample size group ($t_{32} = 3.01$, $p = 0.005$), were the only two factors associated with the overall quality of reporting. For each additional year between 2005 and 2014, the overall quality of reporting score increased on average, by an estimated 1.26 points (95 % CI: 0.76, 1.76)(Refer to Table 5). Compared to the smaller sample size group ($n = 1$–100), the larger sample size group ($n > 100$) scored on average 4.19 points higher (95 % CI: 1.36, 7.02) (Refer to Table 5).

Table 5 Univariate and multivariate regression analysis for overall quality of reporting score vs exploratory variables ($N = 35$)

Univariate Regression Analysis					
Exploratory Variables	Mean Difference	SE	t	p-value	95 % CI
Year of Publication	1.35	0.27	4.99	0.000 [a]	0.80, 1.90
Journal Type	5.81	1.77	3.28	0.002 [a]	2.21, 9.42
Sample Size Group	5.05	1.84	2.75	0.010 [a]	1.31, 8.80
Industry Funding	2.35	2.02	1.16	0.253	−1.76, 6.46
Positive Finding	3.30	2.18	1.51	0.140	−1.14, 7.74
Multivariate Regression Analysis					
Year of Publication (1)	1.26	0.24	5.17	0.000 [a]	0.76, 1.76
Sample Size Group (1)	4.19	1.39	3.01	0.005 [a]	1.36, 7.02
Year of Publication Grp (2)	8.16	1.73	4.73	0.000 [a]	4.64, 11.67
Sample Size Group (2)	4.56	1.45	3.15	0.004 [a]	1.61, 7.51

Legend: [a] statistically significant result; SE Standard Error; t t-test statistic; CI Confidence Interval; Grp Group; (1) Multivariate Analysis; (2) Additional analysis

The additional multivariate regression analysis conducted with the two time periods for the year of publication, revealed that, compared to the period 2005–2007, chiropractic RCTs published between 2008–2014, scored on average 8.16 points higher (95 % CI: 4.64, 11.67) (Refer to Table 5 and Fig. 5). The outcome was not affected by this additional analysis, as the multivariate regression analysis revealed that year of publication and sample size were the only two factors associated with the overall quality of reporting.

The final model in the multivariate regression analysis, revealed that 56 % of the variability in the reporting quality of the included RCTs can be explained by later year of publication and larger sample size (Adjusted $R^2 = 0.556$).

Discussion

This appears to be the first study investigating the quality of reporting of chiropractic RCTs relative to the CONSORT checklist. This study suggests, that there has been a significant improvement in the reporting quality of chiropractic RCTs between 2005 and 2014. This may be explained by an increased uptake of the CONSORT guidelines by journal editors and authors, but also by an increasingly professional cadre of chiropractic researchers. Furthermore, studies with sample sizes with $n > 100$, also revealed this trend. This is understandable, as studies with larger sample sizes are associated with greater resources. Furthermore, studies with larger sample sizes are also more likely to be adequately powered in order to find a statistically significant result, if in fact one exists.

While recent publications were more likely to adhere to the CONSORT 2010 criteria, the same cannot be said

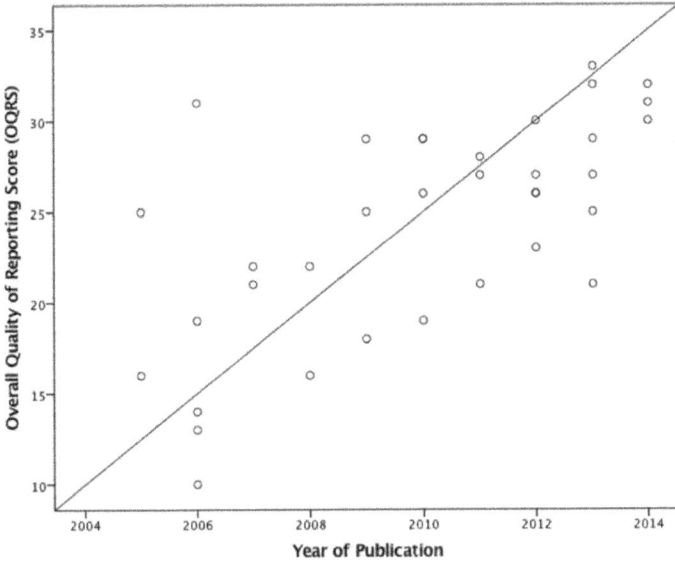

Fig. 2 Scatterplot of the correlation between the Overall Quality of Reporting Score and Year of Publication(N = 35)

for the CONSORT Extension for Non-Pharmacological Treatments criteria. Some specific areas, such as: describing items related to care providers and centers, details of adherence to protocols, and how interventions were standardised and if training was administered as prescribed, were very poorly reported. Perhaps this is due to a lack of awareness within the chiropractic research community of these extension criteria.

Under-reported items from the CONSORT 2010 statement included: blinding; explanation of losses and

exclusions after randomization with reasons on the flow chart; adverse event reporting; and analysis according to ITT principles, despite the fact these criteria have been established since the 2001 CONSORT statement [40].

Factors such as publishing in non-chiropractic journals showed a trend towards improved quality of reporting scores, although this was not statistically significant in the multivariate regression analysis.

Industry funding was not associated with improved quality of reporting of chiropractic RCTs. In contrast with

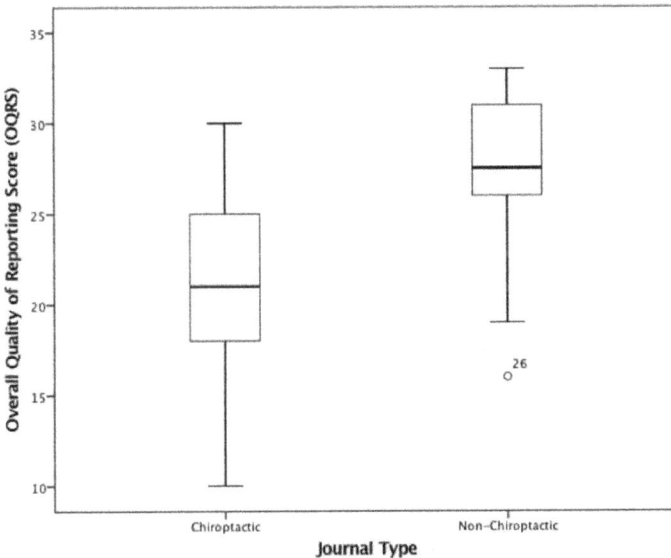

Fig. 3 Boxplot of the distribution of Overall Quality of Reporting Scores for Chiropractic vs Non-Chiropractic Journals (N = 35)

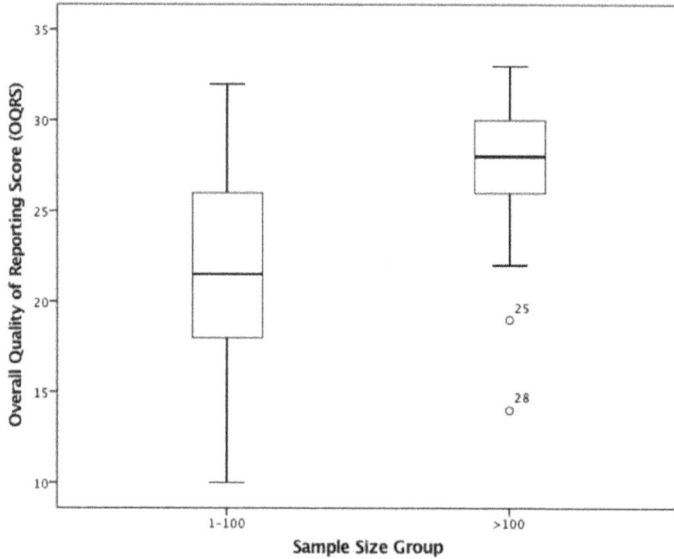

Fig. 4 Boxplot of the distribution of Overall Quality of Reporting Scores for Sample Size 1–100 vs >100 (N = 35)

several medical studies [7, 16, 18, 24, 39, 43], and some reviews [44, 45], which reported concerns that industry funding may be associated with publication bias [44–47].

We also found that a positive finding, was also not associated with the overall quality of reporting within the 35 chiropractic RCTs analysed. This was in contrast to several medical studies that reported that, improved quality of reporting was associated with positive findings [7, 39, 48]. One particular review

found that there was a positive association between reporting of favorable outcomes among pharmaceutical trials registered in ClinicalTrials.gov and industry funding [48].

Transparency and accuracy of RCT reporting contributes to the evidence-based information for the profession and will make assessing the validity of RCT results easier. This in turn can lead to better decision-making, helping chiropractic professionals improve their clinical decision making and thus providing better outcomes for patients

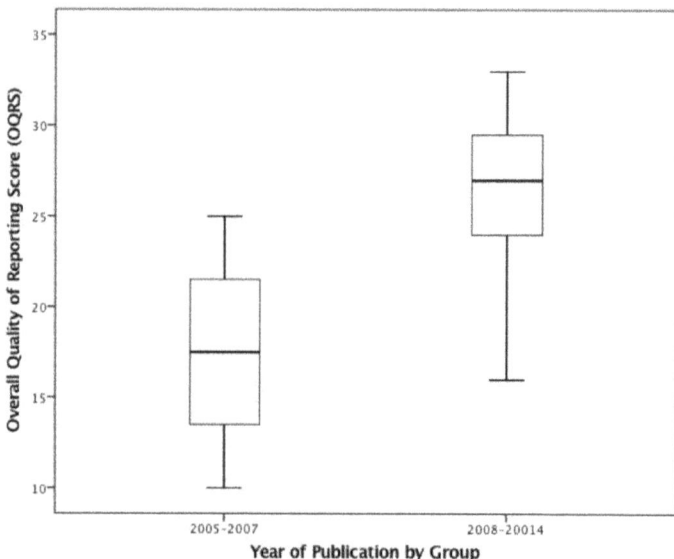

Fig. 5 Boxplot of the distribution of Overall Quality of Reporting Scores for Year of Publication by group, 2005–2007 vs 2008–2014 (N = 35)

[49]. As the chiropractic profession is the largest non-medical healthcare profession [50, 51], it is important to continue developing the evidence base so as to inform evidence-based practices. This in turn, will enable the profession to maintain and broaden acceptance from the public, mainstream healthcare and policy makers.

The insights gained from this study should be viewed as an opportunity for improved reporting of RCTs and increased awareness as to the importance of using the CONSORT for Non-Pharmacologic Treatments statement amongst chiropractic researchers. To enhance the practice of evidence-based chiropractic care, researchers are encouraged to implement the CONSORT guidelines with greater rigor, especially in reporting of key methodological items, such as allocation concealment, blinding, and the use of ITT analysis. As these key methodological items can safeguard against bias in the execution and the reporting of future RCTs.

It has been known for some time that the quality of reporting has significantly improved in the medical literature with the adoption of the CONSORT guidelines [10]. Similar outcomes have been reported in a physiotherapy review [52], and a chiropractic review investigating low back and neck pain studies [53]. Our present study suggests that the quality of reporting in chiropractic spinal and non-musculoskeletal studies has also followed this trend.

Limitations

One limitation to this study was that it is possible that our search strategy did not capture every available chiropractic RCT. We searched ten Clinical Trial registries and two databases and only included published full-text articles in the English language. Additionally, we could not always verify the trial methodology from authors or check their protocols.

Our assessment does not offer any insight into the external validity of the RCTs analysed, as it was too challenging to rate the reporting of such items [7], as there have not yet been any scales developed that have been validated to accomplish this task [39].

Although the CONSORT Extension for Non-Pharmacological Treatments statement was published in 2008 [12], we decided to use time periods starting in 2005, because that was the year the International Committee of Medical Journal Editors published guidelines that required trials to be registered prior to participant enrolment as a precondition for publishing [54]. Furthermore, the original CONSORT was published in 1996 [6], revised in 2001 [55], and again in 2010 [13], and the original CONSORT items continue to exist in all the versions of the CONSORT statements.

Another limitation to the study is that we cannot generalize the results to all forms of chiropractic. We have included studies, which used adjunctive techniques as long as those RCTs also employed an HVLA procedure.

A potential weakness of this study is that, we created a sum score for the overall quality of reporting and used it for both descriptive purposes and as the dependent (outcome) variable for the regression analysis. A problem may be that the attributes we were adding are multidimensional and it may not be appropriate to simply add their scores together, as some items in the CONSORT carry greater importance than others. Furthermore, two RCTs may receive the same score but differ in the areas considered deficient with respect to reporting. This can make the overall quality of reporting score somewhat difficult to interpret between studies.

Conclusion

Reporting quality of RCTs varies widely in chiropractic research. While steady improvement has been observed over the last decade, the chronological improvement observed in this study appears to reflect a more thorough and stringent adoption of the CONSORT criteria. This study suggests that quality reporting was influenced by year of publication and sample size and may also have been be influenced by factors such as journal choice, but not funding source or outcome positivity. This should be regarded as a reassuring finding for the profession and scientific community.

Recommendations

In light of these findings, we have made some simple recommendations for the improvement of reporting of future chiropractic RCTs.

1: Researchers are encouraged to design and fully report studies to meet the requirements of CONSORT 2010 statement, with extra emphasis on key methodological items:- allocation concealment, blinding of participants and assessors and the use of ITT analysis.

2: Researchers are encouraged to incorporate items from the CONSORT Extension for Non-Pharmacological Treatments statement.

3: Researchers must register their clinical trials, which is in alignment with the standards established by the International Committee of Medical Journal Editors in 2005.

4: Chiropractic journals could exhort researchers to publish the protocols for RCTs in their respective journals for assessment of the study and statistical review, with the understanding that their results are more likely to be published if the protocol meets the CONSORT criteria. (The Lancet is just one of several medical journals that encourages this practice)

Additional files

Additional file 1: *Characteristics of the 35 RCTs included in Overall Quality of Reporting Score Analysis.* Legend: Chiro: Chiropractic; JMPT: Journal of Manipulative and Physiological Therapeutics; CJA Chiropractic Journal of Australia; JCCA Journal of the Canadian Chiropractic Association. [29–36, 56–82]. (DOCX 28 kb)

Additional file 2: *Characteristics of the 50 RCTs excluded from Overall Quality of Reporting Analysis.* [83–100]. (DOCX 25 kb)

Abbreviations

CONSORT: Consolidated Standards of Reporting Trials; HVLA: High-Velocity, Low-Amplitude; ITT: Intention-to-Treat; RCTs: Randomised Controlled Trials; VIFs: Variation Inflation Factors.

Competing interests

The authors declare that they have no competing interests.

Authors' contributions

FK conceived the study. FK conducted the statistical analyses. FK, BB, and RB designed the assessment tool. BB, FK, RB, AK and MP all sourced and scored the studies, and contributed to the writing and review of the manuscript. All authors read and approved the final manuscript.

Author details

[1]PO Box 2108, Rose Bay Nth 2030, NSW, Australia. [2]School of Health Professions, Murdoch University, South St., Murdoch 6150, WA, Australia. [3]Department of Chiropractic, Macquarie University, Balaclava Rd., North Ryde 2109, NSW, Australia.

References

1. Cartwright N. Are RCTs the gold standard? BioSocieties. 2007;2:11–20. doi:10.1017/S1745855207005029.
2. Rothwell P. External validity of randomised controlled trials: "To whom do the results apply?". Lancet. 2005;365(9453):82–93.
3. Keech A, Gebski V, Pike R. Interpreting and reporting clinical trials. A guide to the CONSORT statement and the principles of randomised controlled trials. Sydney: MJA Books, Australasian Medical Publishing Company; 2007.
4. Moher D, Jones A, Lepage L, for the CONSORT Group. Use of the CONSORT Statement and quality of reports of randomised trials: a comparative before-and after-evaluation. JAMA. 2001;285(15):1992–5.
5. Altman D, Schulz K, Moher D, Egger M, Davidoff F, Elbourne D, Gotzsche P, Lang T, for the CONSORT Group. The revised CONSORT statement for reporting randomized trials: Explanation and elaboration. Ann Intern Med. 2001;134(8):663–94.
6. Begg C, Cho M, Eastwood S, Horton R, Moher D, Olkin I, Pitkin R, Rennie D, Schulz K, Simel D, et al. Improving the quality of reporting of randomized controlled trials: the CONSORT statement. JAMA. 1996;276(8):637–9.
7. Péron J, Pond GR, Gan HK, Chen EX, Almufti R, Maillet D, et al. Quality of reporting of modern randomized controlled trials in medical oncology: a systematic review. J Natl Cancer Inst. 2012;104(13):982–9.
8. Ntala C, Birmpili P, Worth A, Anderson NH, Sheikh A. The quality of reporting of randomised controlled trials in asthma: Systematic review protocol. Prim Care Respir J. 2013;22(1):S1–PS8.
9. Borg-Debono V, Zhang S, Ye C, Paul J, Arya A, Hurlburt L, Murthy Y, Thabane L. The quality of reporting of RCTs used within a postoperative pain management meta-analysis, using the CONSORT statement. BMC Anesthesiol. 2012;12:13.
10. Plint AC, Moher D, Morrison A, Schulz KF, Altman DG, Hill C, Gaboury I. Does the CONSORT checklist improve the quality of reports of randomised controlled trials? A systematic review. Med J Aust. 2006;185(5):263–7.
11. The CONSORT 2010 Statement [http://www.consort-statement.org/consort-2010].
12. Boutron I, Moher D, Altman DG, Schulz KF, Ravaud P, for the CONSORT Group. Extending the CONSORT Statement to randomized trials of nonpharmacologic treatments: Explanation and elaboration. Ann Intern Med. 2008;148:295–309.
13. Schulz KF, Altman DG, Moher D, for the CONSORT Group. CONSORT 2010 Statement: updated guidelines for reporting parallel group randomised trials. Br Med J. 2010;340(c332):698–702.
14. Tiruvoipati R, Balasubramanian SP, Atturu G, Peek GJ, Elbourne D. Improving the quality of reporting randomized controlled trials in cardiothoracic surgery: The way forward. J Thorac Cardiovasc Surg. 2006;132(2):233–40.
15. Partsinevelou A, Zintzaras E. Quality of reporting of randomized controlled trials in polycystic ovary syndrome. Trials. 2009;10:106.
16. Chen B, Liu J, Zhang C, Li M. A retrospective survey of quality of reporting on randomized controlled trials of metformin for polycystic ovary syndrome. Trials. 2014;15:128.
17. Kim KH, Kang JW, Lee MS, Lee J-D. Assessment of the quality of reporting for treatment components in Cochrane reviews of acupuncture. r Open. 2014;4:e004136.
18. Rios LP, Odueyungbo A, Moitri MO, Rahman MO, Thabane L. Quality of reporting of randomized controlled trials in general endocrinology literature. J Clin Endocr Metab. 2008;93:3810–6.
19. Lu L, Luo G, Xiao F. A retrospective survey of the quality of reports and their correlates among randomised controlled trials of immunotherapy for Guillian-Barre syndrome. Immunotherapy. 2013;5(8):829–36.
20. Bo C, Xue Z, Yoi G, Zelin C, Yang B, Zixu W, Yajun W. Assessing the quality of reports about randomized controlled trials of acupuncture treatment on Diabetic Peripheral Neuropathy. Plos ONE. 2012;7(7):e38461.
21. Sjögren P, Halling A. Quality of reporting randomised clinical trials in dental and medical research. Br Dent J. 2002;192(2):100–4.
22. Zhuang L, He J, Zhuang X, Lu L. Quality of reporting on randomized controlled trials of acupuncture for stroke rehabilitation. BMC Compl Alternative Med. 2014;14:151.
23. DeMauro SB, Giaccone A, Kirpalani H, Schmidt B. Quality of reporting of neonatal and infant trials in high-impact journals. Pediatrics. 2011;128:e639.
24. Montori VM, Alonso-Coello P, Wang YG, Bhagra S. Systematic evaluation of the quality of randomized controlled trials in Diabetes. Diabetes Care. 2006;29(8):1833–8.
25. Moberg-Mogren E, Nelson DL. Evaluating the quality of reporting occupational therapy randomized controlled trials by expanding the CONSORT criteria. Am J Occup Ther. 2006;60(2):226–35.
26. Adetugbo K, Williams H. How well are randomized controlled trials reported in the dermatology literature? Arch Dermatol. 2000;136(3):381–5.
27. Karpouzis F, Brown BT, Kalamir A, Pribicevic M, Bonello R. Quality of reporting of randomized controlled trials in chiropractic using the CONSORT checklist: A protocol for a review. Chiropr J Aust. 2016;44(1):17–32.
28. Christensen MG, Kerkoff D, Kollasch MW. Job Analysis of Chiropractic: A Project Report, Survey Analysis, and Summary of the Practice of Chiropractic within the United States. Greeley, Colo: National Board of Chiropractic Examiners; 2000.
29. Brennan GP, Fritz JM, Hunter SJ, Thackeray A, Delitto A, Erhard RE. Identifying subgroups of patients with acute/subacute "nonspecific" low back pain: Results of a randomized clinical trial. Spine. 2006;31(6):623–31.
30. Juni P, Battaglia M, Nuesch E, Hammerle G, Eser P, van Beers R, Vils D, Bernhard J, Ziswiler H-R, Reichenbach S, et al. A randomised controlled trial of spinal manipulative therapy in acute low back pain. Ann Rheum Dis. 2008;68:142–27.
31. Leaver AM, Maher CG, Herbert RD, Latimer J, McAuley JH, Jull G, Refshauge KM. A randomized controlled trial comparing manipulation with mobilization for recent onset neck pain. Arch Phys Med Rehabil. 2010;91:1313–8.
32. Eisenberg DM, Post DE, Davis RB, Connelly MT, Legedza ATR, Hrbek AL, Prosser LA, Buring JE, Inui TS, Cherkin DC. Addition of choice of complementary therapies to usual care for acute low back pain: a randomized controlled trial. Spine. 2007;32(2):151–8.
33. Rosner AL, Conable KM, Edelmann T. Influence of foot orthotics upon duration of effects of spinal manipulation in chronic back pain patients: A randomized clinical trial. J Manipulative Physiol Ther. 2014;37:124–40.
34. Petersen T, Larsen K, Nordsteen J, Olsen S, Fournier G, Jacobsen S. The McKenzie Method compared with manipulation when used adjunctive to information and advice in low back pain patients presenting with centralization or peripheralization: A randomized controlled trial. Spine. 2011;36(24):1999–2010.
35. Parkin-Smith GF, Norman IJ, Briggs E, Angier E, Wood TG, Brantingham JW. A structured protocol of evidence-based conservative care compared with usual care for acute nonspecific low back pain: A randomized clinical trial. Arch Phys Med Rehabil. 2012;93:11–20.

36. Poulsen E, Hartvigsen J, Christensen HW, Roos EM, Vach W, Overgaard S. Patient education with or without manual therapy compared to a control grou. in patients with osteoarthritis of the hip. A proof-of- principle three-arm parallel group randomized clinical trial. Osteoarthritis Cartilage. 2013;21:494e1503.

37. Piggott M, McGee H, Feuer D. Has CONSORT improved the reporting of randomized controlled trials in the palliative care literature? A systematic review. Palliat Med. 2004;18(1):32–8.

38. Huwiler-Muntener K, Juni P, Junker C, Egger M. Quality of reporting of randomized trials as a measure of methodologic quality. JAMA. 2002; 287(21):2801–4.

39. Lai R, Chu R, Fraumeni M, Thabane L. Quality of randomized controlled trials reporting in the primary treatment of brain tumors. J Clin Oncol. 2006;24(7):1136–44.

40. Moher D, Schulz KF, Altman D, for the CONSORT Group. The CONSORT statement: revised recommendations for improving the quality of reports of parallel-group randomized trials. BMC Med Res Method. 2001;1:2.

41. Boutron I, Moher D, Altman D, Schulz K, Ravaud P, for the CONSORT Group. Methods and processes of the CONSORT group: example of an extension for trials assessing nonpharmacologic treatments: explanation and elaboration. Ann Intern Med. 2008;148(4):295–309.

42. Rubinstein SM, van Middelkoop M, Assendelft WJ, de Boer MR, van Tulder MW: Spinal manipulative therapy for chronic low-back pain. *Cochrane Database of Syst Rev* 2011, Issue 2(Art. No.: CD008112).

43. Bhandari M, Richards RR, Sprague S, Schemitsch EH. The quality of reporting of randomized trials in the journal of bone and joint surgery from 1988 through 2000. J Bone Joint Surg Am. 2002;84(3):388–96.

44. Lexchin J, Bero LA, Djulbegovic B, Clark O. Pharmaceutical industry sponsorship and research outcome and quality: systematic review. Br Med J. 2003;326(7400):1167–70.

45. Okike K, Kocher MS, Mehlman CT, Bhandari M. Industry-sponsored research. Injury. 2008;39(6):666–80.

46. Djulbegovic B, Lacevic M, Cantor A, Fields KK, Benett CL, Adams JR, Kuderer NM, Lyman GH. The uncertainty principle and industry-sponsored research. Lancet. 2000;356(9230):635–8.

47. Easterbrook PJ, Berlin JA, Gopalan R, Matthews DR. Publication Bias in clinical research. Lancet. 1991;337(8746):867–72.

48. Bourgeois FT, Murthy S, Mandl KD. Outcome reporting among drug trials registered in ClinicalTrials.gov. Ann Intern Med. 2010;153(3):158–66.

49. Mansholt BA, Stites JS, Derby DC, Boesch RJ, Salsbury SA. Essential literature for the chiropractic profession: a survey of chiropractic research leaders. Chiropr Man Therap. 2013;21:33.

50. Coulter ID, Hurwitz EL, Adams AH, Genovese BJ, Hays R, Shekelle PG. Patients using chiropractors in North America: who are they, and why are they in chiropractic care? Spine (Phila Pa 1976). 2002;27:291–6.

51. Davis MA, Davis AM, Luan J, Weeks WB. The supply and demand of chiropractors in the United States from 1996 to 2005. Altern Ther Health Med. 2009;15(3):36–40.

52. Moseley AM, Herbert RD, Maher CG, Sherrington C, Elkins MR. Reported quality of randomized controlled trials of physiotherapy interventions has improved over time. J Clin Epidemiol. 2011;64(6):594–601.

53. Rubinstein SM, van Eekelen R, Oosterhuis T, de Boer MR, Ostelo RWJG, van Tulder MW. The risk of bias and sample size of trials of spinal manipulative therapy for low back and neck pain: analysis and recommendations. J Manipulative Physiol Ther. 2014;37(8):523–41.

54. DeAngelis C, Drazen J, Frizelle F, Haug C, Hoey J, Horton R, Kotzin S, Laine C, Marusic A, Overbeke A, et al. Clinical trial registration: a statement from the International Committee of Medical Journal Editors. JAMA. 2004;292(11):1363–4.

55. Moher D, Schulz K, Altman D. The CONSORT statement: revised recommendations for improving the quality of reports of parallel-group randomiized trials. JAMA. 2001;285(15):1987–91.

56. Maiers M, Bronfort G, Evans R, Hartvigsen J, Svendsen K, Bracha Y, Schulz C, Schulz K, Grimm R. Spinal manipulative therapy and exercise for seniors with chronic neck pain. Spine. 2014;14(9):1879–89.

57. Brantingham JW, Parkin-Smith GF, Cassa TK, Globe GA, Globe D, Pollard H, deLuca K, Jensen M, Mayer S, Korporaal C. Full kinetic chain manual and manipulative therapy plus exercise compared with targeted manual and manipulative therapy plus exercise for symptomatic osteoarthritis of the hip: a randomized controlled trial. Arch Phys Med Rehabil. 2012; 93:259–67.

58. Haas M, Vavrek D, Peterson D, Polissar N, Neradilek MB. Dose-response and efficacy of spinal manipulation for care of chronic low back pain: a randomized controlled trial. Spine J. 2014;14:1106–16.

59. Pollard H, Ward G, Hoskins W, Hardy K. The effect of a manual therapy knee protocol on osteoarthritic knee pain: a randomised controlled trial. J Can Chiropr Assoc. 2008;52(4):229–42.

60. Hondras MA, Long CR, Cao Y, Rowell RM, Meeker WC. A randomised controlled trial comparing 2 types of spinal manipulation and minimal conservative medical care for adults 55 years and older with subacute or chronic low back pain. J Manipulative Physiol Ther. 2009;32(5):330–43.

61. Roy RA, Boucher JP, Comtois AS. Heart rate variability modulation after manipulation in pain free patients vs patients in pain. J Manipulative Physiol Ther. 2009;32(4):277–86.

62. Evans R, Bronfort G, Schulz C, Maiers M, Bracha Y, Svendsen K, Grimm J, Richard , Garvey T, Transfeldt E. Supervised exercise with and without spinal manipulation performs similarly and better than home exercise for chronic neck pain: a randomized controlled trial. Spine. 2012;37(11):903–14.

63. Bronfort G, Maiers MJ, Evans RL, Schulz CA, Bracha Y, Svendsen KH, Grimm J, Richard H, Owens JEF, Garvey TA, Transfeldt EE. Supervised exercise, spinal manipulation, and home exercise for chronic low back pain: a randomized clinical trial. Spine J. 2011;11:585–98.

64. McMorland G, Suter E, Casha S, du Plessis SJ, Hurlbert JR. Manipulation or microdiskectomy for sciatica? a prospective randomized clinical study. J Manipulative Physiol Ther. 2010;33(8):576–84.

65. Srbely JZ, Vernon H, Lee D, Polgar M. Immediate effects of spinal manipulative therapy on regional antinociceptive effects in myofascial tissues in healthy young adults. J Manipulative Physiol Ther. 2013;36(6):333–41.

66. Walker BF, Hebert J, Stomski NJ, Losco B, French S. Short-term usual chiropractic care for spinal pain: a randomized controlled trial. Spine (Phila PA 1976). 2013;38(24):2071–8.

67. Walker BF, Hebert JJ, Clarke BR, Bowden RS, Losco BM, French SD. Outcomes of usual chiropractic. The OUCH randomized controlled trial of adverse events. Spine (Phila PA 1976). 2013;38(20):1723–9.

68. Holt K, Beck R, Sexton S, Taylor HH. Reflex effects of a spinal adjustment on blood pressure. Chiropr J Aust. 2010;40(3):95–9.

69. Engel RM, Vemulpad SR. The effect of combining spinal manipulation with exercise on the respiratory function of normal individuals: a randomized control trial. J Manipulative Physiol Ther. 2007;30(7):509–13.

70. Ward J, Coats J, Tyer K, Weigand S, Williams G. Immediate effects of anterior upper thoracic spine manipulation on cardiovascular response. J Manipulative Physiol Ther. 2013;36(2):101–10.

71. Stochkendahl MJ, Christensen HW, Vach W, Høilund-Carlsen PF, Haghfelt T, Hartvigsen J. Chiropractic treatment vs self-management in patients with acute chest pain: a randomized controlled trial of patients without acute coronary syndrome. J Manipulative Physiol Ther. 2012;35:7–17.

72. Goertz CM, Long CR, Hondras MA, Petri R, Delgado R, Lawrence DJ, Owens JEF, Meeker WC. Adding chiropractic manipulative therapy to standard medical care for patients with acute low back pain. Spine. 2013;38(8):627–34.

73. Muller R, Giles LG. Long-term follow-up of a randomized clinical trial assessing the efficacy of medication, acupuncture, and spinal manipulation for chronic mechanical spinal pain syndromes. J Manipulative Physiol Ther. 2005;28(1):3–11.

74. Bishop PB, Quon JA, Fisher CG, Dvorak MFS. The chiropractic hospital-based interventions research outcomes (CHIRO) study: a randomized controlled trial on the effectiveness of clinical practice guidelines in the medical and chiropractic management of patients with acute mechanical low back pain. Spine J. 2010;10:1055–64.

75. Shearar KA, Colloca CJ, White HL. A randomized clinical trial of manual versus mechanical force manipulation in the treatment of sacroiliac syndrome. J Manipulative Physiol Ther. 2005;28:493–501.

76. Wilkey A, Gregory M, Byfield D, McCarthy P. A comparison between chiropractic management and pain clinic management for chronic low-back pain in a national health service outpatient clinic. J Altern Complement Med. 2008;14(5):465–73.

77. Beyerman KL, Palmerino MB, Zohn LE, Kane GM, Foster KA. Efficacy of treating low back pain and dysfunction secondary to osteoarthritis: chiropractic care compared with moist heat alone. J Manipulative Physiol Ther. 2006;29:107–14.

78. Santilli V, Beghi E, Finucci S. Chiropractic manipulation in the treatment of acute back pain and sciatica with disc protrusion: a randomized double-

blind clinical trial of active and simulated spinal manipulations. Spine J. 2006;6:131–7.

79. Teodorczyk-Injeyan JA, Injeyan SH, Ruegg R. Spinal manipulative therapy reduces inflammatory cytokines but not substanc P production in normal subjects. J Manipulative Physiol Ther. 2006;29:14–21.

80. Palmgren PJ, Sandstrom PJ, Lundqvist FJ, Heikkila H. Improvement after chiropractic care in cervicocephalic kinesthetic sensibility and subjective pain intensity in patients with nontraumatic chronic pain. J Manipulative Physiol Ther. 2006;29:100–6.

81. Saayman L, Hay C, Abrahamse H. Chiropractic manipulative therapy and low-level laser therapy in the management of cervical facet dysfunction: a randomised controlled study. J Manipulative Physiol Ther. 2011;34:153–63.

82. Puhl AA, Injeyan SH. Short-term effects of manipulation to the upper thoracic spine of asymptomatic subjects on plasma concentrations of epinephrine and norepinephrine-a randomized and controlled observational study. J Manipulative Physiol Ther. 2012;35(3):209–15.

83. Schenk R, Dionne C, Simon C, Johnson R. Effectiveness of mechanical diagnosis and therapy in patients with back pain who meet a clinical prediction rule for spinal manipulation. J Man Manip Ther. 2012;20(1):43–9.

84. Schulz C, Leininger B, Evans R, Vavrek D, Peterson D, Haas M, Bronfort G. Spinal manipulation and exercise for low back pain in adolescents: study protocol for a randomized controlled trial. Chiropr Man Therap. 2014;22(21):1–9.

85. Schneider MJ, Brach J, Irrgang JJ, Abbott KV, Wisniewski SR, Delitto A. Mechanical vs manual manipulation for low back pain: an observational cohort study. J Manipulative Physiol Ther. 2010;33(3):193–200.

86. Miller JE, Newell D, Bolton JE. Efficacy of chiropractic manual therapy on infant colic: A pragmatic single-blind, randomized controlled trial. J Manipulative Physiol Ther. 2012;35:600–7.

87. Goertz CM, Salsbury SA, Vining RD, Long CR, Andresen AA, Jones ME, Lyons KJ, Hondras MA, Killinger LZ, Wolinsky FD, et al. Collaborative care for older adults with low back pain by family medicine physicians and doctors of chiropractic (COCOA): study protocol for a randomized controlled trial. Trials. 2013;14:18. doi:10.1186/1745-6215-14-18.

88. Brantingham JW, Globe GA, Cassa TK, Globe D, de Luca K, Pollard H, Jensen ML, Bates C, Jensen M, Mayer S, et al. A single-group pretest posttest design using full kinetic chain manipulative therapy with rehabilitation in the treatment of 18 patients with hip osteoarthritis. J Manipulative Physiol Ther. 2010;33(6):445–57.

89. Brantingham JW, Globe GA, Jensen ML, Cassa TK, Globe D, Price JL, Mayer SN, Lee FT. A feasibility study comparing two chiropractic protocols in the treatment of patellofemoral pain syndrome. J Manipulative Physiol Ther. 2009;32(7):536–48.

90. Rowe DE, Feise RJ, Crowther ER, Grod JP, Menke MJ, Goldsmith CH, Stoline MR, Souza TA, Kambach B. Chiropractic manipulation in adolescent idiopathic scoliosis: a pilot study. Chiropr Osteopat. 2006;14(15):1–10.

91. UK BEAM Trial Team: United Kingdom back pain exercise and manipulation (UK BEAM) randomised trial: effectiveness of physical treatments for back pain in primary care. BMJ online 2004.

92. Thorman P, Dixner A, Sundberg T. Effects of chiropractic care on pain and function in patients with hip osteoarthritis waiting for arthroplasty: a clinical pilot trial. J Manipulative Physiol Ther. 2010;33(6):438–44.

93. Hawk C, Pfefer MT, Strunk R, Ramcharan M, Uhl N. Feasibility study of short-term effects of chiropractic manipulation on older adults with impaired balance. J Chiropr Med. 2007;6:121–31.

94. Westrom KK, Maiers MJ, Evans RL, Bronfort G. Individualized chiropractic and integrative care for low back pain: the design of a randomized clinical trial using a mixed-methods approach. Trials. 2010;8(11):24.

95. Engel R, Vemulpad SR, Beath K. Short-term effects of a course of manual therapy and exercise in people with moderate chronic obstructive pulmonary disease: a prelimay clinical trial. J Manipulative Physiol Ther. 2013;36(8):490–6.

96. Botelho MB, Andrade BB. "Effect of cervical spine manipulative therapy on judo athletes' grip strength". J Manipulative Physiol Ther. 2012;35(1):38–44.

97. Strunk RG, Hondras Maria A. A feasibility study assessing manual therapies to different regions of the spine for patients with subacute or chronic neck pain. J Chiropr Med. 2008;7:1–8.

98. Eisenberg DM, Buring JE, Hrbek AL, Davis RB, Connelly MT, Cherkin DC, Levy DB, Cunningham M, O'Connor B, Post DE. A model of integrative care for low-back pain. J Altern Complement Med. 2012;18(4):354–62.

99. Vavrek D, Haas M, Peterson D. Physical examination and self-reported pain outcomes from a randomized trial on chronic cervicogenic headache. J Manipulative Physiol Ther. 2010;33:338–48.

100. Hurwitz EL, Morgenstern H, Kominski GF, Yu F, Chiang L-M. A randomized trial of chiropractic and medical care for patients with low back pain: eighteen-month follow-up outcomes from UCLA low back pain study. Spine. 2006;31(6):611–21.

22

Importance of psychological factors for the recovery from a first episode of acute non-specific neck pain - a longitudinal observational study

Brigitte Wirth[1*], B. Kim Humphreys[1] and Cynthia Peterson[1,2]

Abstract

Background: The influence of psychological factors on acute neck pain is sparsely studied. In a secondary analysis of prospectively collected data, this study investigated how several psychological factors develop in the first three months of acute neck pain and how these factors influence self-perceived recovery.

Methods: Patients were recruited in various chiropractic practices throughout Switzerland between 2010 and 2014. The follow-up telephone interviews were conducted for all patients by research assistants in the coordinating university hospital following a standardized procedure. The population of this study consisted of 103 patients (68 female; mean age = 38.3 ± 13.8 years) with a first episode of acute (<4 weeks) neck pain. Prior to the first treatment, the patients filled in the Bournemouth Questionnaire (BQ). One week and 1 and 3 months later, they completed the BQ again along with the Patient Global Impression of Change (PGIC). The temporal development (repeated measure ANOVA) of the BQ questions 4 (anxiety), 5 (depression), 6 (fear-avoidance) and 7 (pain locus of control) as well as the influence of these scores on the PGIC were investigated (binary logistic regression analyses, receiver operating curves (ROC)).

Results: All psychological parameters showed significant reduction within the first month. The parameter 'anxiety' was associated with outcome at 1 and 3 months ($p = 0.013$, $R^2 = 0.40$ and $p = 0.039$, $R^2 = 0.63$, respectively). Baseline depression ($p = 0.037$, $R^2 = 0.21$), but not baseline anxiety, was a predictor for poor outcome. A high reduction in anxiety within the first month was a significant predictor for favorable outcome after 1 month ($p < 0.001$; $R^2 = 0.57$).

Conclusions: Psychological factors emerged from this study as relevant in the early phase of acute neck pain. Particularly persistent anxiety and depression at baseline might be risk factors for a transition to chronic pain that should be addressed in the early management of neck pain patients.

Keywords: Acute, Neck pain, Psychological factors, Recovery

Background

Neck pain is one of the leading causes for global years lived with a disability [1]. In the general population, its 12 months prevalence ranges from 4.8 to 79.5 % (mean 25.8 %) [2]. Its course is typically fluctuating, but the majority of patients do not completely recover from their symptoms [3] and about 5–10 % of all neck problems become chronic [4].

It is widely established that psychological factors play an important role in chronic non-specific neck pain. Particularly anxiety, depression and catastrophizing seem to negatively affect pain intensity and disability in this patient group [5]. Although different psychological variables might be crucial at different time points in the course of neck pain, patient populations are often rather heterogeneous in terms of symptom duration [6], and only very little is known about this temporal aspect [7]. In patients

* Correspondence: brigitte.wirth@balgrist.ch
[1]Chiropractic Medicine Department, Faculty of Medicine, University of Zurich and University Hospital Balgrist, Forchstr. 340, CH-8008 Zurich, Switzerland
Full list of author information is available at the end of the article

with sub-acute (and chronic) neck pain, coping strategies that involved self-assurance resulted in better disability outcomes after 6 months [8], while fear of movement hindered short-term (3 months) and long-term (12 months) outcome of sub-acute neck pain as assessed by global perceived recovery, pain and disability [4]. Prognostic factors in acute neck pain are widely investigated in whiplash, but studies in acute non-specific neck pain are sparse. An overview of systematic reviews on prognostic factors for the outcome of a current neck pain episode [9] found two reviews that addressed non-specific neck pain. These reviews [10, 11] revealed two studies that included psychological factors [12, 13]. Bot et al. studied patients with a new episode of neck and shoulder symptoms in general practice and found that pain intensity at baseline, the duration of symptoms before seeking health care, a history of previous neck or shoulder symptoms, reduced vitality and more resting negatively affected self-perceived outcome after 3 months [12]. After 12 months, also more worrying and multiple musculoskeletal symptoms hindered recovery. Hill et al. investigated patients with neck pain in the last month [13]. The strongest risk factor for persistent neck pain after 12 months was age. Further main risk factors were mainly not working at the time of baseline, comorbid low back pain, but also poor general and psychological health were significantly associated with pain persistence. Thus, there is little data available on the impact of psychological factors in the early phase of a non-specific neck pain episode. This might be the reason why Walton et al. concluded in their overview of systematic reviews that in non-whiplash-related neck pain, only older age and other musculoskeletal disorders could be regarded as risk factors for poor recovery, while inconsistent results existed for pain intensity at baseline [14]. The outcome parameters of most studies on psychological risk factors for neck pain were either pain intensity, disability or return to work [7]. However, global ratings of change such as the 'Patient global impression of change' (PGIC), which allow the patient to integrate different aspects into one single rating [15] were shown to be more sensitive and to correlate better with the patient's satisfaction than serial assessments such as pain rating by a visual analogue scale [16]. The above mentioned studies by Bot et al. and Hill et al. assessed global recovery, but used non-validated recovery measures [12, 13].

Thus, in order to prevent acute neck pain from becoming chronic, the goals of this study were to investigate how psychological factors (anxiety, depression, fear avoidance, health locus of control) develop in the first 3 months after a first episode of acute neck pain, and how these psychological factors are associated with self-perceived recovery (assessed by PGIC). We hypothesized that i) the investigated psychological variables decreased in the first 3 months, ii) high psychological distress co-

occurred with poor outcome, iii) high scores in the psychological variables at baseline were predictive for poor outcome, and iv) reduction in psychological distress led to favorable outcome.

Methods

Participants

This study is based on the secondary analysis of data that were prospectively collected between 2010 and 2014 [17]. For the prospective cohort study with 1 year follow-up, neck pain patients over 18 years with pain of any duration were recruited from various chiropractic practices in Switzerland. Patients with specific pathologies that are contraindications for chiropractic treatment (e.g. tumors, infections) were not included. In total, 850 patients were recruited. For the present observational study that focused on acute non-specific neck pain, only patients who reported that they had no previous episode of neck pain and whose present pain episode lasted for less than 4 weeks were included. Whiplash and any signs of radiculopathy were exclusion criteria. These rather rigid criteria were chosen in order to minimize bias by previous history of neck complaints and duration of symptoms. Thus, the sample of this study consisted of 103 patients (68 female; mean age = 38.3 ± 13.8 years) suffering from the first episode of acute, non-specific neck pain (Table 1).

Ethics and consent

Ethical approval was obtained from the ethics committee from the Canton of Zurich, Switzerland (EK-19/2009) and all participants gave written informed consent prior to participation.

Baseline data and outcome measures

Immediately prior to the first treatment, a numerical rating scale (NRS) for neck pain and a separate NRS (0 = no pain, 10 = worst pain imaginable) for arm pain were filled in by the patients. Furthermore, they answered a validated German version of the Bournemouth questionnaire (BQ) for neck pain [18–20]. The BQ is a valid and reliable outcome measure that considers the multidimensionality of musculoskeletal pain. It covers seven dimensions of the bio-psycho-social pain model: 1) pain, 2) disability (activities of daily living), 3) disability (social activities), 4) anxiety, 5) depression, 6) fear-avoidance (work-related) and 7) pain locus of control. External validity of every single item was shown by significant correlations to its established counterpart external measure [18]. At 1 week, 1 month and 3 months after the first consultation, the same data were collected in a short telephone interview that was conducted for all patients by research assistants in the coordinating university hospital following a standardized procedure. In these

Table 1 Characteristics of the study population

	All patients (N = 103)	Patients with improvement after 1 month (N = 70)	Patients without improvement after 1 month (N = 14)	Patients with improvement after 3 months (N = 71)	Patients without improvement after 3 months (N = 11)
Age (SD)	38.3 (±13.8)	37.5 (±13.8)	47.5 (±15.0)	38.6 (±13.8)	47.3 (±16.2)
Gender (m/f)	35/68	22/48	4/10	27/44	2/9
Pain at baseline (SD)	6.4 (±1.9)	6.5 (±1.8)	5.5 (±2.1)	6.2 (±2.0)	7.2 (±1.7)
BQ 4: anxiety BL/1 m/3 m (SD)	5.5 (±2.9)	5.6 (±2.8)	4.3 (±2.9)	5.3 (±3.0)	6.7 (±1.7)
	2.1 (±2.7)	1.6 (±2.2)	5.0 (±2.9)	1.7 (±2.4)	5.3 (±2.7)
	1.7 (±2.6)	1.4 (±2.2)	2.5 (±2.9)	1.0 (±1.9)	6.0 (±2.0)
BQ 5: depression BL/1 m/3 m (SD)	3.6 (±3.2)	3.5 (±3.2)	3.1 (±2.9)	3.1 (±3.2)	5.9 (±2.3)
	1.6 (±2.7)	1.0 (±2.1)	3.9 (±3.6)	1.2 (±2.3)	4.3 (±3.5)
	0.8 (±2.0)	0.5 (±1.2)	1.9 (±3.0)	0.4 (±1.3)	3.7 (±2.9)
BQ 6: fear avoidance BL/1 m/3 m (SD)	4.7 (±3.1)	4.6 (±3.1)	4.6 (±2.6)	4.5 (±3.2)	5.7 (±1.6)
	2.0 (±2.7)	1.5 (±2.1)	4.4 (±3.8)	1.6 (±2.5)	4.7 (±2.5)
	1.7 (±2.6)	1.5 (±2.5)	2.3 (±3.0)	1.2 (±2.3)	5.2 (±2.4)
BQ 7: locus of control BL/1 m/3 m (SD)	5.0 (±2.8)	5.2 (±3.0)	4.0 (±2.4)	5.0 (±3.0)	4.5 (±1.7)
	2.8 (±3.3)	2.5 (±3.3)	3.9 (±3.4)	2.6 (±3.3)	5.0 (±2.9)
	2.2 (±2.9)	1.6 (±2.3)	4.2 (±4.0)	1.6 (±2.6)	5.7 (±2.5)

BQ Bournemouth questionnaire
BL baseline
f female
m male
SD standard deviation
1 m 1 month
3 m 3 months

consecutive assessments, a German version of the PGIC was also presented to the patients. The PGIC is a retrospective seven-point Likert scale that asks the patients how they feel now compared to before the onset of treatment [16]. Its extreme scores are "much better" and "much worse", respectively.

Data analysis and statistics

The BQ questions 4 (anxiety), 5 (depression), 6 (fear-avoidance) and 7 (pain locus of control) were entered into the models as independent variables and were analyzed as continuous data. As for the PGIC, only the two scores "much better" and "better", but not "somewhat better", were considered a clinically significant change [21]. Thus, the PGIC data were analyzed as binomial data (0 = not improved, 1 = improved). To determine the development of the psychological factors over time, a repeated measure ANOVA was conducted for each of the four BQ questions. In the posthoc tests (Bonferroni), only the differences between two consecutive time points were of interest. To investigate the importance of the psychological factors for self-perceived recovery, a series of logistic regression analyses with the PGIC as dependent variable was conducted in order to avoid over-fitting the models [22]. Into a first model (model 1), only the psychological variables were entered as independent variables. Thereby, to assess the co-occurrence

of these factors with self-perceived recovery, the BQ questions at each concurrent time point were used. To determine their predictive value, the BQ questions at baseline were entered into the model. Lastly, to study the impact of changes in these factors on recovery, the changes in the BQ questions (value of baseline – value of the concurrent time point) were used as independent variables. Then, a further logistic regression model (model 2) was run to estimate the importance of the findings in the context of the literature. This model included the significant factors, if any, emerging from model 1, together with age and pain intensity at baseline [12, 14]. Lastly, the receiver operating curve (ROC) was calculated and the area under the curve (AUC) was determined as a measure for accuracy in discriminating between patients who reported clinically significant improvement and the rest. To test for multicollinearity, we calculated the tolerance and variance inflation factor (VIF) values by running a linear regression analysis with the same outcome and predictors, as recommended by Field [23] (p. 297). According to Field [23] (p. 224), we regarded VIF values >10 and tolerance values <0.1 as critical. No multicollinearity was detected (Tables. 2, 3 and 4). Only complete data sets were included in the regression analyses (complete-case analysis). For all other analyses, data sets with missing values were excluded from the corresponding analyses only (available case

Table 2 Co-occurrence of psychological factors with self-perceived recovery

	B (SE)	Exp B (Odds Ratio)	95 % CI Exp B	p
PGIC 1 week (N = 76):				
Nagelkerke R^2 = 0.05; AUC = 0.62 (95 % CI 0.48–0.75; p = 0.126)				
BQ4: anxiety	−0.18 (0.13)	0.83	0.64–1.08	0.171
BQ5: depression	−0.01 (0.11)	0.99	0.80–1.23	0.901
BQ6: fear avoidance	0.06 (0.13)	1.06	0.82–1.36	0.667
BQ7: locus of control	0.04 (0.10)	1.04	0.86–1.25	0.717
PGIC 1 month (N = 82):				
Nagelkerke R^2 = 0.40; AUC = 0.85 (95 % CI 0.73–0.97; p < 0.001)				
BQ4: anxiety	−0.55 (0.22)	**0.58**	0.38–0.89	**0.013**
BQ5: depression	0.13 (0.21)	1.14	0.76–1.71	0.540
BQ6: fear avoidance	−0.25 (0.16)	0.78	0.57–1.06	0.110
BQ7: locus of control	0.17 (0.16)	1.19	0.87–1.63	0.286
PGIC 3 months (N = 77):				
Nagelkerke R^2 = 0.63; AUC = 0.98 (95 % CI 0.94–1.00; p < 0.001)				
BQ4: anxiety	−0.60 (0.29)	**0.55**	0.31–0.97	**0.039**
BQ5: depression	−0.13 (0.23)	0.88	0.56–1.39	0.579
BQ6: fear avoidance	−0.17 (0.18)	0.84	0.59–1.21	0.353
BQ7: locus of control	−0.20 (0.20)	0.82	0.55–1.22	0.325

Logistic regressions with PGIC (0 = not improved, 1 = improved) of each time point as dependent variable and the psychological factors of the same time point as independent variables. Multicollinearity diagnostics: Tolerance: 0.27-0.72, VIF: 1.38-3.65. Numbers in bold indicate significant results.
AUC area under the receiver operating curve
BQ Bournemouth questionnaire
PGIC patient global impression of change

analysis). The significance level α was set at 0.05 for all analyses. All analyses used IBM SPSS Statistics 21.0 (SPSS, Chicago, IL, USA).

Results
One week after the first consultation, 75.6 % (25 missing values) of the patients reported clinically significant improvement. The percentage increased to 83.3 % (19 missing values) after 1 month and to 86.6 % (21 missing values) after 3 months.

All tested psychological parameters showed significant reduction within the first month after onset of treatment, but only the parameter 'depression' further improved afterwards (Fig. 1). Anxiety (F(2.70,169.78) = 33.54; $p < 0.001$) significantly decreased from baseline to 1 week ($p = 0.009$) and from 1 week to 1 month ($p = 0.001$). Depression (F(2.37,149.44) = 17.25; $p < 0.001$) significantly declined between baseline and 1 week ($p = 0.022$) and 1 month to 3 months ($p = 0.025$). Fear avoidance (F(2.58,146.96) = 25.43; $p < 0.001$) and pain locus of control (F(2.75,167.77) = 17.15; $p < 0.001$) showed a significant reduction from

1 week to 1 month after onset of treatment ($p < 0.001$ and $p = 0.001$, respectively).

The regression model with the psychological factors at each time point as independent variables and the concurrent self-reported outcome as dependent variable explained an increasing proportion of data variability up to 3 months. At 1 and 3 months after the first consultation, high scores in the parameter 'anxiety' were concurrent with poor self-reported outcome. The models showed good accuracy for discrimination between improved and unimproved patients at 1 month (AUC = 0.85) and excellent accuracy at 3 months (AUC = 0.98) (Table 2).

The psychological factors at baseline had no influence on the self-reported outcome at 1 week and 1 month. In the model that included only the psychological variables, high level of anxiety at baseline was somewhat predictive for favorable outcome at 1 month (AUC = 0.76). However, anxiety level at baseline became insignificant in the model that included age and baseline pain, where higher age emerged as a predictor for poor recovery (AUC = 0.74) (Table 3). Conversely, depression at baseline emerged from both

Table 3 Prediction of self-perceived recovery by psychological factors at baseline

	B (SE)	Exp B (Odds Ratio)	95 % CI Exp B	p
Model 1: psychological factors as independent variables				
PGIC 1 week (N = 77):				
Nagelkerke R^2 = 0.02; AUC = 0.58 (95 % CI 0.43–0.72; p = 0.321)				
BQ4: anxiety	−0.09 (0.15)	0.92	0.68–1.24	0.572
BQ5: depression	0.07 (0.12)	1.07	0.85–1.35	0.579
BQ6: fear avoidance	−0.01 (0.12)	0.99	0.78–1.25	0.928
BQ7: locus of control	0.09 (0.12)	1.09	0.87–1.36	0.459
PGIC 1 month (N = 82):				
Nagelkerke R^2 = 0.17; AUC = 0.76 (95 % CI 0.62–0.90; p = 0.002)				
BQ4: anxiety	0.44 (0.21)	**1.55**	1.04–2.32	**0.033**
BQ5: depression	−0.18 (0.16)	0.83	0.61–1.14	0.247
BQ6: fear avoidance	−0.33 (0.18)	0.72	0.51–1.02	0.061
BQ7: locus of control	0.25 (0.16)	1.28	0.93–1.77	0.529
PGIC 3 months (N = 80):				
Nagelkerke R^2 = 0.22; AUC= 0.83 (95 % CI 0.72–0.93; p = 0.001)				
BQ4: anxiety	0.14 (0.22)	1.15	0.74–1.78	0.529
BQ5: depression	−0.41 (0.21)	**0.67**	0.45–1.00	**0.049**
BQ6: fear avoidance	−0.09 (0.18)	0.91	0.64–1.29	0.597
BQ7: locus of control	0.25 (0.18)	1.28	0.91–1.81	0.163
Model 2: signifiant factors of model 1 and age and baseline pain as independent variables				
PGIC 1 week (N = 77):				
Nagelkerke R^2 = 0.001; AUC= 0.52 (95 % CI 0.39–0.66; p = 0.763)				
Age	−0.001 (0.02)	1.00	0.96–1.04	0.938
Pain at baseline	0.03 (0.14)	0.97	0.74–1.28	0.841
PGIC 1 month (N = 83):				
Nagelkerke R^2 = 0.18; AUC= 0.74 (95 % CI 0.58–0.90; p = 0.005)				
BQ 4: anxiety	0.12 (0.12)	1.12	0.89–1.41	0.321
Age	−0.05 (0.02)	**0.95**	0.91–0.99	**0.021**
Pain at baseline	0.20 (0.16)	1.22	0.89–1.68	0.225
PGIC 3 months (N = 81):				
Nagelkerke R^2 = 0.21; AUC= 0.80 (95 % CI 0.69–0.91; p = 0.002)				
BQ 5: depression	−0.26 (0.12)	**0.77**	0.61–0.98	**0.037**
Age	−0.04 (0.03)	0.97	0.92–1.02	0.163
Pain at baseline	−0.13 (0.20)	0.88	0.60–1.31	0.536

Logistic regressions with PGIC (0 = not improved, 1 = improved) of each time point as dependent variable and the psychological factors at baseline as independent variables. Multicollinearity diagnostics model 1/model 2: Tolerance: 0.39-0.76/0.89-1.00, VIF: 1.31-2.59/1.00-1.13. Numbers in bold indicate significant results.

AUC area under the receiver operating curve
BQ Bournemouth questionnaire
PGIC patient global impression of change

models as a significant predictor for poor outcome at 3 months (AUC = 0.83 and 0.80, respectively). Pain at baseline could not predict outcome at any point in time.

A high reduction in anxiety between 1 week and 1 month after the first consultation was linked to a significantly higher chance for self-reported improvement at 1 month in both models (Table 4) and the models showed excellent discrimination accuracy (AUC = 0.97 and 0.92, respectively). Self-reported improvement at 3 months was not related to changes in any of the psychological variables.

Table 4 Prediction of self-perceived recovery by changes in psychological factors

	B (SE)	Exp B (Odds Ratio)	95 % CI Exp B	p
Model 1: psychological factors as independent variables				
PGIC 1 week (N = 75):				
Nagelkerke R^2 = 0.05; AUC = 0.62 (95 % CI 0.48–0.76; p = 0.119)				
BQ4: anxiety	0.07 (0.10)	1.07	0.88–1.29	0.488
BQ5: depression	0.16 (0.13)	1.17	0.90–1.53	0.235
BQ6: fear avoidance	−0.06 (0.11)	0.95	0.76–1.17	0.603
BQ7: locus of control	0.02 (0.08)	1.02	0.87–1.20	0.806
PGIC 1 month (N = 80):				
Nagelkerke R^2 = 0.71; AUC = 0.97 (95 % CI 0.94–1.00; p < 0.001)				
BQ4: anxiety	0.93 (0.31)	**2.53**	1.37–4.67	**0.003**
BQ5: depression	0.44 (0.36)	1.56	0.77–3.15	0.218
BQ6: fear avoidance	0.35 (0.28)	1.42	0.83–2.45	0.204
BQ7: locus of control	0.09 (0.16)	1.09	0.79–1.50	0.598
PGIC 3 months (N = 75):				
Nagelkerke R^2 = 0.36; AUC = 0.90 (95 % CI 0.82–0.98; p < 0.001)				
BQ4: anxiety	0.30 (0.20)	1.35	0.92–1.99	0.123
BQ5: depression	−0.17 (0.18)	0.85	0.85 0.60–1.20	0.352
BQ6: fear avoidance	0.02 (0.15)	1.02	0.76–1.37	0.074
BQ7: locus of control	0.23 (0.13)	1.26	0.98–1.63	0.163
Model 2: signifiant factors of model 1 and age and baseline pain as independent variables				
PGIC 1 week (N = 77):				
Nagelkerke R^2 = 0.001; AUC = 0.52 (95 % CI 0.39–0.66; p = 0.763)				
Age	−0.001 (0.02)	1.00	1.44–3.54	<0.001
Pain at baseline	0.03 (0.14)	0.97	0.74–1.28	0.841
PGIC 1 month (N = 83):				
Nagelkerke R^2 = 0.57; AUC = 0.92 (95 % CI 0.85–0.99; p < 0.001)				
BQ 4: anxiety	0.81 (0.23)	**2.26**	1.44–3.54	**<0.001**
Age	−0.01 (0.03)	1.00	0.95–1.05	0.851
Pain at baseline	0.16 (0.21)	1.17	0.77–1.78	0.454
PGIC 3 months (N = 82):				
Nagelkerke R^2 = 0.12; AUC = 0.75 (95 % CI 0.63–0.86; p = 0.009)				
Age	−0.04 (0.02)	0.96	0.92–1.01	0.111
Pain at baseline	−0.27 (0.19)	0.76	0.53–1.10	0.152

Logistic regressions with PGIC (0 = not improved, 1 = improved) of each time point as dependent variable and the *changes* in the psychological factors as independent variables. Multicollinearity diagnostics model 1/model 2: Tolerance: 0.42-0.83/0.85-0.97, VIF: 1.20-2.38/1.00-1.18. Numbers in bold indicate significant results.
AUC area under the receiver operating curve
BQ Bournemouth questionnaire
PGIC patient global impression of change

Discussion

All psychological parameters that were investigated in this study improved during the first month. Depression declined only somewhat during the first week, but was the only parameter that still improved after the first month. Poor outcome at 1 and 3 months went along with high levels of anxiety. High baseline anxiety was not a risk factor for poor outcome, but its reduction during the first month was highly related to favorable recovery. In contrast, high level of depression at baseline was fairly related to poor recovery at 3 months.

In order to prevent an acute neck pain episode from developing into a chronic problem, the reduction of anxiety at the beginning seems to be a key point in treatment even in this sample of patients who had not previously experienced neck pain. For recovery at 3 months, anxiety was of

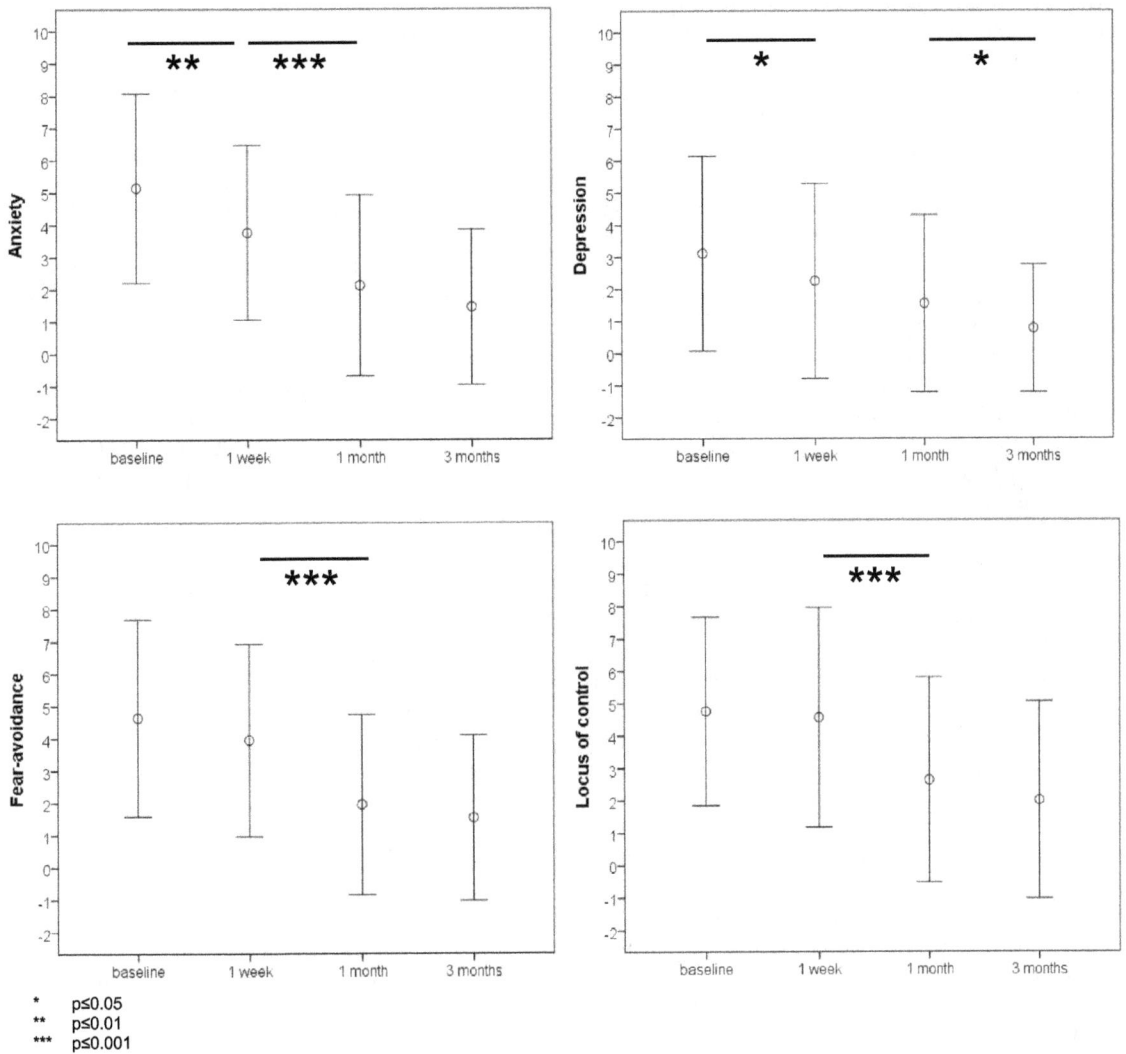

Fig. 1 Changes in psychological factors during the first three months of a first neck pain episode. The figure shows the development of anxiety, depression, fear avoidance and pain locus of control during the first three months of a first episode of acute neck pain (mean ± standard deviation). * $p \leq 0.05$. ** $p \leq 0.01$. *** $p \leq 0.001$

minor importance, but the factor depression became meaningful. Linton brought up in his review the temporal aspect of the influence of psychological factors on pain and hypothesized that different factors might be relevant at different time points in the course of neck and back pain [7]. The findings of the present study support this developmental approach and bring the patient management in the early phase of treatment into focus. High anxiety at baseline per se does not seem to hinder recovery, provided that it decreases early in the course of treatment. A significant correlation between the reduction in anxiety and in somatic complaints was also reported in a study with orthopedic patients in a rehabilitation setting [24]. This

finding suggests that the clinicians should also focus on the changes in the psychological parameters rather than only on their levels at baseline. It further stresses that also in patients with acute neck pain, the multidimensional approach of pain management should be present from the onset of treatment in order to improve outcome, which might not always be the case in daily clinical practice. In the management of acute low back pain, general practitioners were reported to understand pain as a direct representation of tissue injury, and therefore, assessment or management of attitudes and beliefs was of low priority [25]. However, it is well known that appropriate information and the patient's understanding of pain is crucial in the treatment of acute LBP [26]. A recent qualitative study on attitudes and beliefs of LBP patients found that most participants felt depressed by their pain [27]. This might in most cases not lead into severe depression, which should, in case, promptly be evaluated by a psychiatrist. Nevertheless, the clinicians should be aware that this might result in an attention bias of the patient towards negative information indicating that threatening information might be particularly harmful [27]. Thus, patients with acute non-specific neck pain might benefit from adequate information and communication that targets at reducing anxiety by encouraging self-management of the problem. Cognitive-behavioral therapy (CBT) that focuses on improving coping strategies by diminishing negative thoughts is such an approach. A study that compared usual physiotherapy with a short hands-off intervention by specifically trained physiotherapists using CBT principles could not detect any difference in the effects on sub-acute and chronic neck pain [28]. Similarly, a recent Cochrane Review reported no beneficial effects of CBT for patients with chronic neck pain. For patients with sub-acute neck pain, however, this review found a significantly higher pain reduction at short-term by CBT compared to other interventions [29]. No study was found that investigated the effects of CBT in the management of acute neck pain. The results of the present study, however, encourage the application of CBT principles before neck pain turns into sub-acute or chronic pain. With a view to medication, most pharmacological studies focus on LBP. Non-steroidal anti-inflammatory drugs and muscle relaxants were reported to be effective in acute LBP [30], while the adjunction of an anxiolytic medication (antihistamine) to morphine analgesia did not show an additional benefit in the acute phase of LBP [31].

Anxiety and depression emerged from this study as the most important psychological factors for self-perceived recovery in the first 3 months of a first episode of acute neck pain. Accordingly, the study by Bot et al. on patients with acute neck and shoulder complaints reported that less vitality, which might be seen as a symptom of a depressive disorder, was related to poor recovery after 3 months [12]. Contrary to that study, however, pain at baseline was not a predictor for outcome in the present study. Also fear-avoidance did not emerge as risk factor for poor prognosis for acute neck pain, but was reported to hinder recovery in patients with sub-acute neck pain [4]. In chronic patients, in turn, anxiety and depression were the two main factors related to pain and disability [5]. These findings might partly be explained by the temporal aspect of the psychological variables, but also by the variety of outcomes that were used in these studies. The studies on acute neck pain [12, 13] patients assessed recovery by simple, non–validated questions, while the majority of studies

on the role of psychological factors on the course of neck pain used pain, disability or work status as outcome variables [7]. The PGIC as a single-item overall assessment has recently been shown to reflect different specific domains to different degrees. In chronic patients, the overall PGIC particularly reflected improvements in physical activities and mood, rather than improvements in pain and social functioning [32]. Thus, the patient's impression of change might not linearly influence e.g. socioeconomic relevant variables. Therefore, the impact of anxiety and its reduction in the early phase of acute neck pain on other parameters, such as e.g. sick leave, needs further investigation.

The proportion of patients who reported clinically significant improvement was high (87 %), but well comparable with the numbers in the literature (5 to 10 % of neck problems become chronic [4]). However, it was much higher than reported in a comparable study by Bot et al. [12], which might be explained by differences in the study design: In the latter study, the patients were simply asked whether their symptoms still bothered them. Consequently, patients who answered in the present study that they felt much better or better compared to the beginning, could still have been bothered by their symptoms, which might be the reason for the better outcome in the present study. Nevertheless, the observed proportion of patients with improvement was still small compared to a sample of patients with various acute problems, of whom 97 % reported significant improvement after physiotherapy [33]. This result reflects the persistency of neck pain [3] and emphasizes the need for early attempts to prevent an acute neck pain from transition to a chronic problem.

The strength of this study was that its data design allowed for analyzing not only the influence of psychological factors at certain time points, but also their development over time. Furthermore, the rather rigid inclusion criteria provided a homogeneous patient population and reduced bias resulting from symptom duration and previous pain episodes. However, of course, there were also several limitations. The major limitation of this study was the small number of patients that did not report improvement, which reduced power and might have hidden some findings. This limits generalizability of the results and implies that a confirmation of the results is needed. A second limitation was that the study did not control for the number and type of treatment that the patients underwent during the timespan when they were followed. However, the goal of this study was not to attribute the observed outcome to a certain treatment. The collected data rather reflect clinical practice, where the patients undergo individual treatment according to their needs. In addition, particularly in this sample of acute patients, the observed improvement might at least partly be attributed to natural history. Furthermore, this study did not assess information about other musculoskeletal complaints, although this is a known predictor for an unfavorable course of neck pain [14]. Lastly, the BQ is a valid and reliable questionnaire that reflects the multidimensionality of musculoskeletal pain [18, 20]. Its large advantage is its shortness that allows its use in routine clinical practice. Its items were validated with their counterpart established measures. Nevertheless, the BQ might not be capable of assessing psychological factors in-depth. Thus, the results of this study need to be confirmed by future investigations on the importance of psychological factors in acute non-specific neck pain using separate questionnaires that assess anxiety and depression in more detail. These studies should include a larger number of patients with poor recovery and might investigate strategies to reduce anxiety and depression in the acute phase of neck pain, such as the application of CBT principles by specifically trained health professionals.

Conclusion

Psychological factors emerged from this study as relevant in the early phase of treatment of patients with a first episode of acute non-specific neck pain. A temporal development of these factors and their influence on self-reported outcome could be observed. Persisting anxiety in the early phase of an acute neck pain problem and depression at baseline emerged as risk factors for poor self-reported recovery and might thus contribute to the transition from acute to chronic pain. The clinical message of this study is that acute neck pain should be regarded as multidimensional. Clinicians should be aware that baseline depression and persisting anxiety might be risk factors for poor prognosis, which should be addressed in the early management of patients with acute non-specific neck pain.

Competing interests
The authors declare that they have no competing interests.

Authors' contributions
BW was involved in study conception, analyzed the data and wrote the manuscript. KH was involved in study design and revised the manuscript critically for important intellectual content. CK was involved in study conception, in data acquisition and analysis and revised the manuscript critically for important intellectual content. All authors finally approved this manuscript.

Acknowledgments
We thank all involved chiropractors for participation.
The authors would like to thank the Balgrist Hospital Foundation, the Chirosuisse Foundation, the Uniscientia Stiftung and the European Academy for Chiropractic for providing funding for this study.

Author details
[1]Chiropractic Medicine Department, Faculty of Medicine, University of Zurich and University Hospital Balgrist, Forchstr. 340, CH-8008 Zurich, Switzerland. [2]Radiology Department, University Hospital Balgrist, Forchstr. 340, 8008 Zurich, Switzerland.

References
1. Vos T, Flaxman AD, Naghavi M, Lozano R, Michaud C, Ezzati M, et al. Years lived with disability (YLDs) for 1160 sequelae of 289 diseases and injuries 1990–2010: a systematic analysis for the Global Burden of Disease Study 2010. Lancet. 2012;380:2163–96.
2. Hoy DG, Protani M, De R, Buchbinder R. The epidemiology of neck pain. Best Pract Res Clin Rheumatol. 2010;24:783–92.
3. Cote P, Cassidy JD, Carroll LJ, Kristman V. The annual incidence and course of neck pain in the general population: a population-based cohort study. Pain. 2004;112:267–73.
4. Pool JJ, Ostelo RW, Knol D, Bouter LM, de Vet HC. Are psychological factors prognostic indicators of outcome in patients with sub-acute neck pain? Man Ther. 2010;15:111–6.
5. Dimitriadis Z, Kapreli E, Strimpakos N, Oldham J. Do psychological states associate with pain and disability in chronic neck pain patients? J Back Musculoskelet Rehabil. 2015;28(4):797–802.
6. Ailliet L, Rubinstein SM, Knol D, Van Tulder MW, De Vet HC. Somatization is associated with worse outcome in a chiropractic patient population with neck pain and low back pain. Man Ther. 2016;21:170–6.
7. Linton SJ. A review of psychological risk factors in back and neck pain. Spine. 2000;25:1148–56.
8. Hurwitz EL, Goldstein MS, Morgenstern H, Chiang LM. The impact of psychosocial factors on neck pain and disability outcomes among primary care patients: results from the UCLA Neck Pain Study. Disabil Rehabil. 2006; 28:1319–29.
9. Walton DM, Carroll LJ, Kasch H, Sterling M, Verhagen AP, Macdermid JC, et al. An overview of systematic reviews on prognostic factors in neck pain: results from the International Collaboration on Neck Pain (ICON) Project. Open Orthop J. 2013;7:494–505.
10. Carroll LJ, Hogg-Johnson S, van der Velde G, Haldeman S, Holm LW, Carragee EJ, et al. Course and prognostic factors for neck pain in the general population: results of the bone and joint decade 2000–2010 task force on neck pain and its associated disorders. J Manipulative Physiol Ther. 2009;32:S87–96.
11. McLean S, May S, Klaber Moffett J, MacFie Sharp D. E G. Prognostic factors for progressive non-specific neck pain: a systematic review. Phys Ther Rev. 2007;12:207–20.
12. Bot SD, van der Waal JM, Terwee CB, van der Windt DA, Scholten RJ, Bouter LM, et al. Predictors of outcome in neck and shoulder symptoms: a cohort study in general practice. Spine. 2005;30:E459–70.
13. Hill J, Lewis M, Papageorgiou AC, Dziedzic K, Croft P. Predicting persistent neck pain: a 1-year follow-up of a population cohort. Spine. 2004;29:1648–54.
14. Walton DM, Macdermid JC, Giorgianni AA, Mascarenhas JC, West SC, Zammit CA. Risk factors for persistent problems following acute whiplash injury: update of a systematic review and meta-analysis. J Orthop Sports Phys Ther. 2013;43:31–43.
15. Dworkin RH, Turk DC, Wyrwich KW, Beaton D, Cleeland CS, Farrar JT, et al. Interpreting the clinical importance of treatment outcomes in chronic pain clinical trials: IMMPACT recommendations. J Pain. 2008;9:105–21.
16. Fischer D, Stewart AL, Bloch DA, Lorig K, Laurent D, Holman H. Capturing the patient's view of change as a clinical outcome measure. JAMA. 1999; 282:1157–62.
17. Peterson C, Bolton J, Humphreys BK. Predictors of outcome in neck pain patients undergoing chiropractic care: comparison of acute and chronic patients. Chiropr Man Therap. 2012;20:27.
18. Bolton JE, Humphreys BK. The Bournemouth Questionnaire: a short-form comprehensive outcome measure. II. Psychometric properties in neck pain patients. J Manipulative Physiol Ther. 2002;25:141–8.
19. Soklic M, Peterson C, Humphreys BK. Translation and validation of the German version of the Bournemouth questionnaire for neck pain. Chiropr Man Therap. 2012;20:2.
20. Bolton JE, Breen AC. The Bournemouth Questionnaire: a short-form comprehensive outcome measure. I. Psychometric properties in back pain patients. J Manipulative Physiol Ther. 1999;22:503–10.
21. Hurst H, Bolton J. Assessing the clinical significance of change scores recorded on subjective outcome measures. J Manipulative Physiol Ther. 2004;27:26–35.

22. Williamson E, Williams MA, Gates S, Lamb SE. Risk factors for chronic disability in a cohort of patients with acute whiplash associated disorders seeking physiotherapy treatment for persisting symptoms. Physiotherapy. 2015;101:34–43.

23. Field A. Discovering statistics using SPSS. 3rd ed. London: SAGE Publications; 2009.

24. Michalski D, Zweynert U, Kuppers-Tiedt L, Hinz A. Physical complaints, emotional stress and locus of control in the course of orthopaedic rehabilitation. Rehabilitation. 2008;47:299–307.

25. Darlow B, Dean S, Perry M, Mathieson F, Baxter GD, Dowell A. Acute low back pain management in general practice: uncertainty and conflicting certainties. Fam Pract. 2014;31:723–32.

26. Henrotin Y, Moyse D, Bazin T, Cedraschi C, Duplan B, Duquesnoy B, et al. Study of the information delivery by general practitioners and rheumatologists to patients with acute low back pain. Eur Spine J. 2011;20: 720–30.

27. Darlow B, Dean S, Perry M, Mathieson F, Baxter GD, Dowell A. Easy to harm, hard to heal: patient views about the back. Spine. 2015;40:842–50.

28. Klaber Moffett JA, Jackson DA, Richmond S, Hahn S, Coulton S, Farrin A, et al. Randomised trial of a brief physiotherapy intervention compared with usual physiotherapy for neck pain patients: outcomes and patients' preference. BMJ. 2005;330:75.

29. Monticone M, Ambrosini E, Cedraschi C, Rocca B, Fiorentini R, Restelli M, et al. Cognitive-behavioral treatment for subacute and chronic neck pain: a cochrane review. Spine. 2015;40:1495–504.

30. Schnitzer TJ, Ferraro A, Hunsche E, Kong SX. A comprehensive review of clinical trials on the efficacy and safety of drugs for the treatment of low back pain. J Pain Symptom Manage. 2004;28:72–95.

31. Behrbalk E, Halpern P, Boszczyk BM, Parks RM, Chechik O, Rosen N, et al. Anxiolytic medication as an adjunct to morphine analgesia for acute low back pain management in the emergency department: a prospective randomized trial. Spine. 2014;39:17–22.

32. Scott W, McCracken LM. Patients' impression of change following treatment for chronic pain: global, specific, a single dimension, or many? J Pain. 2015; 16(6):518–26.

33. Swanenburg J, Gruber C, Brunner F, Wirth B. Patients' and therapists' perception of change following physiotherapy in an orthopedic hospital's outpatient clinic. Physiother Theory Pract. 2015;31:293–8.

Permissions

All chapters in this book were first published in CMT, by BioMed Central; hereby published with permission under the Creative Commons Attribution License or equivalent. Every chapter published in this book has been scrutinized by our experts. Their significance has been extensively debated. The topics covered herein carry significant findings which will fuel the growth of the discipline. They may even be implemented as practical applications or may be referred to as a beginning point for another development.

The contributors of this book come from diverse backgrounds, making this book a truly international effort. This book will bring forth new frontiers with its revolutionizing research information and detailed analysis of the nascent developments around the world.

We would like to thank all the contributing authors for lending their expertise to make the book truly unique. They have played a crucial role in the development of this book. Without their invaluable contributions this book wouldn't have been possible. They have made vital efforts to compile up to date information on the varied aspects of this subject to make this book a valuable addition to the collection of many professionals and students.

This book was conceptualized with the vision of imparting up-to-date information and advanced data in this field. To ensure the same, a matchless editorial board was set up. Every individual on the board went through rigorous rounds of assessment to prove their worth. After which they invested a large part of their time researching and compiling the most relevant data for our readers.

The editorial board has been involved in producing this book since its inception. They have spent rigorous hours researching and exploring the diverse topics which have resulted in the successful publishing of this book. They have passed on their knowledge of decades through this book. To expedite this challenging task, the publisher supported the team at every step. A small team of assistant editors was also appointed to further simplify the editing procedure and attain best results for the readers.

Apart from the editorial board, the designing team has also invested a significant amount of their time in understanding the subject and creating the most relevant covers. They scrutinized every image to scout for the most suitable representation of the subject and create an appropriate cover for the book.

The publishing team has been an ardent support to the editorial, designing and production team. Their endless efforts to recruit the best for this project, has resulted in the accomplishment of this book. They are a veteran in the field of academics and their pool of knowledge is as vast as their experience in printing. Their expertise and guidance has proved useful at every step. Their uncompromising quality standards have made this book an exceptional effort. Their encouragement from time to time has been an inspiration for everyone.

The publisher and the editorial board hope that this book will prove to be a valuable piece of knowledge for researchers, students, practitioners and scholars across the globe.

List of Contributors

Jane Mulcahy
Centre for Chronic Disease Prevention & Management, College of Health & Biomedicine, Victoria University, Melbourne, Australia

Brett Vaughan
Centre for Chronic Disease Prevention & Management, College of Health & Biomedicine, Victoria University, Melbourne, Australia
Institute of Sport, Exercise & Active Living, Victoria University, Melbourne, Australia
School of Health & Human Sciences, Southern Cross University, Lismore, Australia

Amir M Arab
Department of Physical Therapy, University of Social Welfare and Rehabilitation Sciences, Velenjak, Tehran, Iran

Ailin Talimkhani, Noureddin Karimi and Fetemeh Ehsani
University of Social Welfare and Rehabilitation Sciences, Velenjak, Tehran, Iran

Rikke K. Jensen
Research Department, Spine Centre of Southern Denmark, Hospital Lillebaelt, Institute of Regional Health Research, University of Southern Denmark, Oestre Hougvej 55, 5500 Middelfart, Denmark
Department of Sports Science and Clinical Biomechanics, University of Southern Denmark, Campusvej 55, 5230 Odense M, Denmark

Peter Kent
Research Department, Spine Centre of Southern Denmark, Hospital Lillebaelt, Institute of Regional Health Research, University of Southern Denmark, Oestre Hougvej 55, 5500 Middelfart, Denmark
Department of Sports Science and Clinical Biomechanics, University of Southern Denmark, Campusvej 55, 5230 Odense M, Denmark

Mark Hancock
Faculty of Human Sciences, Macquarie University, Balaclava Rd, North Ryde 2113NSW, Australia

Stacie A Salsbury, James W DeVocht, Michael B Seidman and Christine M Goertz
Palmer College of Chiropractic, Palmer Center for Chiropractic Research, 741 Brady Street, Davenport, IA 52803, USA

Maria A Hondras
Institute of Sports Science and Clinical Biomechanics, University of Southern Denmark, Odense, Denmark

Clark M Stanford
The University of Illinois, 801 South Paulina Street, 102c (MC621), Chicago, IL 60612, USA

Sara Glithro, Adrian Hunnisett and Christina Cunliffe
McTimoney College of Chiropractic, Abingdon, UK

David Newell
Anglo European College of Chiropractic (AECC) and Bournemouth University, Dorset, UK

Lorna Burrows
Salisbury NHS Foundation Trust, Salisbury, UK

Lisa C Carlesso
Toronto Western Research Institute, University Health Network, 399 Bathurst Street - MP11-328, Toronto, Ontario M5T 2S8, Canada

Joy C MacDermid
School of Rehabilitation Sciences McMaster University, Hamilton, Ontario, Canada
Clinical Research Lab, Hand and Upper Limb Centre, St. Joseph's Health Centre, London, Ontario, Canada

Anita R Gross
School of Rehabilitation Sciences McMaster University, Hamilton, Ontario, Canada

David M Walton
School of Physical Therapy, Western University, London, Ontario, Canada

P Lina Santaguida
Department of Clinical Epidemiology and Biostatistics, Hamilton, Ontario, Canada

Søren O'Neill
Spine Centre of Southern Denmark, Lillebælt Hospital, Østre Hougvej 55, 5500 Middelfart, DK, Denmark
Institute of Regional Health Research, University of Southern Denmark, Campusvej 55, 5230 Odense, DK, Denmark

Øystein Ødegaard-Olsen
Spine Centre of Southern Denmark, Lillebælt Hospital, Østre Hougvej 55, 5500 Middelfart, DK, Denmark

Beate Søvde
Stathelle Healthcentre, Brugata 10, 3960 Stathelle, Norway

Guy Gosselin and Michael Fagan
School of Engineering, University of Hull, Cottingham Road, Kingston-upon-Hull HU6 7RX, UK

Alexander C Breen and Mihai Dupac
School of Design Engineering and Computing, Bournemouth University, Bournemouth, BH1 5BB, UK

Neil Osborne
Anglo-European College of Chiropractic, Bournemouth, BH5 2DF, UK

Peter W. McCarthy and Andrew I. Heusch
Faculty of Life Sciences and Education, University of South Wales, Pontypridd, Mid-Glamorgan, Wales CF37 1DL, UK

Phillip J. Hume
Anglo-European College of Chiropractic, Parkwood Road, Bournemouth, Dorset BH5 2DF, UK

Sally D. Lark
Massey University Wellington, College of Health, P O Box 756, Wellington 6140, New Zealand

Karin Ried, Simon Armstrong and Avni Sali
National Institute of Integrative Medicine, Melbourne VIC 3122, Australia

Patrick McLaughlin
College of Health and Biomedicine, Victoria University, Melbourne VIC 3001, Australia

Salman Afsharpour and Samuel Demons
Basic Science Division, Department of Anatomy, Life University, College of Chiropractic, 1269 Barclay Circle, Marietta, GA 30060, USA

Kathryn T. Hoiriis
Chiropractic Sciences Division, Life University, College of Chiropractic, 1269 Barclay Circle, Marietta, GA, USA

R. Bruce Fox
Clinical Sciences Division, Department of Radiology, Life University, College of Chiropractic, 1269 Barclay Circle, Marietta, GA, USA

Eva Jespersen, Christina T Rexen and Claudia Franz
Research in Childhood Health, Department of Sports Science and Clinical Biomechanics, University of Southern Denmark, Campusvej 55, 5230 Odense, Denmark
The Sport Medicine Clinic, Orthopaedic Department, Hospital of Lillebaelt, Lillebaelt, Denmark

Niels Wedderkopp
Research in Childhood Health, Department of Sports Science and Clinical Biomechanics, University of Southern Denmark, Campusvej 55, 5230 Odense, Denmark
The Sport Medicine Clinic, Orthopaedic Department, Hospital of Lillebaelt, Lillebaelt, Denmark
Research Department, Spine Center of Southern Denmark, Hospital Lillebaelt, Middelfart and Institute of Regional Health

Services Research, University of Southern Denmark, Denmark

Charlotte Leboeuf-Yde
Research Department, Spine Center of Southern Denmark, Hospital Lillebaelt, Middelfart and Institute of Regional Health Services Research, University of Southern Denmark, Denmark

Kyle Colin Deutschmann
M.Tech:Chiropractic, Durban, South Africa

Andrew Douglas Jones
M.Dip:Chiropractic, MMedSci (Sports Science), CCSP, Durban, South Africa

Charmaine Maria Korporaal
Department of Chiropractic and Somatology, Chiropractic Programme, M.Tech:Chiropractic, CCFC, CCSP, ICSSD, Durban University of Technology, Durban, South Africa

Eirik Johan Skeie
MChiro, MSc, Ulriksdal 2, 5009 Bergen, Norway

Jan Arve Borge
DC, MSc, Ulriksdal 2, 5009 Bergen, Norway

Charlotte Leboeuf-Yde
Department Spincenter of Southern Denmark Hospital Lillebælt, Østre Hougvej 55, DK-5500 Middelfart, Denmark

Jenni Bolton
Anglo European College of Chiropractic Research Department, 13-15 Parkwood Road, Bournemouth BH5 2DF England, UK

Niels Wedderkopp
Orthopaedic Department, Center for Spine Surgery, Hospital of Lillebaelt, Institute of Regional Health Service Research and Center for Research in Childhood Health, University of Southern Denmark, Østre Hougvej 55, DK5500 Middelfart, Denmark

Benjamin T. Brown
Department of Chiropractic, Macquarie University, Balaclava Road, North Ryde 2109NSW, Australia

Petra L. Graham
Department of Statistics, Macquarie University, Balaclava Road, North Ryde 2109NSW, Australia

Rod Bonello
School of Health Professions - Murdoch University, 90 South Street, Murdoch 6150WA, Australia

Henry Pollard
Private Practice, 84 Kingsway, Cronulla 2230NSW, Australia

Sandra Grace, Paul Orrock, Raymond Blaich and Rosanne Coutts
School of Health & Human Sciences, Southern Cross University, PO Box 157, Lismore NSW 2480, Australia

Brett Vaughan
College of Health & Biomedicine, Victoria University, 301 Flinders Lane, Melbourne, Australia

Nicoline M. Lambers and Jennifer E. Bolton
Anglo-European College of Chiropractic, 13-15 Parkwood Road, Bournemouth BH5 2DF, UK

Craig A. Bauman and James D. Milligan
Department of Family Medicine, McMaster University, Hamilton, ON, Canada
The Centre for Family Medicine Family Health Team, 25 Joseph Street, Kitchener, ON, CanadaN2G 4X6

Tammy Labreche
School of Optometry and Vision Science, University of Waterloo, Waterloo, ON, Canada

John J. Riva
Department of Family Medicine, McMaster University, Hamilton, ON, Canada
Department of Clinical Epidemiology & Biostatistics, McMaster University, Hamilton, ON, Canada

Amy L. Crothers
Private practice of chiropractic, Geraldton, WA 6530, Australia

Simon D. French
School of Health Professions, Discipline of Chiropractic, Murdoch University, South Street, Murdoch, WA, Australia
School of Rehabilitation Therapy, Faculty of Health Sciences, Queen's University, Ontario, Canada

Jeff J. Hebert
School of Psychology and Exercise Science, Murdoch University, South Street, Murdoch, WA, Australia

Bruce F. Walker
School of Health Professions, Discipline of Chiropractic, Murdoch University, South Street, Murdoch, WA, Australia

Fay Karpouzis
PO Box 2108, Rose Bay Nth 2030, NSW, Australia

Rod Bonello
School of Health Professions, Murdoch University, South St., Murdoch 6150, WA, Australia

Mario Pribicevic, Allan Kalamir and Benjamin T. Brown
Department of Chiropractic, Macquarie University, Balaclava Rd., North Ryde 2109, NSW, Australia

Brigitte Wirth and B. Kim Humphreys
Chiropractic Medicine Department, Faculty of Medicine, University of Zurich and University Hospital Balgrist, Forchstr 340, CH-8008 Zurich, Switzerland

Cynthia Peterson
Chiropractic Medicine Department, Faculty of Medicine, University of Zurich and University Hospital Balgrist, Forchstr 340, CH-8008 Zurich, Switzerland
Radiology Department, University Hospital Balgrist, Forchstr 340, 8008 Zurich, Switzerland

Index